Rehabilitation Robotics: Technology and Applications

Rehabilitation Robotics: Technology and Applications

Editor: Lucille Alvarado

STATES
ACADEMIC PRESS
www.statesacademicpress.com

States Academic Press,
109 South 5th Street,
Brooklyn, NY 11249, USA

Visit us on the World Wide Web at:
www.statesacademicpress.com

ISBN: 978-1-63989-468-0 (Hardback)

Cataloging-in-Publication Data

Rehabilitation robotics : technology and applications /
edited by Lucille Alvarado.
p. cm.
Includes bibliographical references and index.
ISBN 978-1-63989-468-0
1. Rehabilitation technology. 2. Robotics in medicine. 3. Robotics.
4. Robots--Control systems. I. Alvarado, Lucille.
RM950 .R44 2022
617.03--dc23

Table of Contents

Preface

Physical medicine and rehabilitation, also called physiatry, aims to enhance and restore functional ability and quality of life to people with physical impairments or disabilities. Rehabilitation robotics is an area of research dedicated to understanding and enhancing physiatry through the use of robotic devices. It involves the development of robotic devices to assist different sensorimotor functions, different schemes of assisting therapeutic training, and assessment of patient's ability to move. Robots are used mainly as therapy aids instead of assistive devices in rehabilitation robotics. Some of the techniques used within this field are active assisted exercise, active resistive exercise and adaptive exercise. This book elucidates new techniques and their applications in a multidisciplinary manner. The ever growing need of advanced technology is the reason that has fueled the research in the field of rehabilitation robotics in recent times. As this field is emerging at a rapid pace, the contents of this book will help the readers understand the technology and applications of the subject.

Significant researches are present in this book. Intensive efforts have been employed by authors to make this book an outstanding discourse. This book contains the enlightening chapters which have been written on the basis of significant researches done by the experts.

Finally, I would also like to thank all the members involved in this book for being a team and meeting all the deadlines for the submission of their respective works. I would also like to thank my friends and family for being supportive in my efforts.

Editor

1

Work Assistive Mobile Robot for the Disabled in a Real Work Environment

Hyun Seok Hong, Jung Won Kang and Myung Jin Chung
KAIST
Republic of Korea

1. Introduction

Previous works related to welfare service robotics have mainly focused on assisting the disabled in their daily life. Robot systems such as the Intelligent Bed-Robot System (Kim et al. 2002) and Care Robot System (Yoo, 2003a) are designed to help the disabled in performing daily activities in specialized indoor environments. Human-machine interfaces such as Eye Gaze Estimation System (Yoo, 2003b) have been developed to facilitate easy control of the robot system. FRIEND (Martens, 2001) and KARES II (Bien, 2003) are wheelchair-based rehabilitation robotic systems equipped with a robot arm and are designed to help the disabled manipulate small objects such as food, drink, books, etc.
It is important that human beings have the opportunity to feel self-worth and happiness by living productive lives through their own vocation. Therefore, the development of a vocational robotic system has important implications with respect to welfare. Although some vocational assistive robots have been developed, they are limited to office environments. The robot RAID (Eftring, 1993), which was developed at the Rehabilitation Engineering Research Center in Sweden, assists in removing books from a bookshelf, bringing documents, and serving drinks in a office environment. The robot known as WALKY (Neveryd, 1994) can avoid obstacles while it maneuvers to deliver objects in a laboratory environment. The robot ProVAR (Van der Loos, 1999) receives orders via a speech recognition system and helps to process office tasks such as serving drinks and delivering documents, diskettes, video tapes, etc. In addition, the current status of the robot is displayed through a monitor.

Due to regional differences in industrial structures, the types of tasks that the disabled can perform differ from country to country. As a result, robots assisting the disabled in a real manufacturing environment can be more useful than robots providing assistance in office environments in some countries.

However, there has been relatively little research reported on the development of vocational robotic systems in real manufacturing environments. The objective of the present work is to develop mobile robot systems that assist the disabled to work in real manufacturing factories. Specifically, the assistive robot is targeted for the disabled in Korea, where the authors dwell. In this research, to clearly determine the objectives of developing assistive mobile robots, a mission statement is addressed based on statistical data. Furthermore, the target manufacturing environment is surveyed to specify the dimensions and working algorithm of the work assistive mobile robot. Two work assistive mobile robots are proposed and developed according to slightly different function definitions. User trials are performed for the two work assistive mobile systems. The robot systems are expected to provide practical assistance to disabled workers and help satisfy their desires and fulfill their capabilities so that they can become productive members of society. We expect that this will result in an increase in the working population of the disabled.

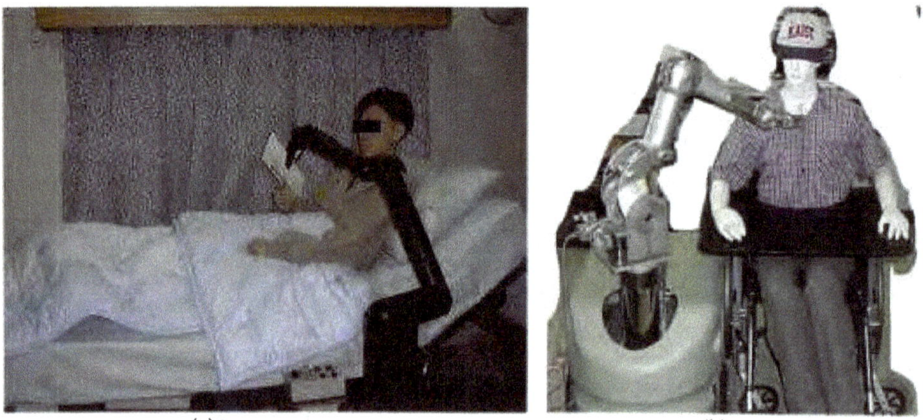

(a) (b)

Fig. 1. Examples of robots for daily activities of the disabled; (a) Intelligent bed-robot system, (b) KARES II.

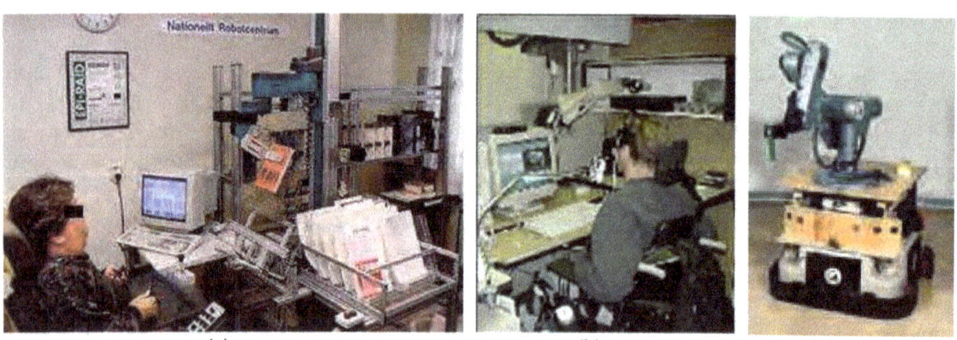

(a) (b) (c)

Fig. 2. Examples of robots for desktop vocational activities of the disabled; (a) RAID, (b) ProVAR, (c) WALKY.

2. Derivation of Mission Statements

Our objective in developing the present robot systems is to assist the disabled as much as possible in real employment situations. For determining our specific mission, we surveyed an abundance of data pertaining to people with disabilities in real employment situations. We categorized the survey results into three criteria, 'A. to assist the disabled as much as possible,' 'B. to consider the real situation of employment for the disabled and 'C. to provide assistance for the most necessary tasks for the disabled in the work space'.

2.1 Survey based on Criterion A

In order to assist the disabled as much as possible, we investigated disability types and the type of work presently being performed in Korea by workers with disabilities. To this end, we surveyed data[1] on the disabled in Korea. Among people with disabilities, 55.1%suffer from limb impairment, 8.7% cerebral paralysis, 10.5% visual disorder, 8.8% hearing disorder, and 0.8% speech disorder. On the other hand, there were relatively few people with internal organ impediments or cognitive disabilities.

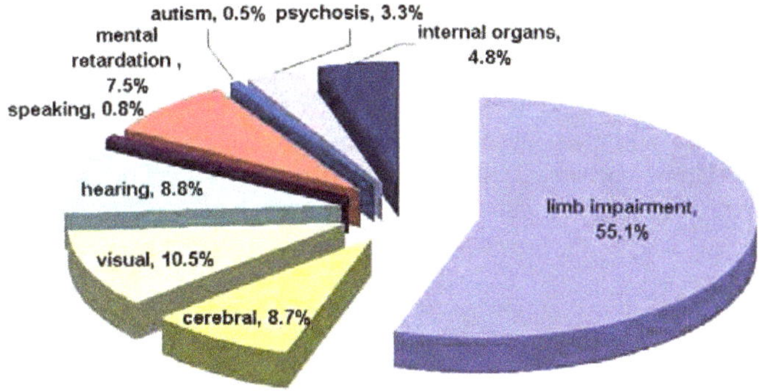

Fig. 3 Distribution of the disabled

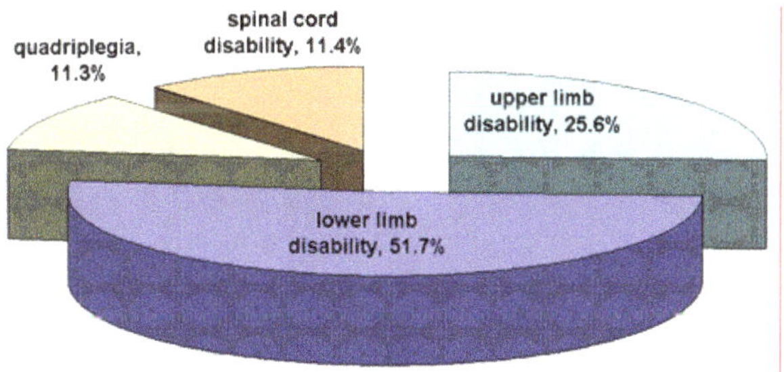

Fig. 4 Distribution of limb impairment and cerebral paralysis

Types of disorder	Large workshop	Small workshop
Limb impairment	82.0%	81.0%
Cerebral paralysis	0.2%	0.2%
Visual disorder	4.4%	3.1%
Hearing disorder	9.8%	6.2%
Speech disorder	1.2%	1.1%
Other	2.4%	8.4%

Table 1. Distribution of actual employment for the disabled. Companies with more than 300 employees are classified as a large workshop.

[1] Statistical data from reports (written in Korean): "The present condition of registered disable people," published by the Korea Ministry of Health and Welfare, Sep. 2004, "Research on the actual conditions of the disabled in 2000," published by the Korea Institute for Health and Social Affairs, 2000, "Research on the actual conditions of disabled workers in 2000," published by the Korea Employment Promotion Agency for the Disabled, 2000.

Fig. 3 shows the distribution of the disabled, and Fig. 4 describes the disability distribution of people who suffer from limb impairment or cerebral paralysis. From the distributions, it is noted that the percentage of disabled having leg impediments is large. Table 1 shows that most people with disabilities who have entered the workforce have limb impairment regardless of the scale of the workshop. Therefore, it is desirable to develop a robot system that assists workers who suffer from limb impairment.

2.2 Survey based on Criterion B

In order to assess the real employment situation of the disabled, we visited vocational education facilities[2] and companies[3] that hire disabled workers. As shown in Fig. 5, our survey results show that the physically disabled tend to prefer computer-oriented jobs, as there are numerous occupations in this field and these jobs require little spatial movement. According to the results, they are also interested in mechanical jobs, primarily because there is huge industrial demand for labor and the other is that they can gain expertise in performing these jobs.

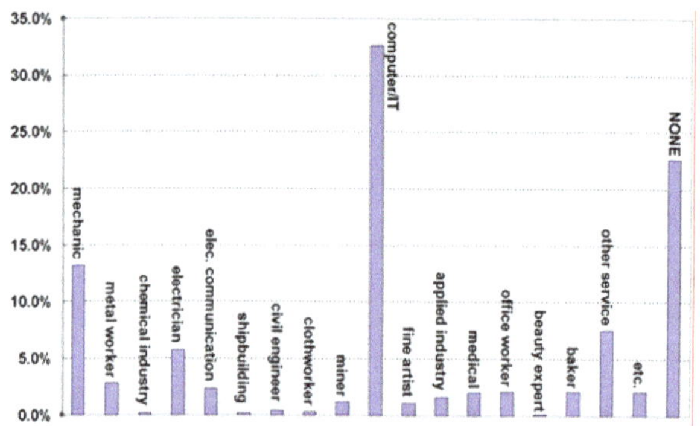

Fig. 5. Vocational fields in which the disabled desire training.

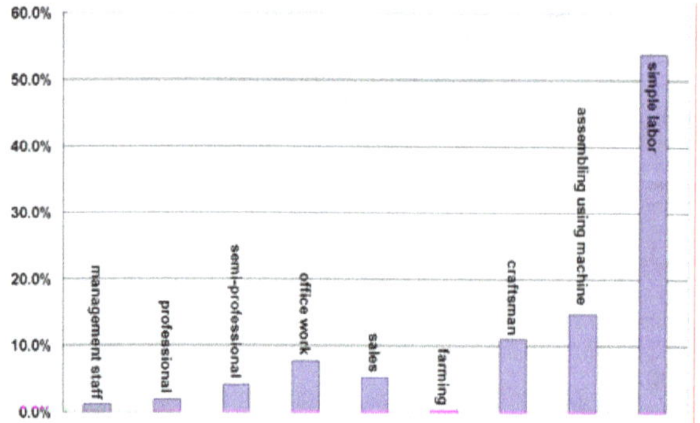

Fig. 6. Vocational fields for which the employers seek workers; 'simple labor' and 'assembling using a machine' include assembling and classifying circuit parts, moving boxes, packing, delivering, and cleaning up.

---

2 Bundang branch of the Korea Employment Promotion Agency for the disabled and vocational schools in Daejeon and Ilsan.

3 Eleven factories including Mugunghwa Electronics and Immanuel Electronics, which mainly make electronic products, and Boram-Dongsan, which mainly assembles mechanical parts.

However, vocational fields[4] for which employers wish to hire disabled workers mainly involve simple labor, as shown in Fig. 6. According to these investigations, there are huge gaps between occupations that people with disabilities want and occupations that companies need to fill. As a result, although many social organizations provide vocational education to the disabled, due to the actual employment situation the disabled mainly perform simple labor. Therefore, it is desirable to develop an assistive robot system that can help the disabled work in performing physical and simple labor such as assembling and classifying circuit parts, moving boxes, and packing and delivering goods.

2.3 Survey based on Criterion C

According to the survey results shown in Table 2, disabled laborers experience difficulties when they should carry heavy materials.

Situations	Large workshop	Small workshop
Transferring goods	55.4%	33.8%
Moving around the workshop	14.5%	31.5%
Operating machines	27.9%	20.0%
Difficulty to understand instructions	24.4%	22.3%
Operating speed	20.0%	31.5%

Table 2. Situations where a disabled worker requires help. Duplicated answers are permitted. Companies with more than 300 employees are classified as a large workshop.

Survey results also show that those who have upper limb impediments desire a robot system that can help perform movements normally performed by the arms (fixing, loading, fine motion, etc). Those with leg impediments meanwhile require a system to substitute the functions of the leg (movement, loading, etc) and those who have both impediments would like a system that would provide assistance when they should carry heavy materials. Target objects for transferring goods are divided into heavy and light objects[5]. In the case of fine motion tasks, the assistive robot system cooperates with the human and supports roller inserting and PCB inspection tasks. Therefore, it is necessary to design a work assistive robot that can transfer goods, perform dexterous tasks, and move around freely.

From the above survey results, our mission has been determined. The following is our mission statement: to develop a work assistive mobile robot to help the disabled who have lower limb(s) or upper limb disabilities, or lower limb(s) and upper limb disabilities obtain employment in manufacturing factories involving the performance of simple physical labor.

3. Work Space Environment of Real Manufacturing Factories

3.1 Work Space Environment of Real Manufacturing Factories

As described earlier, our work assistive robot helps the disabled person to work in a real manufacturing factory. Before designing this assistive robot, the environments of real

[4] Statistical data from the report (written in Korean): "Classified statistics on the disabled in the first quarter of 2002," published by the Korea Employment Promotion Agency for the Disabled, 2002.

[5] Boxes used in a real factory are investigated and classified into two groups: heavy boxes (maximum size: 65×35×40cm, shape: box, maximum weight: 30kg), and light boxes (maximum size: 30×25×10cm, shape: box or bag, maximum weight: 3kg).

manufacturing factories should be known. We surveyed several manufacturing factories that employ workers with disabilities. Through the survey, we defined the general environment to help the disabled. Manufacturing factory environment survey results are described in Fig. 7 ~ Fig. 10.

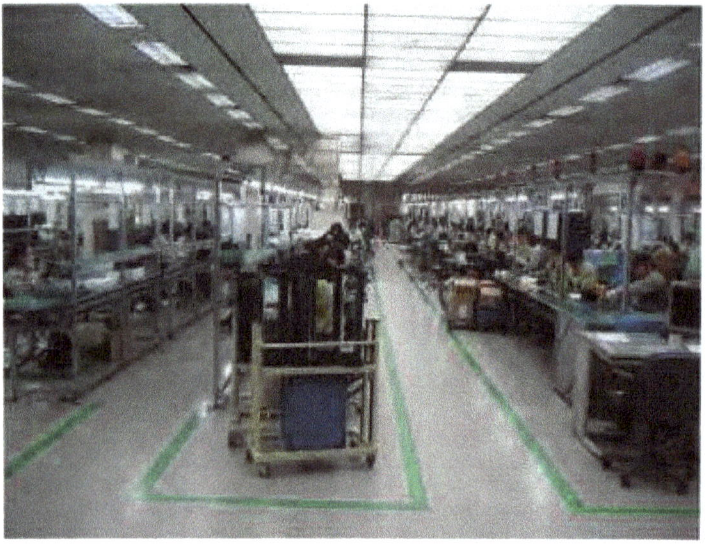

Fig. 7. Whole view of general environment of manufacturing factory. Safety lines are painted around work tables.

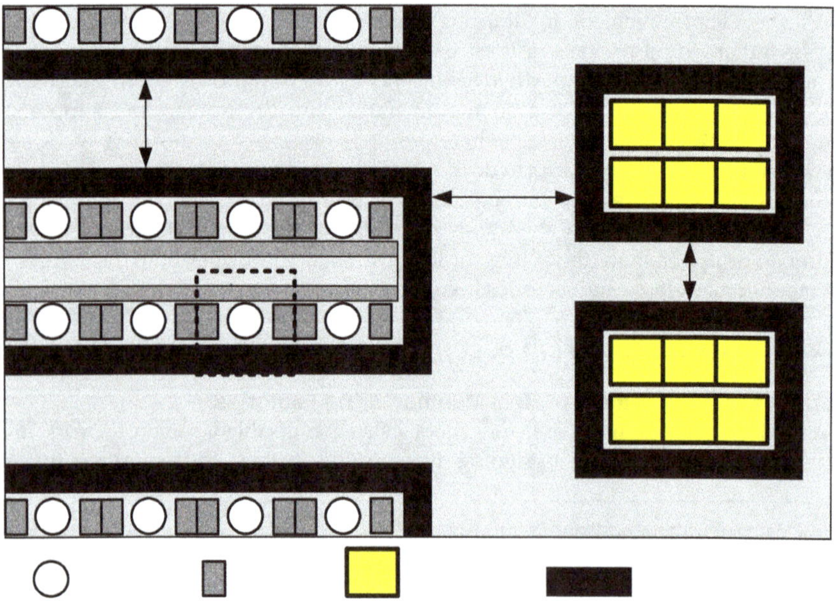

Fig. 8. Top view of general environment of manufacturing factory (dimensions in [cm]).

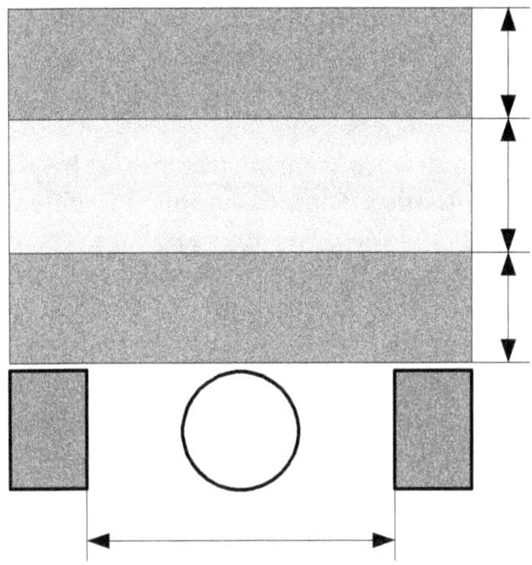

Fig. 9. Top view of space allocated for an employee working at worktable in manufacturing factories (dimensions in [cm]).

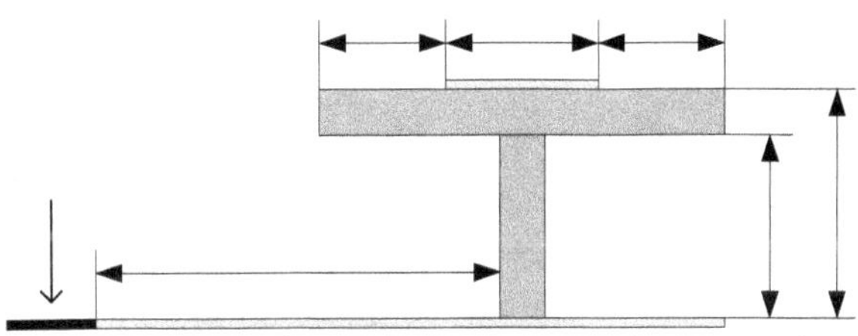

Fig. 10. Side view of space allocated for an employee working at worktable in manufacturing factories (dimensions in [cm]).

The major work in the factories is making electronic products such as battery chargers, vacuum cleaners and circuits that require soldering, and assembling task. For the tasks, as described in Fig. 8, most manufacturing factories are composed of long tables equipped with a conveyor, a warehouse containing parts in boxes on palettes, safety lines around these elements, and aisles between tables and storage areas. There are aisles with various widths, excluding the safety line width (10cm):

-between tables: min. 120cm, max. 140cm

-between storage areas: min. 80cm, max. 120cm

-between tables and storage areas: 210cm

Allocated space for a worker who works at a worktable is expressed in the dotted box in Fig. 8 while Fig. 9 and Fig. 10 show top and side views of the space, respectively. For each worker doing table tasks, boxes containing parts are stacked at the left and right sides, and the width between the boxes is 75cm at the minimum and 90cm at the maximum. The table height of the lower side is 70cm and the width between the safety line and table is about 100cm.

In the environment, workers perform dexterous tasks such as soldering and assembling at the work table. When workers do not have enough parts, they move to the warehouse, and pick up boxes that contain parts. After returning to the work table, they resume working.

3.2 Required Specification of Work Assistive Mobile Robot System

The purpose of our robot system is to help the disabled to work in a factory environment. Therefore, the robot should have function on behalf of the legs and arms of the disabled worker. In a factory, workers carry boxes including assembled parts, load and unload boxes from a warehouse, and perform dexterous tasks. In order to help the disabled worker, we adopted a mobile platform with four wheels and equipped it with a forklift and a robot arm. The forklift helps to load and unload the boxes that contain parts to be assembled. Also, the robot arm helps to move light parts and to perform dexterous jobs such as providing aid when soldering.

From the environment survey results and task analysis, the required specifications for the mobile robot system are determined. The robot arm should be able to perform various dexterous tasks such as soldering, assembling, and moving light goods. The forklift should be able to lift up boxes that are more than 30kg. The mobile platform should be small enough to move through narrow aisles between tables in factories. The size of the robot system should be less than 1500mm in length and 700mm in width. The robot should be able to carry a payload of 120kg, including 80kg for the worker's weight and 30~40kg for a box.

By using this robot, the worker can easily move around, even in a confined area. The worker can also load, unload, and transfer boxes without difficulty. The robot arm also helps in performing dexterous tasks.

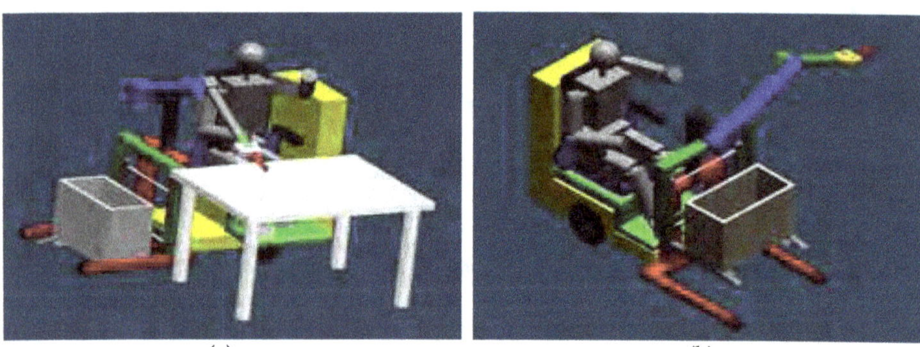

(a) (b)

Fig. 11. Basic concept of work assistive mobile robot system type I; (a) assisting table tasks, (b) moving objects.

4. Development of Work Assistive Robot Systems

After a survey of general factories environments, we developed two work assistive robot systems. Work assistive mobile robot system type I is focused on versatility and work assistive robot system type II is mainly focused on mobility. Each robot system was developed after defining tasks and functions. We also conducted user-trials with the robot systems in a real factory to obtain feedback from real workers.

4.1 Work Assistive Mobile Robot System Type I

4.1.1 Design of Work Assistive Mobile Robot System Type I

We assume that the disabled user works sitting on the chair of the work assistive mobile robot. Therefore, the height of the robot chair should be designed to be lower than that of a desk. Furthermore, the chair should be designed to rotate up to a right angle to work at a desk. When parts to be assembled are needed or it is necessary to transfer goods, the person moves the robot and picks up and puts down the objects. Therefore, a fork-lift system is adopted in the robot system. When the robot moves, obstacle avoidance is employed and a related alarm is used for safety. The basic concept of the work assistive mobile robot system is described in Fig. 11. Fig. 11 describes a scenario to help the disabled person to work at their table tasks (soldering, assembling, etc.) and to move boxes containing parts. To support table tasks, the mobile robot is parked parallel with the table, and the chair of the robot is rotated toward the table. This setting makes it easy to use the robot arm to perform a task, and the fork-lift can be employed to load the box at the proper height.

The driving mechanism for the work assistive mobile robot is an important issue because the fork-lift must move heavy boxes. We considered two driving mechanisms: forward wheel steering/backward wheel driving and forward wheel driving/backward wheel steering. A forward wheel steering/backward wheel driving mechanism is a popular mechanism for three or four wheel scooters. However, this mechanism is not appropriate for a work assistive robot that has a fork-lift at its front area, especially with regard to steering. A forward wheel driving/backward wheel steering mechanism is also a popular mechanism for commercial forklift trucks, and is more appropriate. Therefore, we adopted a forward wheel driving/backward wheel steering mechanism.

4.1.2 Development of Work Assistive Mobile Robot Type I

Based on the design result of the robot, we developed work assistive mobile robot type I, as shown in Fig. 12. As noted earlier, the work assistive mobile robot type I is based on a forward wheel driving/backward wheel steering mechanism. For this mechanism, the robot has two motors, one for driving and another for steering. The mobile platform is basically controlled by a DSP controller and several peripherals. It also has four limit switches for emergency stopping, and ten ultrasonic sensors to detect obstacles to the rear for collision avoidance. Additionally, a camera is set up in the rear area and a monitor connected with it displays rear objects. The fork-lift system has two actuators to place and lift objects. A MANUS arm is equipped in front of the mobile platform. All components are controlled and communicated through the main system, which is run by a personal computer. Each component of work assistive mobile robot type I such as the robot arm, mobile platform, and fork lift is controlled by a 2-axis joystick, with several operation modes for controlling each component.

Size	650×1400× 550[mm] (width×length×height)
Speed	12[km/h]
Max. Load (Robot)	200 kg
Max. Load (Lift)	60 kg

Table 3. Specifications of work assistive mobile robot type I

From a structural point of view, we divided the work assistive mobile robot system into one main system and three subsystems according to their functions. Fig. 13 shows each module configuration of the robot system.

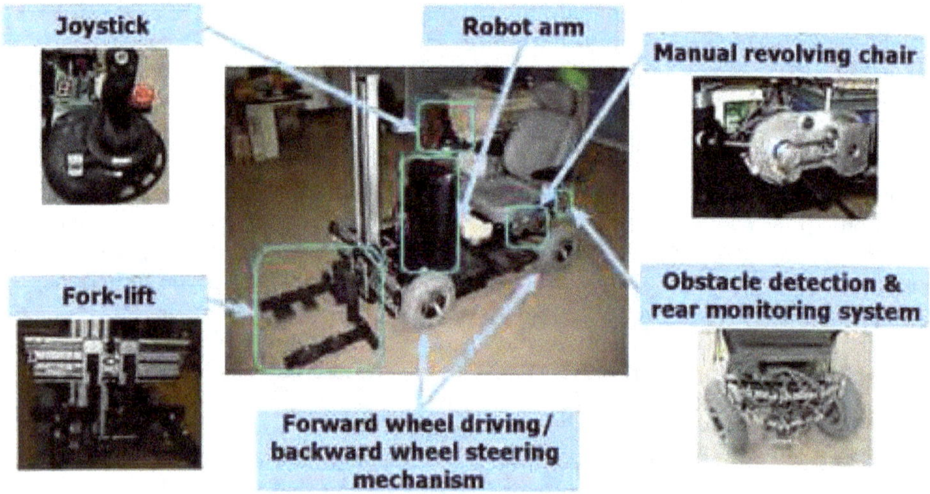

Fig. 12. Developed work assistive mobile robot type I.

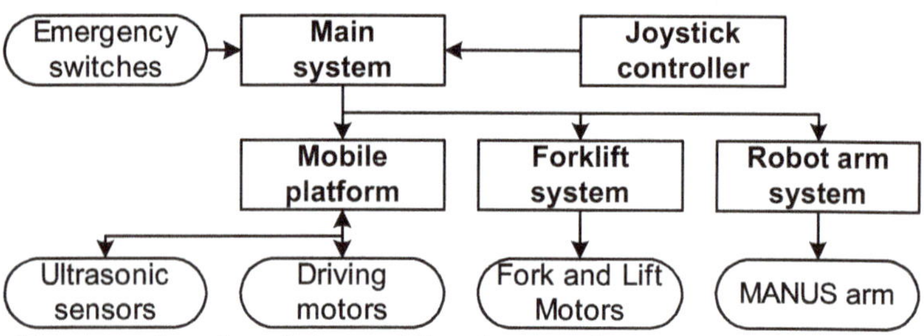

Fig. 13. Architecture of work assistive mobile robot type I.

The main system is a PC that runs RTAI-linux for real-time control. It is connected to subsystems, i.e., the mobile platform, fork-lift system, robot arm system, and the joystick controller. The joystick connection uses a USB communication port of the main computer, whereas others connections are through the RS232 port. Command data is composed of a start byte, data bytes, and an end byte. The number of data bytes corresponds with the number of actuators in each subsystem. For example, a command data from the main system to the mobile platform has one start byte (eight bits), two data bytes, and one end byte. Each data byte has a value between -125 and 125. The start byte value is 126, and the value of the end byte is 127. This short data length speeds up communication.

4.1.3 User-trials

We conducted a series of user-trials of the developed work assistive mobile robot system with the participation of disabled persons who work in actual manufacturing factories, Boram-Dongsan and Mugungwha Electronics in Korea. We gathered their feedback about the robot. The participants were randomly selected among factory workers who have lower-limb or upper-limb impairments or lower-limb and upper-limb impairments. Fig. 14 shows pictures describing the user-trials of work assistive mobile robot system type I.

After conducting the user-trials of work assistive mobile robot system type I, we asked the subjects questions pertaining to the velocities of driving and steering, the convenience of the joystick interface, ease of riding, the risk during driving, and the need for the rear camera. The velocities of moving forward and reversing were confirmed by the respondents as being appropriate. However, they pointed out that the steering speed was slightly slow. This problem was caused by a high reduction ratio gearbox to generate high torque, and was fixed by using a gearbox with a lower gear ratio and a motor with higher torque. The respondents also said the joystick interface was very easy to use. They also reported that they felt safe while moving. This is due to the intuitive joystick control method and the ultrasonic sensor system to avoid collision with obstacles. However, they habitually did not use the rear monitoring system.
Additionally, we identified some shortcomings: (1) the robot arm system is hard to control, and should be smaller or be installed on a work desk; (2) the mobile base and the radius of turning of the robot need to be smaller and the chair needs to be rotated electrically and its should be height lower; and (3) the fork of the fork-lift system should smaller or capable of being folded electrically. We considered these problems for developing the next version, type II.

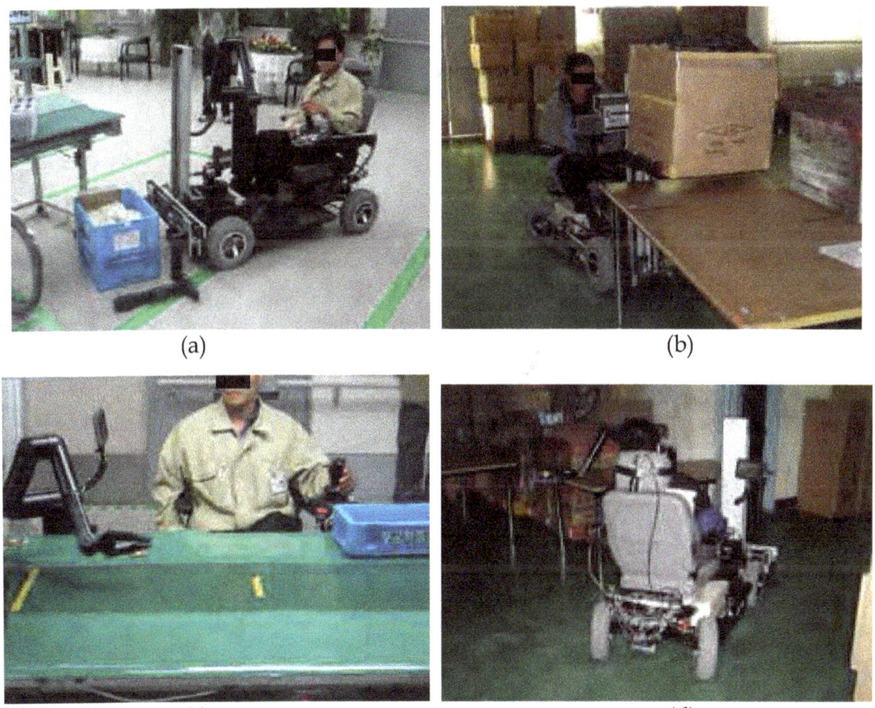

Fig. 14. User trials for Work Assistive Mobile Robot System Type I; (a) Moving objects - lifting up, (b) Moving objects - lowering, (c) Working at a desk, (d) Moving around.

4.2 Work Assistive Mobile Robot System Type II

Based on the results of the user-trials of work assistive mobile robot system type I, we developed work assistive mobile robot system type II. The basic function, control system architecture, and the method of user-trials are basically the same as those of type I.

4.2.1 Design of Work Assistive Mobile Robot System Type II

Since a robot arm is chiefly used in table tasks and is not used when the robot moves around, the robot arm is installed on the table, and a foldable fork-lift is incorporated in order to reduce the size of the robot. One very important issue is the driving mechanism. The robot should be capable of moving in a confined space. For this, we adopted an omni-directional wheel driving mechanism. Among the available omni-directional wheels, we use four omni-directional wheels called 'mecanum wheels'. A mecanum wheel consists of one active main wheel and several passive rollers around the main wheel. When the main wheel rotates, a force vector along the wheel and a force vector perpendicular to the wheel are created. The net force, which determines the moving direction of the robot, is created by combining each force vector of the four wheels. By simply controlling the rotation of each wheel without steering them, the robot can move in any direction. Although the power efficiency of the omni-directional mechanism is relatively low and it is difficult to fabricate mecanum wheels, we choose this mechanism since the use of four wheels will guarantee stability. By using the omni-directional wheel driving mechanism, positioning tasks become much easier, especially in narrow aisles, for upper limb impaired workers.

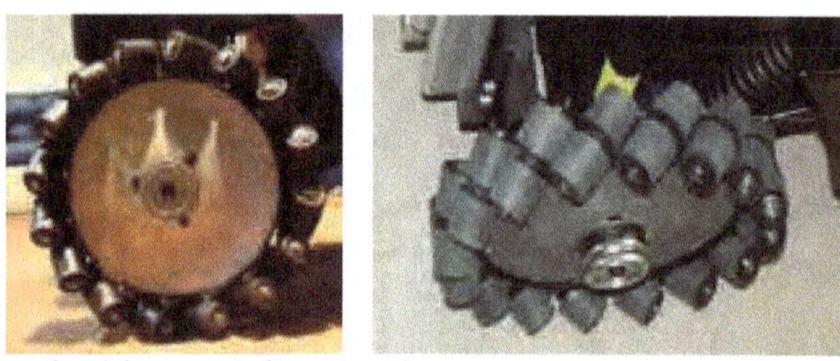

Fig. 15. Mecanum wheel for omni-directional movement.

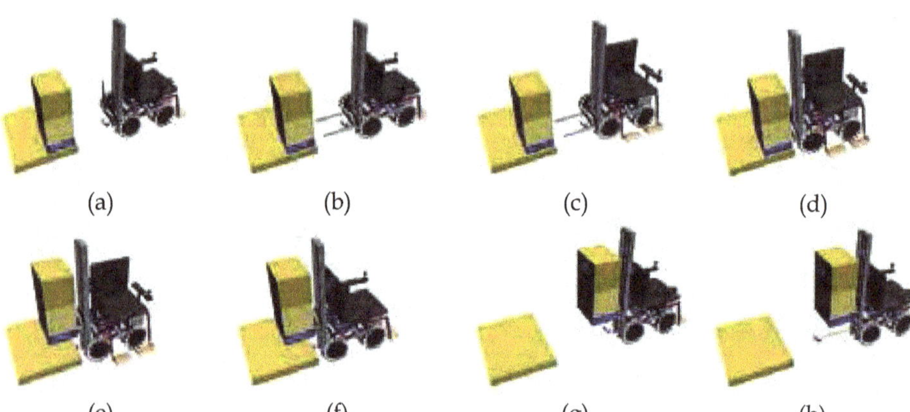

Fig. 16. Scenario of work assistive mobile robot type II; (a) robot moves to the warehouse and orients the rear side to a box on a pallet in the warehouse; (b) the user unfolds the fork using switch; (c) the user rotates the chair using a switch and prepares to extract the box; (d) the robot moves toward the box, and grips the pallet; (e) the user makes the robot raise the fork using a switch; (f) the user rotates the chair using the switch toward forward; (g) the robot moves toward the table; (h) when moving boxes, two sonar sensors are stretched out by DC motors so as not to interfere with boxes on the fork-lift.

Fig. 16 describes the task of moving a box from a warehouse to a work table. When the user simply moves around, the fork is folded, and thus the actual size of the robot is relatively small. When the user picks up boxes, he/she unfolds the fork. While lifting objects, the user can vary the rotation angle to see and check the objects of interest by revolving the chair electrically.

During the transfer of objects, the robot can be used in a confined environment since its steering radius is actually zero. When the user works at a table, the chair can be rotated toward the table.

4.2.2 Development of Work Assistive Mobile Robot System Type II

Fig. 17 shows the developed work assistive mobile robot type II. As noted earlier, for in order to realize a robot with a smaller size and smaller turning radius, we used an omni-directional driving mechanism at the cost of efficiency and excluded the robot arm subsystem. We adopted a foldable fork controlled by motors and equipped the fork-lift system at the rear side. We also adopted an electrically revolving chair so that the user can face the forklift when operating it. Two sonar sensors are used to detect obstacles in the rear. All these components are controlled by a 3-axis joystick and several switches and buttons.

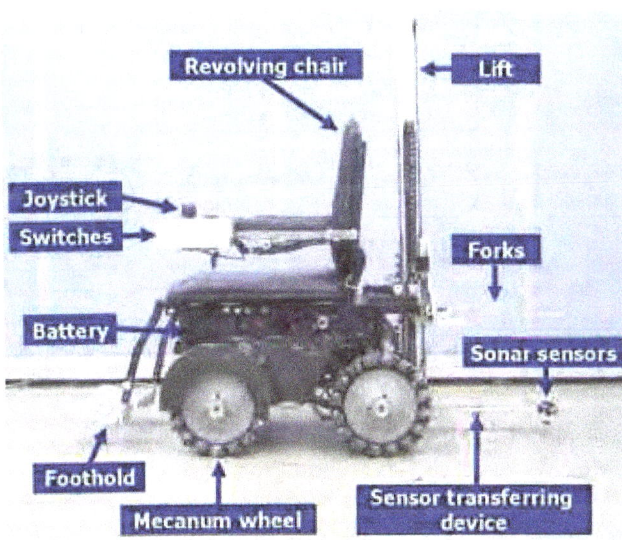

Fig. 17. Developed work assistive mobile robot type II.

Size	760 x 1140 x 510[mm](WxLxH)		
Speed(Robot)	Translation	Slow Mode	2.5 ~ 3[km/h]
		Fast Mode	5[km/h]
	Rotation	45 [deg/s]	
Speed(Chair)	Rotation	18.4 [deg/s]	
Max. Load(Robot)	120 kg		
Max. Load(Lift)	35 kg		

Table 4. Specifications of work assistive mobile robot type II.

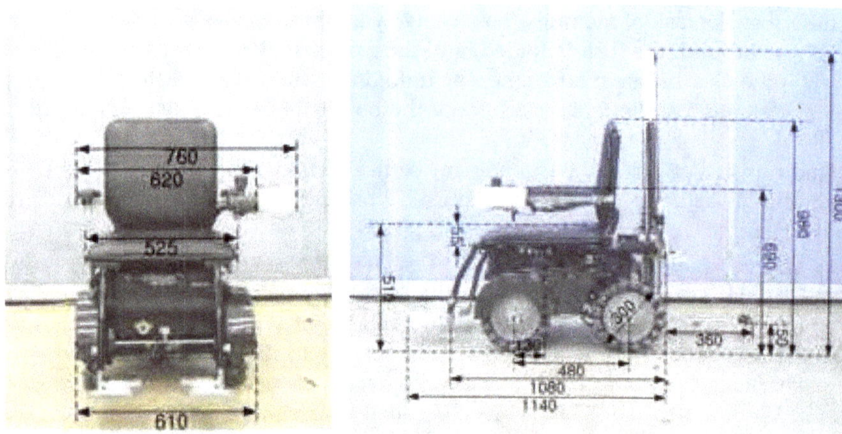

Fig. 18. Developed work assistive mobile robot type II (dimensions in [mm]).

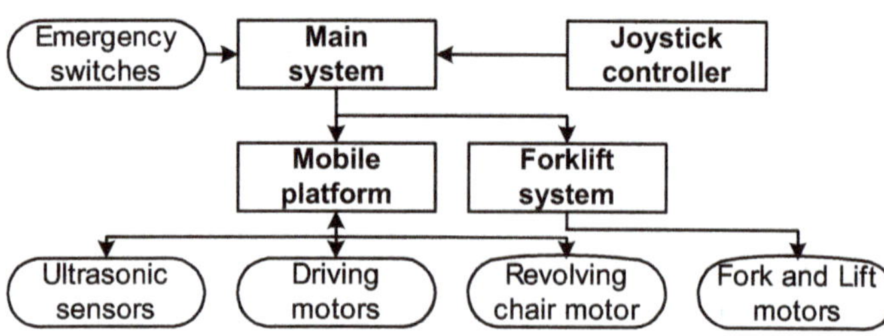

Fig. 19. Architecture of work assistive mobile robot type II.

Fig. 18 shows the developed work assistive mobile robot type II along with its size. The developed robot is small enough to assist in the performance of table tasks. Furthermore, the robot can be parked parallel with the table, and the chair can be rotated to face the table. In addition, the fork is foldable, and the fork-lift can be used as a box feeding device.

The work assistive mobile robot system type II consists of one main system and two subsystems, a mobile platform and a fork lift system. Fig. 19 shows each module configuration. The main system, which is based on FPGA (Field Programmable Gate Array) circuit, receives user input from the joystick controller and emergency switches. According to the user input, the main system gives commands to the mobile platform components such as four driving motors, the revolving chair motor, ultrasonic sensors, and the fork lift system components.

4.2.3 User-trials

Among the enhancements of the work assistive mobile robot system type II, many users applauded the omni-directional mechanism because of its ease of control. Fig. 20 shows pictures of the user-trials.

The participants commented that, "it is very good idea to move boxes when moving around", "the robot is small enough, having a similar size to an electrical wheelchair", "due to the small size, table work is possible without transferring to the table chair", "due to the omni-directional wheel driving mechanism and joystick, it is very easy to control the mobile robot", and "the collision avoidance device helps avoid collisions". However, some participants said, "to avoid collisions in the rear, a rear monitoring system may be needed". This is because the work assistive mobile robot type II does not adopt a rear monitoring system.

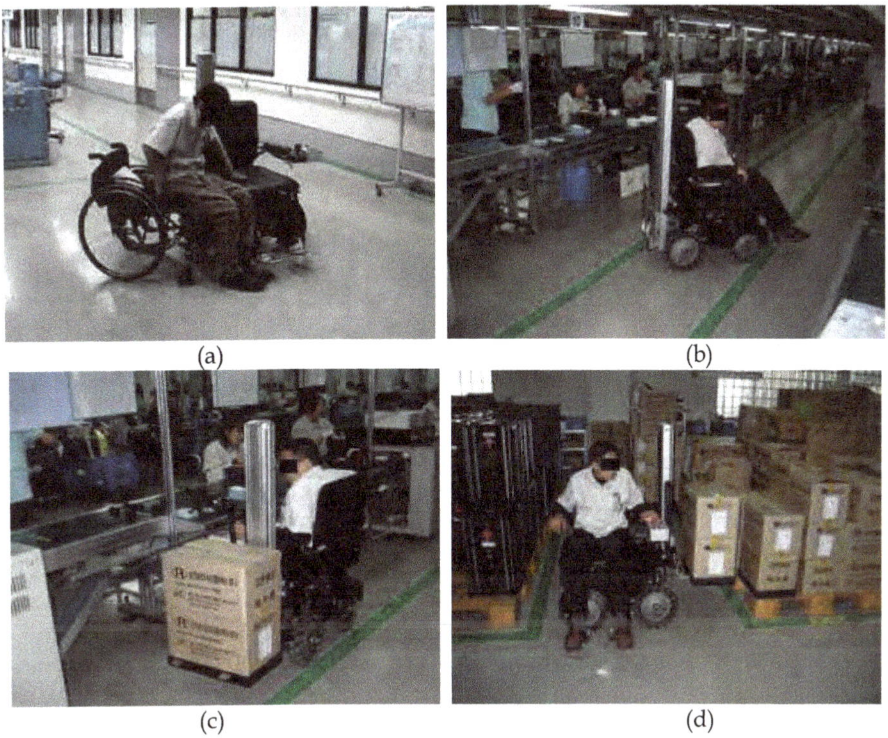

Fig. 20. User trials for Work Assistive Mobile Robot System Type II; (a) Transferring boxes, (b) Moving around, (c) Working at a desk, (d) Moving boxes.

5. Conclusion

Considering the real employment situation of the disabled, it was concluded that there is demand for a robot system that can be used in a real manufacturing environment. To derive our mission statement, we conducted a survey with three criteria: 'A. to assist the disabled as much as possible'; 'B. to consider the real situation of employment for the disabled'; and 'C. to provide assistance for the most necessary tasks for the disabled in the work space'. Based on the survey results, our goal can be stated as follows: To develop work assistive mobile robots to help persons with limb disabilities obtain jobs in manufacturing environments where they can perform simple manual labor. Here, simple labor includes such tasks as circuit inspection and moving boxes.

For our goal, we developed two types of work assistive mobile robots, which are small enough to work in the confined environments of real factories. Work assistive mobile robot type I is equipped with a forklift to move boxes and a robotic arm to help with jobs requiring more dexterity. Robot type II is compact in size, adopting an omni-wheel driving mechanism, and is equipped with a lift having a foldable fork. We gathered feedback from empirical work done on the two robots.

It has been verified by user-trials and feedback that the proposed work assistive robot is capable of assisting a person with a disability to work in a manufacturing environment and perform the same tasks as a normally-abled worker. Further study should be carried out to make the proposed robot more convenient to operate and smaller in size.

6. Acknowledgment

This work was supported by the SRC/ERC program of MOST/KOSEF (grant #R11- 1999-008).

7. References

Bien, Z.; Kim, D. J.; Chung, M. J.; Kwon, D. S. & Chang, P. H. (2003). Development of a wheelchair-based rehab robotic system(KARES II) with various human-robot interaction interfaces for the disabled, *Proceedings of the 2003 IEEE/ASME International Conference on Advanced Intelligent Mechatronics (AIM2003)*, ISBN 0-7803-7759-1, Kobe, Japan, Jul. 2003.

Chang, P. H.; Park , S. R.; Cho, G. R.; Jung, J. H. & Park, S. H. (2005). Development of a robot arm assisting people with disabilities at working place using task-oriented design, *Proceedings of the 9th International Conference on Rehabilitation Robotics (ICORR 2005)*, pp. 482–487, ISBN 0-7803-9004-0, Chicago, IL, USA, Jun. 28 - Jul 1, 2005.

Eftring, H. & Bolmsjö, G. (1993). RAID - A robotic workstation for the disabled, *Proceedings of the 2nd European Conference on the Advancement of Rehabilitation Technology*, pp 24.3, ISBN 91-88336-19-0, Stockholm, Sweden, May 1993.

Hong, H. S.; Jung, S. Y.; Jung, J. H.; Lee, B. G.; Kang, J. W.; Park, D. J. & Chung, M. J. (2005). Development of work assistive mobile robot system for the handicapped in a real manufacturing environment, *Proceedings of the 9th International Conference on Rehabilitation Robotics (ICORR 2005)*, pp. 197–200, ISBN 0-7803-9004-0, Chicago, IL, USA, Jun. 28 - Jul 1, 2005.

Kim, Y.; Park, K. H.; Bang, W. C.; Kim, M. J.; Han, J. S. & Bien, Z. (2002). Development of intelligent bed-robot system for the elderly or the disabled, *Proceedings of 3rd International Workshop on Human-friendly Welfare Robotic Systems(HWRS 2002)*, pp. 94-98, Daejeon, Korea, Jan. 20-22, 2002.

Martens, C.; Ruchel, N.; Lang, O.; Ivlev, O. & Graser, A. (2001). A FRIEND for assisting handicapped people, *Robotics & Automation Magazine*, Vol. 8, issue 1, Mar. 2001, pp. 57-65, ISSN 1070-9932.

Neveryd, H. & Bolmsjö, G. (1994). WALKY, a mobile robot system for the disabled, *Proceedings of the Fourth International Conference on Rehabilitation Robotics (ICORR 1994)*, pp. 137-141, Wilmington, Delaware, USA, Jun. 1994.

Van der Loos, H. F. M.; Wagner, J. J.; Smaby, N.; Chang, K.; Madrigal, O.; Leifer, L. J. & Khatib, O. (1999). ProVAR assistive robot system architecture, *Proceedings of the 1999 IEEE International Conference on Robotics and Automation (ICRA 1999)*, Detroit, pp. 741–746, ISBN 0-7803-5180-0, Michigan, USA, May 1999.

Yoo, D. H.; Hong, H. S.; Kwon, H. J. & Chung, M. J. (2003). Human-friendly care robot system for the elderly, *Proceedings of the 8th International Conference on Rehabilitation Robotics (ICORR 2003)*, pp. 188-191, ISBN 89-88366-09-3, Daejeon, Korea, Apr. 2003.

Yoo, D. H. & Chung, M. J. (2003). Non-contact eye gaze estimation system using robust feature extraction and mapping of corneal reflections, *Proceedings of International Conference of Advanced Robotics (ICAR 2003)*, pp. 911-913, ISBN 972-96889-8-2, Coimbra, Portugal, Jun. 2003.

2

Passive-type Intelligent Walker Controlled Based on Caster-like Dynamics

Yasuhisa Hirata, Asami Muraki & Kazuhiro Kosuge
Department of Bioengineering and Robotics, Tohoku University
Japan

1. Introduction

With the coming of aging societies, many elderly people have serious problems for their locomotion, because of the decline of the physical strength for walking. If they could not use their legs for walking, their physical strength would be weak gradually and they could not walk finally without assistance of other people or some assist system such as wheel chairs, etc. The walking using legs of themselves is very important for improving the quality of their lives, even if they use several kinds of tools for walking such as cane, walker, etc.

In this paper, we pay attention to the walker which support the human based on the physical interaction between the human and the walker. The simple walkers, which consist of support frame, wheels/casters and hand-brakes, are used commercially in many fields such as home, hospital, outside, and so on. On the other hand, to develop the intelligent walkers, many researchers have been proposed several kinds of walkers. Manuel et al. have proposed non-holonomic navigation system of a walking-aid robot referred to as "Care-O-bot II" [1]. Savaniti et al. have developed the motorized "Rollator" [2]. Dubowsky et al. have proposed "PAMM" system to provide a mobility assistance and monitoring for the health status of the user [3]. Fujie et al. have developed the power assisted walker for physical support during walking [4]. We have developed the motion control algorithm of intelligent walker with omni-directional mobile base in which the system is moved based on the intentional force/moment applied by user [5]. Kotani et al. have also proposed "HITOMI" system for permitting outdoor navigation of blind people [6].

The most of the conventional intelligent walkers utilize the servo motors and control them by using the information of sensors such as force/torque sensor, ultra sonic sensor, laser range finder, and so on, to realize the several kinds of functions. Although the active-type walkers using servo motors could realize many functions such as collision avoidance, path following, variable motion characteristics, and so on for supporting the user, the safety issues of this active-type system should also be considered. If we can not control the servo motors of the active-type walker appropriately, the system would move unintentionally and be a dangerous system for human being. In addition, the active-type system might be heavy and its structure might be complicated, because it consists of servo motors, reduction gears, sensors, controller, batteries, and so on. The battery problem is also very severe for its long time working, because the servo motors need much electricity to work. Therefore, the active-type systems still have many problems for their practical use.

To overcome these problems, we have introduced a concept of the passive robotics, in which the systems are developed without using the actuators for mobility. Most of the conventional passive-type walkers based on the passive robotics controlled its heading direction by using the servo motors attached to a steering wheel which can not generate the driving force of walkers [7], [8]. In these systems, the navigation function using sensors such as ultra sonic sensor, laser range finder, etc. could be realized by controlling the steering wheel. Since these kinds of system cannot move by themselves, and can only move when the user applies the force/moment to it, it is intrinsically safe system to support the user in walking similar to the simple walkers which consist of support frame and wheels/casters.

We have also proposed a passive type walker referred to as RT Walker in [9]. Different from the conventional passive-type walkers, RT Walker dose not have servo motors for steering wheel. In stead of it, the servo brakes are attached to the wheels of RT Walker as shown in Figure 1, which can change the brake torques of rear wheels proportionally with respect to the input current. By changing the brake torques of wheels appropriately, the motion of RT Walker could be controlled based on a condition of user and/or environmental information. The brake system is very important and essential functions for most of walkers to adjust their speed from the safety point of view. The controlling of the brakes is effective for developing the intelligent walkers without attaching the active device like servo motors.

Different from the conventional passive-type walkers, RT Walker could realize not only the navigation functions but also its variable motion characteristics by controlling the servo brakes of wheels without using the servo motors [9]. In this paper, we especially propose a motion control algorithm of RT Walker based on the caster-like dynamics, so that the maneuverability of the RT Walker could be improved. In the following part of this paper, first, we introduce the concept of passive robotics and the passive-type intelligent walker referred to as RT Walker developed based on the passive robotics concept. Next, we explain the fundamental motion control algorithm of RT Walker briefly and extend it to the motion control algorithm based on the caster-like dynamics for improving its maneuverability. Finally, we implement its motion control algorithm in RT Walker and illustrate its validity through the experiments.

2. Passive Robotics

For utilizing the intelligent systems practically in the real world environment, we have to consider two points mainly. One is the high performance of them and the other is the safety for users. Most of the conventional intelligent systems have servo motors and they are controlled based on the sensory information such as the force/torque sensor, ultrasonic sensor, laser range finder, etc. Therefore, the high performances for intelligent systems are realized based on the many functions such as power assist, collision avoidance, navigation, variable motion characteristics, and so on.

However, if we can not control the servo motors of the intelligent systems appropriately, they would move unintentionally and be a dangerous system for human being. Especially, in Japan, the legislation has to be formulated for using them in a living environment practically. On the other hand, Goswami et al. have proposed a concept of the passive robotics [10], in which the system moves passively based on the external force/moment without using the actuators, and have dealt with the

passive wrist, whose components are springs, hydraulic cylinders, dampers, and so on. The passive wrist computes a particular motion in response to every applied force and changes the physical parameters of the components for realizing the desired motion.
A robot for direct physical interaction with a human operator within a shared workspace, referred to as COBOT, has been invented as an industrial application of the passive robotics especially for automobile industries [11]. A passive robot is intrinsically safe and its concept has been extended to many fields. PADyC, Passive Arm with Dynamic Constraints, has been proposed as an assistant tool for surgeons [12]. Other applications for surgical robots are seen in [13]. Applications to rehabilitation have been also considered by many researchers. One example is shown in [14]. Applications of the concept to haptic display have been proposed in [15], [16] etc.
In the fields of research on walker system, Wasson et al. [7] and Mac Namara et al. [8] have proposed passive-type intelligent walkers. In the most of them, the servo motor was attached to the steering wheel similar to Cobot system in order to control only the steering angle based on the information of an environment for navigating the user. RT Walker proposed in this paper also has a passive dynamics with respect to the force/moment applied to it. Different from the other passive-type walkers, RT Walker controls the servo brakes appropriately to realize the several functions without using any servo motors.
Many systems have been developed based on the concept of the passive robotics. These passive-type systems are intrinsically safe, since they do not move unintentionally. The passive robotics is a key concept when we consider real-world applications of the advanced robot technology.

3. RT Walker

The passive-type intelligent walker referred to as RT Walker developed based on the passive robotics concept is shown in Figure 1 (a). This prototype consists of a support frame, two passive casters, two wheels with powder brakes, laser range finders, tilt angle sensors, and controller. The part of the rear wheel with powder brake is shown in Figure 1 (b). The powder brakes can change the brake torques of rear wheels of RT Walker proportionally with respect to the input current as shown in Figure 1 (c) and they are transferred to the axes of wheels directly. RT Walker needs little electricity to work by using the servo brakes and is light weight, since its structure is relatively simple compared to the active-type walkers which utilize servo motors for controlling their motions.
By changing the brake torques of two rear wheels appropriately, the motion of RT Walker is controlled based on conditions of users. In addition, RT Walker could get environment information by using the laser range finder and the tilt angle sensors. Based on the information of the environment, RT Walker could realize a collision avoidance function, gravity compensation function, and so on.
In addition to the laser range finder for detecting the environment information, RT Walker has the other laser range finders for measuring the motion of the user, which is attached to the rear part of RT Walker. Based on the motion of the user, we could estimate the user state and change the several functions realized for the intelligent walkers [17].

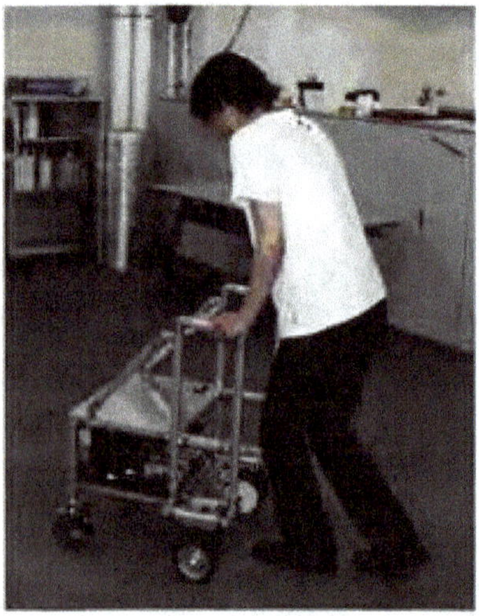

(a) RT Walker

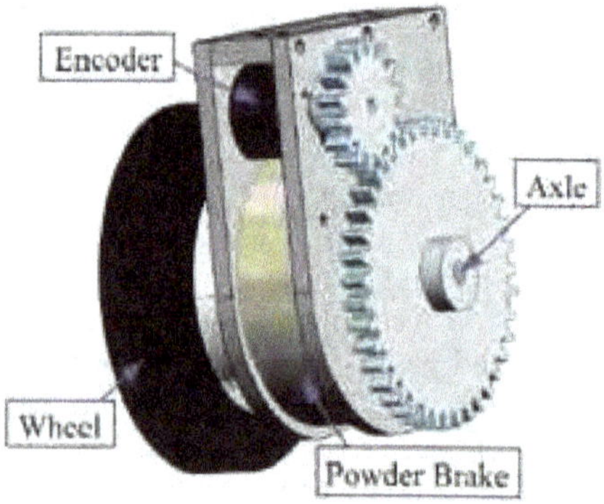

(b) Wheel with Servo Brake

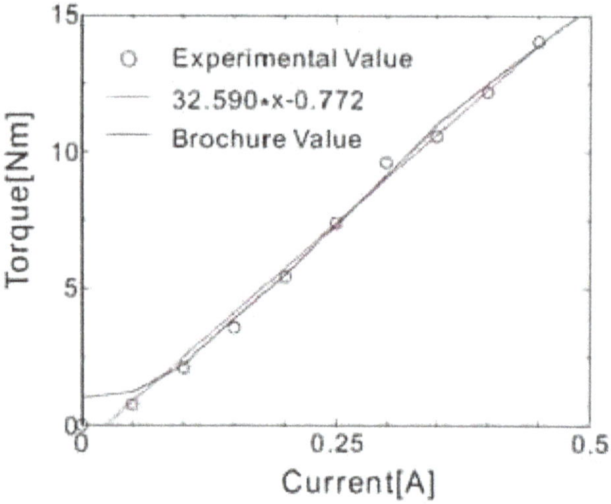

(c) Brake Torque Control based on Input Current

Fig. 1. Prototype of RT Walker.

4. Fundamental Motion Control Algorithm for RT Walker

First, we explain relationships among the brake torque, angular velocity, and applied torque of the wheel with servo brake for realizing the motion control of RT Walker. RT Walker can only move based on the external force/moment applied to it, because it does not have any actuators such as servo motors. To control the motion of RT Walker based on the external force f_{ew} applied to the wheel with servo brake, we can derive the following relationships with respect to the angular velocity of the wheel with servo brakes ω_w.

for $\omega_w \neq 0$

$$t_{bw} = -k_b I_b \operatorname{sgn}(\omega_w) \tag{1}$$

for $\omega_w = 0$

$$t_{bw} = \begin{cases} -f_{ew} R_w & |f_{ew}| R_w \leq k_b I_b \\ -k_b I_b \operatorname{sgn}(f_{ew}) & |f_{ew}| R_w > k_b I_b \end{cases} \tag{2}$$

where t_{bw} is the brake torque generated by the servo brake of RT Walker, R_w is the radius of the wheel, I_b is the input current for the servo brakes, and k_b is the positive coefficient expressed the relationship between the brake torque and the input current. Different from the control of the servo motor, we can only control the motion of RT Walker under these relationships.

Next, we describe the fundamental motion control algorithm of RT Walker. Under the assumption that m_x and j_θ are the inertia coefficients, d_x and d_θ are the damping coefficients, and the velocity and the acceleration are defined as $\dot{x}$, $\dot{\theta}$ and $\ddot{x}$, $\ddot{\theta}$ respectively, the dynamics of RT Walker based on the force/moment f_h, n_h applied by the user and the brake force/moment f_h, n_h generated by the servo brakes is expressed as follows;

$$\begin{bmatrix} m_x & 0 \\ 0 & j_\theta \end{bmatrix} \begin{bmatrix} \ddot{x} \\ \ddot{\theta} \end{bmatrix} + \begin{bmatrix} d_x & 0 \\ 0 & d_\theta \end{bmatrix} \begin{bmatrix} \dot{x} \\ \dot{\theta} \end{bmatrix} = \begin{bmatrix} f_h \\ n_h \end{bmatrix} - \begin{bmatrix} f_b \\ n_b \end{bmatrix} \tag{3}$$

where x-axis is defined as the heading direction of RT Walker as shwon in Figure 2, and the moment and the rotational motion expressed in eq.(3) are defined around the middle point of the real wheel axis.

In this research, the brake force/moment f_h, n_h generated by the powder brakes is controlled for realizing an arbitrary motion of RT Walker, and we can derive the brake torques t_{br}, t_{bl} of each wheel of RT Walker as follows;

$$\begin{bmatrix} t_{br} \\ t_{bl} \end{bmatrix} = \begin{bmatrix} R_w/2 & R_w/T \\ R_w/2 & -R_w/T \end{bmatrix} \begin{bmatrix} f_b \\ n_b \end{bmatrix} \tag{4}$$

where T express the distance between each wheel with powder brake.

For realizing the variable motion characteristics of RT Walker, we derive the following equation with respect to the brake force/moment;

$$\begin{bmatrix} f_b \\ n_b \end{bmatrix} = \begin{bmatrix} m_{dx} - m_x & 0 \\ 0 & j_{d\theta} - j_\theta \end{bmatrix} \begin{bmatrix} \ddot{x} \\ \ddot{\theta} \end{bmatrix} + \begin{bmatrix} d_{dx} - d_x & 0 \\ 0 & d_{d\theta} - d_\theta \end{bmatrix} \begin{bmatrix} \dot{x} \\ \dot{\theta} \end{bmatrix} \tag{5}$$

where m_{dx}, $j_{d\theta}$ are the apparent inertia of RT Walker and d_{dx}, $d_{d\theta}$ are the apparent damping. When we derive the brake force/moment from eq.(5), and specified the brake torques of the servo brakes of RT Walker as shown in eq.(4), RT Walker could move as if it has the following apparent dynamics expressed by m_{dx}, $j_{d\theta}$, d_{dx} and $d_{d\theta}$.

$$\begin{bmatrix} m_{dx} & 0 \\ 0 & j_{d\theta} \end{bmatrix} \begin{bmatrix} \ddot{x} \\ \ddot{\theta} \end{bmatrix} + \begin{bmatrix} d_{dx} & 0 \\ 0 & d_{d\theta} \end{bmatrix} \begin{bmatrix} \dot{x} \\ \dot{\theta} \end{bmatrix} = \begin{bmatrix} f_h \\ n_h \end{bmatrix} \tag{6}$$

When we change the apparent dynamics of RT Walker using the brake system, we could realize many kinds of motion characteristics of RT Walker.

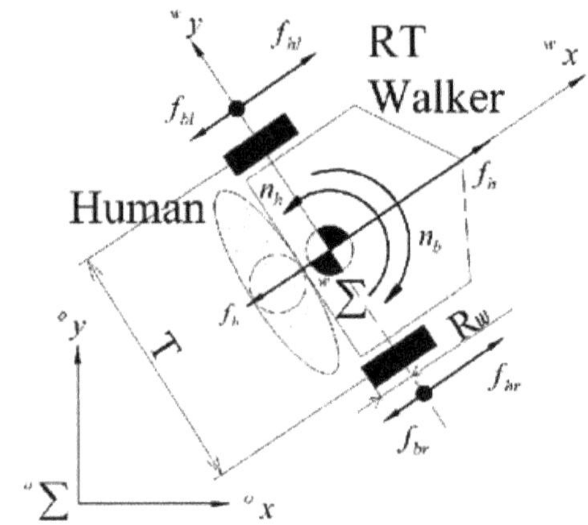

Fig. 2. Model of RT Walker.

5. Caster-like Motion

5.1 Human/Environment-adaptive Motion Control

In the conventional control algorithm of RT Walker proposed in [9], we realize the human-adaptive and the environment-adaptive motion control algorithms. In the human-adaptive motion control algorithm, the apparent dynamics of RT Walker could be specified to it by controlling the servo brakes appropriately, so that we could change its maneuverability, which is explained briefly in the previous section.

However, we have not considered that how RT Walker change its apparent dynamics based on the condition of users, though we have proposed the method for changing the parameters of RT Walker. In this paper, we introduce an example of a method that how we change the apparent dynamics of RT Walker based on its condition, which could be realized by using the caster-like dynamics.

In the environment-adaptive motion control algorithm proposed in [9], we realize the collision avoidance motion of RT Walker using the laser range finder. In this algorithm, to derive the brake torques of servo brakes for avoiding the obstacles, we utilize the method based on an artificial potential field proposed in [18], which is generally utilized by the research of the mobile robot system.

For intelligent walkers, this method is very effective to realize the collision avoidance motion. However, when we consider that intelligent walker utilize in the real world environment including doors, elevators, shelves, walls, and so on, we could not utilize it easily, unless we recognize the object in the real world environment. For example, if RT Walker could not recognize a door, an elevator, a shelf and so on, we could not close to them by using RT Walker implemented in the general collision avoidance methods, because these kinds of object are regarded as obstacles.

To overcome these problems, in this paper, we propose a motion control algorithm based on the caster-like dynamics. By considering the caster-like motion and extending its motion to the advanced motion characteristics of the caster, we could improve the maneuverability of RT Walker in the human-adaptive and the environment-adaptive motion control algorithms.

5.2 Caster-like Dynamics

The concept of the motion control of the robot based on the caster-like dynamics have been proposed in [19] for realizing the coordinative transportation of an object by using multiple mobile robots. In the algorithm proposed in [19], each mobile robot is controlled as if it has a caster-like dynamics as shown in Figure 3, and transports a single object together with other robots based on a intentional force/moment applied by a human. When the human applies the force/moment to the object, the wheel of each virtual caster rotates around the free rotational joint to the direction of the force applied by the human, so that the human could handle a single object together with multiple mobile robots. The caster-like dynamics is also robust against the inevitable positioning error of each robot, even if each robot has a slippage between the wheels of each mobile robot and the ground.

Intelligent walker realizes the physical interaction between the user and walker based on the force/moment applied by the user similar to the case of cooperative transportation of an object by a human and robots. In addition, the robustness with respect to the slippage between wheels of walker and the ground is required. In this paper, we extend the caster-like dynamics proposed in [19] and propose the control algorithm of RT Walker based on its caster-like dynamics for supporting the people who have walking difficulties.

In this section, we consider how the apparent dynamics of RT Walker are changed based on the condition of users or information of an environment. To realize the walker with good maneuverability, we propose Adaptive Caster Action in this paper, which is a control algorithm based on the caster-like dynamics. To realize the caster-like dynamics for RT Walker, first, we consider a motion of a real caster as shown in Figure 3.

The real caster consists of a wheel, a free rotational joint and a wheel support, which connects the wheel and the free rotational joint as shown in Figure 3. The motion of the caster is characterized by three kinds of motion. One is the translational motion of the wheel along the heading direction of its wheel, second one is the rotational motion of the wheel around a point where the wheel contacts with a ground, and third one is the rotational motion of the free rotational joint around its own.

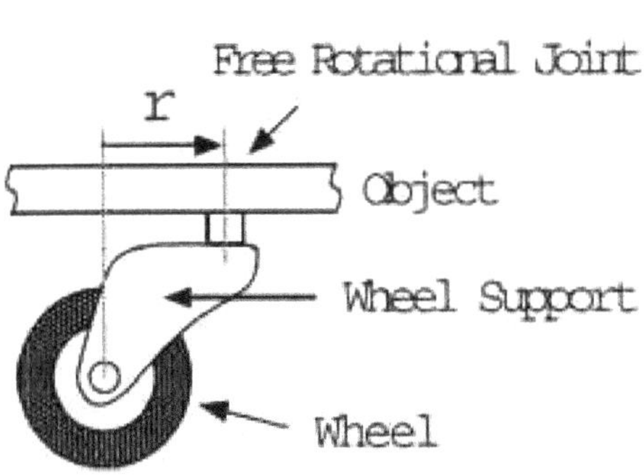

Fig. 3. Real Caster.

In this paper, we control the middle point of the axis of the rear wheels of RT Walker so as to have virtual caster wheel, and the virtual free joint is designed in the forward of RT

Walker along its heading direction as shown in Figure 4. To discuss the motion of the virtual caster, we define two coordinate systems as shown in Figure 4; a wheel coordinate system ${}^{w}\Sigma$ and a free rotational joint coordinate system ${}^{f}\Sigma$. ${}^{w}\Sigma$ is fixed on the virtual caster wheel, and ${}^{f}\Sigma$ is fixed on the virtual free rotational joint. The direction of x-axes of the wheel coordinate system and the free rotational joint coordinate system are defined as the heading direction of the virtual caster wheel as shown in Figure 4. The x-axis of the free rotational joint coordinate system is also defined as the heading direction of RT Walker.

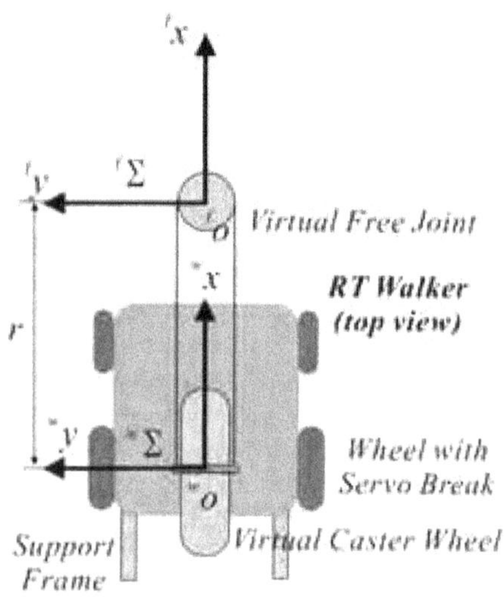

Fig. 4. Coordinate System of RT Walker.

To realize the caster-like dynamics based on two coordinate systems, first, we consider the translational motion of the virtual caster wheel around the free rotational joint based on the force applied to RT Walker along its heading direction as follows;

$${}^{f}f_{hx} = {}^{f}m_{x}\,{}^{f}\ddot{x} + {}^{f}d_{x}\,{}^{f}\dot{x} \tag{7}$$

where ${}^{f}m_{x}, {}^{f}d_{x}$ are positive inertia and damping coefficients and ${}^{f}\ddot{x}, {}^{f}\dot{x}$ are acceleration and velocity of virtual caster wheel with respect to the free rotational joint coordinate system. ${}^{f}f_{hx}$ is a force applied to x-axis of the free rotational joint coordinate system by the human.

Next, to mimic the rotational motion of the caster wheel around a point where the caster wheel contacts with a ground based on the force applied to the virtual free rotational joint perpendicular to the heading direction of RT Walker, we obtain the dynamics of the free rotational joint using the following equation;

$${}^{f}f_{hy} = {}^{f}m_{y}\,{}^{f}\ddot{y} + {}^{f}d_{y}\,{}^{f}\dot{y} \tag{8}$$

where ${}^{f}m_{y}, {}^{f}d_{y}$ are positive inertia and damping coefficients and ${}^{f}\ddot{y}, {}^{f}\dot{y}$ are acceleration and velocity of virtual free rotational joint. ${}^{f}f_{hy}$ is a force applied to y-axis of the free rotational joint coordinate system.

Actually, RT Walker is controlled around the middle of the axis of rear wheels of it, around which the virtual caster wheel is designed, based on the force/moment applied by the user. Therefore, we should derive the dynamics of the virtual caster with respect to the wheel coordinate system. When ${}^{W}f_x$, ${}^{W}n_\theta$, ${}^{W}\ddot{x}$, ${}^{W}\ddot{\theta}$, ${}^{W}\dot{x}$ and ${}^{W}\dot{\theta}$ are force/moment, accelerations, and velocities of the wheel coordinate system, the relations between the force, accelerations and velocities with respect to the free rotational joint coordinate system and the force/moment, accelerations and the velocities with respect to the wheel coordinate system are expressed as follows;

$$ {}^{W}f_h={}^{f}f_{hx},\ {}^{W}n_h={}^{f}f_{hy}r \tag{9}$$

$$ {}^{W}\ddot{x}={}^{f}\ddot{x},\ {}^{W}\ddot{\theta}=\frac{{}^{f}\ddot{y}}{r} \tag{10}$$

$$ {}^{W}\dot{x}={}^{f}\dot{x},\ {}^{W}\dot{\theta}=\frac{{}^{f}\dot{y}}{r} \tag{11}$$

where r is a offset of the virtual caster which is the distance between the virtual caste wheel and the free rotational joint as shown in Figure 4.

From eq.(9)-(11), the caster-like dynamics expressed in eq.(7) and (8) are modified as follows;

$$\begin{bmatrix} {}^{W}m_x & 0 \\ 0 & {}^{W}j_\theta \end{bmatrix}\begin{bmatrix} {}^{W}\ddot{x} \\ {}^{W}\ddot{\theta} \end{bmatrix}+\begin{bmatrix} {}^{W}d_x & 0 \\ 0 & {}^{W}d_\theta \end{bmatrix}\begin{bmatrix} {}^{W}\dot{x} \\ {}^{W}\dot{\theta} \end{bmatrix}=\begin{bmatrix} {}^{W}f_h \\ {}^{W}n_h \end{bmatrix} \tag{12}$$

where

$$ {}^{W}m_x={}^{f}m_x,\ {}^{W}d_x={}^{f}d_x \tag{13}$$

$$ {}^{W}j_\theta=r^2\,{}^{f}m_y,\ {}^{W}d_\theta=r^2\,{}^{f}d_y \tag{14}$$

This equation is similar to eq.(6), so that we could realize the caster-like dynamics by controlling the brake torques of wheels using the method explained in the previous section It should be noted that we do not consider the rotational motion of the free rotational joint of the real caster around its own for implementing the virtual caster, because it dose not effect to the motion of RT Walker actually.

5.3 Adaptive Caster Action

In this section, we consider the maneuverability of RT Walker and propose a control algorithm referred to as Adaptive Caster Action for utilizing it effectively. The apparent dynamics of RT Walker is determined by control parameters such as inertia and damping properties, or offset of virtual caster. Especially, the apparent dynamics is strongly affected by the caster offset r. Adaptive Caster Action adjusts the caster offset based on the condition of users or information of environments

5.3.1 Human-adaptive Control

When the offset is large, the angular acceleration and the velocity of the wheel coordinate system are small as shown in eq.(14) and Figure 5 (a). The larger offset will stabilize the straight line motion of RT Walker against disturbance force perpendicular to the motion direction, but it will make the motion direction change difficult. On the contrary, when the offset is small as shown in Figure 5 (b), the wheel coordinate system rotates to the direction of the intentional force easily, so that RT Walker could rotate to the intentional direction of user.

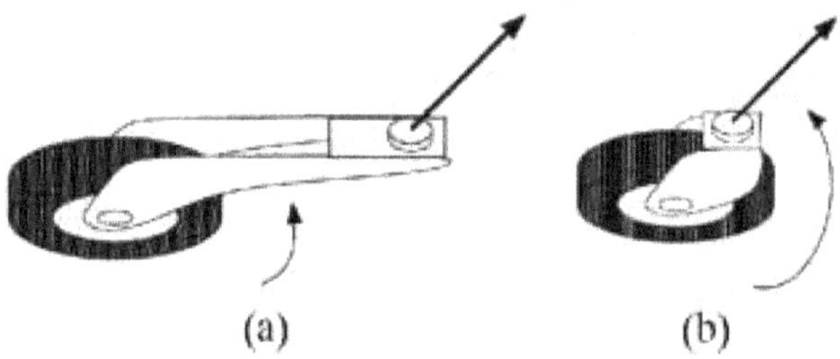

Fig. 5. Adaptive Caster Action.

Let us consider an example of Adaptive Caster Action based on the velocity of RT Walker along its heading direction. When a user moves in narrow space by using RT Walker, its velocity would be low and its easy rotation would be effective. In this case, the smaller caster offset is selected. On the other hand, when the user walks a long distance by using RT Walker, its velocity would be high and the straight line motion of RT Walker would be useful during the walking. In this case, the large caster offset is selected, so that the straight line motion is stabilized and the user could use RT Walker stably, even if the user applies the disturbance force to RT Walker by stumbling. To select the caster offset automatically based on these situations, we change the caster offset according to the velocity of the heading direction of RT Walker, which is expressed by the following equation as an example.

$$r = 0.6\sin({}^{W}\dot{x}) + 0.2 \quad ({}^{W}\dot{x} \geq 0) \tag{15}$$

$$r = -0.2 \quad ({}^{W}\dot{x} < 0) \tag{16}$$

5.3.2 Environment-adaptive Control

To apply the adaptive caster action to the environment-adaptive motion control, we modify eq.(7), (8) as follows;

$${}^{f}f_{hx} - {}^{f}f_{vx} = {}^{f}m_x\, {}^{f}\ddot{x} + {}^{f}d_x\, {}^{f}\dot{x} \tag{17}$$

$${}^{f}f_{hy} - {}^{f}f_{vy} = {}^{f}m_y\, {}^{f}\ddot{y} + {}^{f}d_y\, {}^{f}\dot{y} \tag{18}$$

where ${}^{f}f_{vx}$, ${}^{f}f_{vy}$ are the virtual forces generated based on the information of an environment. By deriving the virtual forces based on the distance between obstacles/steps and the system appropriately and generate the brakes torques by using its virtual force/moment, a user could avoid the collision with obstacles or prevent missing his/her steps in a difference in level [9]. We utilize the method referred to as artificial potential field proposed by Khatib in [18], which is utilized generally in the research on the collision avoidance of the mobile robot.

For measuring the distance between the system and the obstacles or between the system and steps to derive the artificial potential field in the environment, in this research, we utilize the laser range finder which is attached to RT Walker with an angle with respect to the horizontal plan as shown in Figure 6. By attaching the laser range finder with the angle with respect to the horizontal plan, RT Walker could detect the positions of both the obstacles and the steps based on the measured distance.

If the distance is constant d_H, which is derived in advance based on the attached angle and height of the laser range finder from the ground level, this constant measurement means that RT Walker is on the flat ground without obstacles and the steps. When the measured distance is smaller than the constant distance d_H, RT Walker detect the obstacles. In this case, the virtual force/moment is derived based on the measured length d_O, so that the obstacle avoidance motion of RT Walker could be realized. If the measured distance is larger than d_H, RT Walker could detect the steps. In this case, RT Walker generates the map information based on the boundary position of the difference in level, because the length d_S does not change after the detecting the edge of the steps different from the detection of the obstacles. By deriving the virtual force/moment based on the map, the user using RT Walker could avoid the missing his/her steps.

As shown in eq.(17), (18), the virtual force is applied to the free rotational joint of the virtual caster. When we utilize the Adaptive Caster Action, the position of the free joint is changed based on the velocity of RT Walker as shown in Figure 7. When the velocity of RT Walker is high, the larger offset is selected. In this case, RT Walker is influenced by the virtual forces and the avoiding motions with respect to the collision with obstacles and the falling down from the steps could be realized.

On the other hand, when the velocity of RT Walker is low, the smaller offset is selected. In this case, RT Walker would not be influenced by the virtual forces compared with the larger caster offset, so that RT Walker could close to a door, a elevator, a shelf and so on. Even if RT Walker collides with the obstacles with low speed, the dangerousness would also be reduced. It should be noted that the falling down from the step is dangerous situations compared with the collision with obstacles. If RT Walker detects the steps, the control parameters of Adaptive Caster Action should be changed to prevent the falling accident.

6. Experiments

In this research, we implemented Adaptive Caster Action in RT Walker and did several experiments to illustrate the validity of the proposed control algorithm. In this experiment, we move RT Walker to the wall by pushing based on the different kinds of force as shown in Figure 8, so that RT walker closes to the wall in the different kinds of velocity. Motion paths of RT Walker with high speed and low speed are shown in Figure 9 (a), and velocity, caster offset, brake force/moment based on the Adaptive Caster Action during experiments are shown in Figure 9 (b), (c), (d) and (e) respectively.

From these experiments, you can see that RT Walker generates the collision avoiding motion based on the larger caster offset, when its velocity is high. On the other hand, RT Walker can close to the wall, when its velocity is low based on the smaller caster offset. By using Adaptive Caster Action, we could change the apparent dynamics of RT Walker based on its velocity, so that we could use it with good maneuverability in the real world environment.

7. Conclusion

In this paper, we introduce the concept of the passive robotics and the passive-type intelligent walker referred to as RT Walker developed based on the passive robotics concept. For improving the maneuverability of the walker in an environment such as a home, an office, a hospital, etc., we proposed a motion control algorithm referred to as Adaptive Caster Action. The proposed control algorithm is experimentally applied to the developed RT Walker, and the validity of the proposed control algorithm was illustrated by the experimental results.

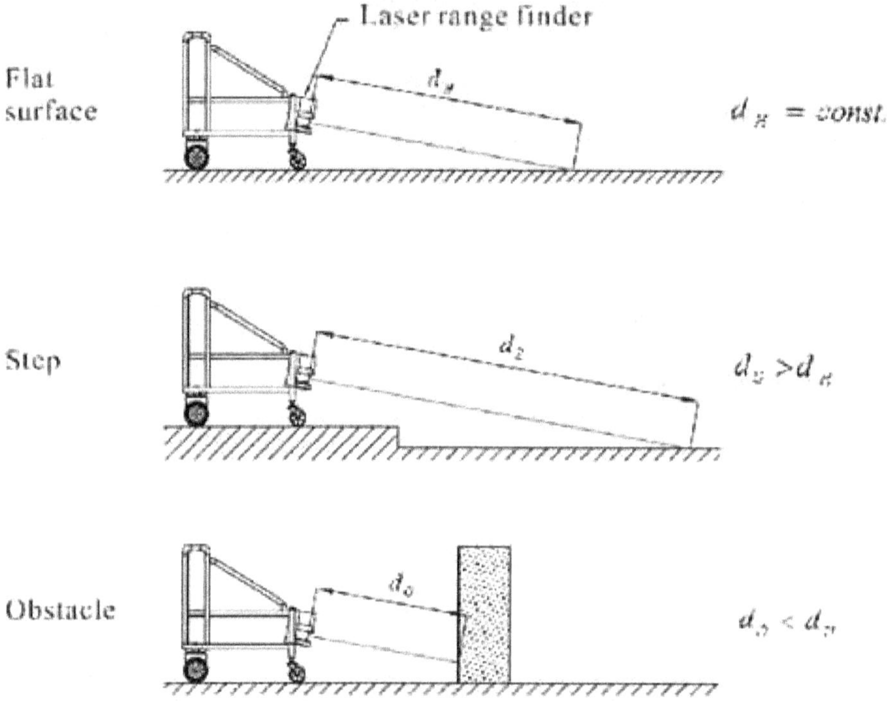

Fig. 6. Detection of Step and Obstacle using Laser Range Finder.

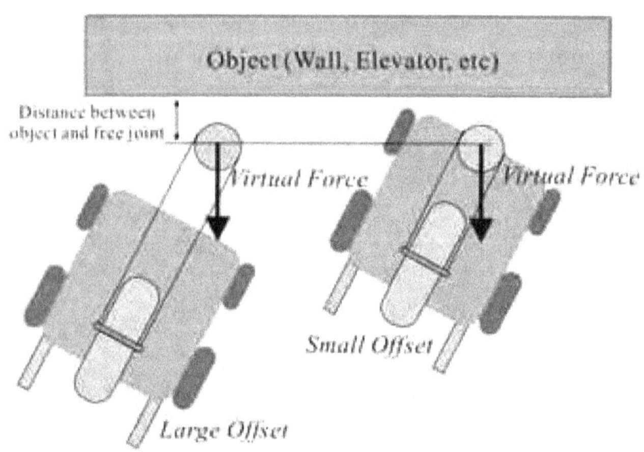

Fig. 7. Environment-adaptive Motion Based on Adaptive Caster Action.

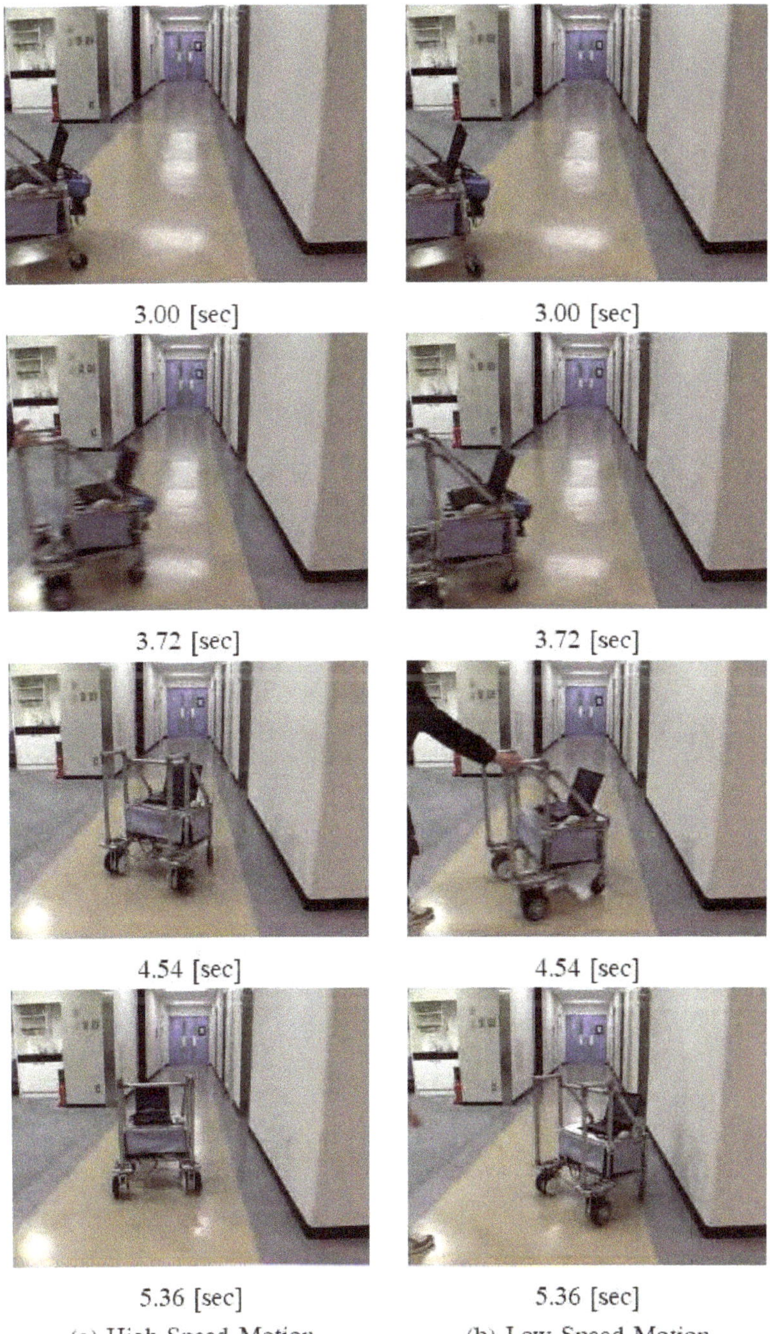

Fig. 8. Motion of RT Walker Based on Adaptive Caster Action.

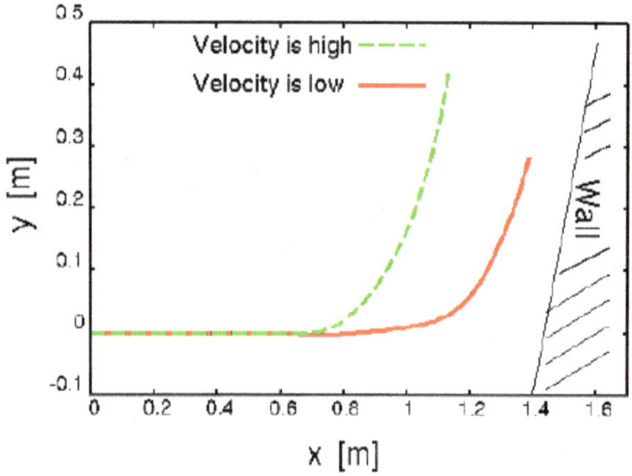

(a) Motion Path of RT Walker

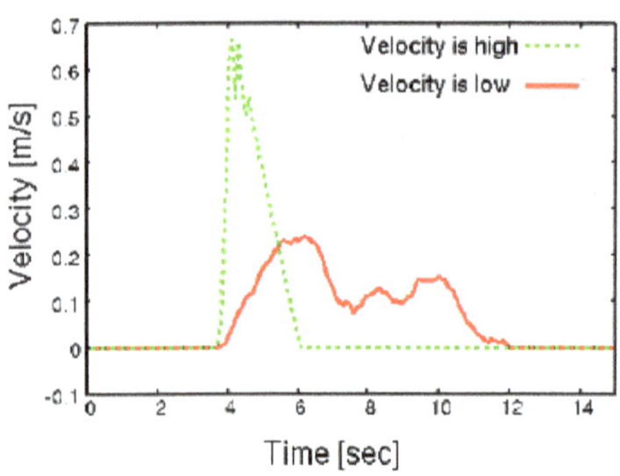

(b) Velocity of Heading Direction

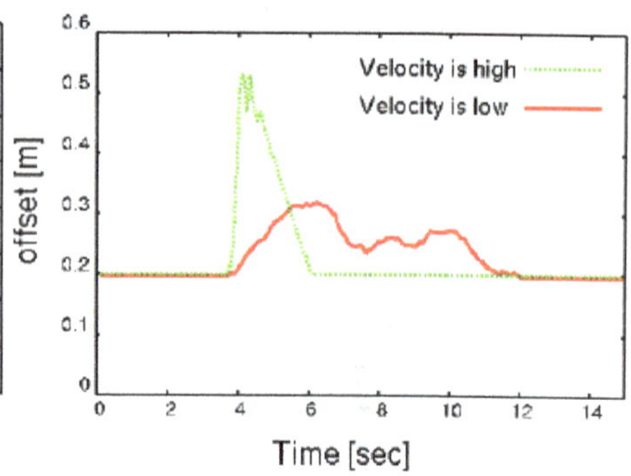

(c) Caster Offset

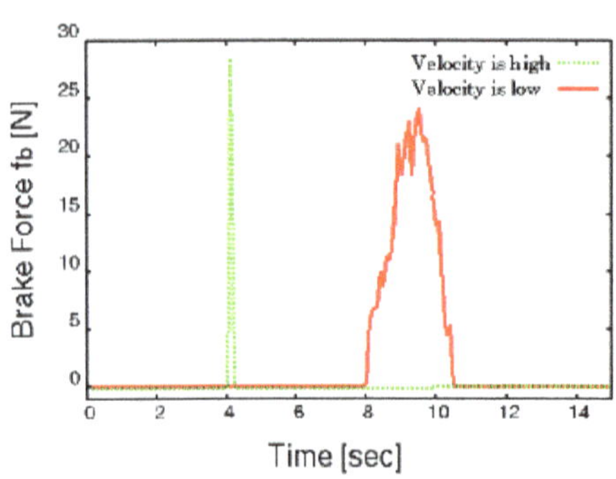

(d) Brake Force

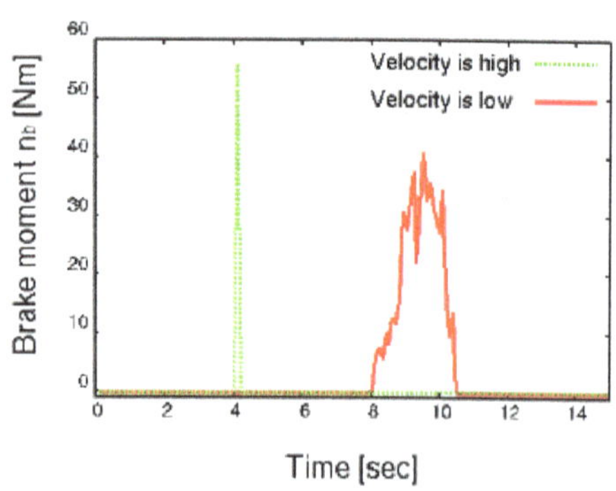

(e) Brake Moment

Fig. 9. Experimental Results.

8. Reference

[1] J. Manuel, H. Wandosell, B. Graf, "Non-Holonomic Navigation System of a walking-Aid Robot", Proc. of IEEE International Workshop on Robot and Human Interactive Communication, pp.518-523, 2002.

[2] A. M. Sabatini, V. Genovese, E. Pacchierotti, "Mobility Aid for the Support to Walking and Object Transportation of People with Motor Impairments", Proc. of IEEE/RSJ International Conference on Intelligent Robots and Systems, pp.1349-1354, 2002.

[3] S. Dubowsky, F. Genot, S Godding, H. Kozono, A. Skwersky, H. Yu, L. S. Yu, "PAMM-A Robotic Aid to the Elderly for Mobility Assistance and Monioring: A "Helping-Hand" for the Elderly", Proc. of IEEE International Conference on Robotics and Automation, pp.570-576, 2000.

[4] M. Fujie, Y. Nemoto, S. Egawa, A. Sakai, S. Hattori, A.Koseki, T. Ishii, "Power Assisted Walking Support and Walk Rehabilitation", Proc. of 1st International Workshop on Humanoid and Human Friendly Robotics, 1998.

[5] Y. Hirata, T. Baba, K. Kosuge, "Motion Control of Omni-directional type Walking Support System "Walking Helper"", Proc. of IEEE Workshop on Robot and Human Interactive Communication, 2A5, 2003

[6] S. Kotani, H. Mori, N. Kyohiro, "Development of the robotic travel aid HITOMI", Proc. of IEEE Int. Conf. on Robotics and Automation, 1990

[7] G. Wasson, P. Sheth, M. Alwan, K. Granata, A. Ledoux, C. Huang, "User Intent in a Shared Control Framework for Pedestrian Mobility Aids", Proc. of the 2003 IEEE/RSJ Intl. Conf. on Intelligent Robots and Systems, 2003

[8] A. J. Rentschler, R. A. Cooper, B. Blaschm M. L. Boninger, "Intelligent walkers for the elderly : Performance and safety testing of VA-PAMAID robotic walker", Journal of Rehabilitation Research and Development, Vol. 40, No. 5, 2003

[9] Y. Hirata, A. Hara, K.Kosuge, "Passive-type Intelligent Walking Support System "RT Walker", Proceedings of the 2004 IEEE/RSJ International Conference on Intelligent Robots and Systems, (2004), pp.3871-3876, 2004.

[10] A. Goswami, M. A. Peshkin, J. Colgate, "Passive robotics: an exploration of mechanical computation (invited) ", Proc. of the IEEE Int. Conf. on Robotics and Automation, pp. 279-284, 1990.

[11] M. A. Peshkin, J. E. Colgate, W. Wannasuphoprasit, C. A. Moore, R. B. Gillespie, P.Akella, "Cobot Architecture", IEEE Transactions on Robotics and Automation, Vol. 17, No.4, 2001

[12] O.Schneider, T.Troccaz, O.Chavanon and D.Blin, "PADyC: a Synergistic Robot for Cardiac Puncturing", Proceedings of 2000 IEEE International Conference on Robotics and Auotmation, 2000.

[13] Jocelyne Troccaz, Peter Berkelman, Philippe Cinquin, Adriana Vilchis-Gonzales, "Surgical robot dependability: propositions and examples", 2nd IARP/IEEE-RAS Joint Workshop on Technical Challenge for Dependable Robots in Human Environments, 2002.

[14] J. Furusho, M. Sakaguchi and N. Takesue: Basic Study for Development of Muscular-Strength Estimation and Training System Using ER Brake --- Development of ER Brake and its Passive Velocity Control---, Journal of RSJ, Vol.20, No.1, pp.77-84 (2002), in Japanese.

[15] Michael A. Peshkin, J. Edward Colgate, Carl Moore, "Passive Robots and Haptic Displays based on Nonholonomic Elements", Proceedings of the 1996 IEEE International Conference on Robotics and Automation, pp.551-556, 1996

[16] Michael A. Peshkin, J. Edward Colgate, Carl Moore, "Passive Robots and Haptic Displays based on Nonholonomic Elements", Proceedings of the 1996 IEEE International Conference on Robotics and Automation, pp.551-556, 1996

[17] Y. Hirata, A. Muraki, K. Kosuge, "Motion Control of Intelligent Passive-type Walker for Fall-prevention Function based on Estimation of User State", Proceedings of the 2006 IEEE International Conference on Robotics and Automation,(2006),3498-3503

[18] Y. Hirata, K. Kosuge, "Distributed Robot Helpers Handling a Single Object in Cooperation with a Human", Proc. of IEEE International Conference on Robotics and Automation, pp.458-463, 2000.

[19] O. Khatib, "Real-Time Obstacle Avoidance for Manipulators and Mobile Robots", Int. Journal of Robotics Research, pp. 90--98, 1986.

3

PLEIA: A Reconfigurable Platform for Evaluation of HCI Acting

Peralta H., Monacelli E., Riman C., Baklouti M., Ben Ouezdou F., Mougharbel I. 1 , Laffont I.[2] & Bouteille J.[2]

LISV, Engineering Systems Laboratory of Versailles, Versailles Saint Quentin en Yvelines University, France.

[1]Lebanon University, Lebanon

New Technologies Platform, Raymond Poincaré Hospital

France

1. Introduction

For people with severe motor disabilities, it is difficult or sometimes impossible to use standard interface devices (mouse, keyboards, joysticks, trackballs, etc ...). The evaluation of their capabilities, the education or re education of abilities and the compensation of their deficiencies is essential. Nowadays, the performance of a person is only determinated by the observation of the trajectory followed by the cursor during the exercises and to facilitated people's accessibility to computer and electrical devices, few exist. Standard test and reliable indicators would bring a better evaluation of the use of peripheral interfaces for motor handicapped people. Two ways of research have been developed: some researchers have focused on defining new peripheral devices, others have focused their works on new rehabilitation process and algorithms to adapt commands. We assume that we are able to associate on the same study of pointing task: computer, wheelchair and environment control.

2. Problem

For the handicapped person, the use of interface controls could be a very complex task. The systems for aiding the person are controlled by an interface. It is founded on the relation between the Human Computer Interactions (HCI). The most important problem in the Human interaction is the adequacy between the user and the interface: computer, wheelchair, remote control... Moreover, the wide range of motor disabilities makes impossible the development of standard solutions. In most cases, a customized interface device is developed to fit to the deficiency of person. Some laboratories focused their researches on the design and the development of a personalized and adjustable Human-Computer Interface (HCI). However, for motor disabilities, few studies based on the interface tasks and quantitative evaluations were conduced. Nowadays, there are few works that present simple and reliable indicators (Buaud A.,2003)(Kadouche R, 2004) for evaluating the performance of impaired users. Usually this task is achieved by a qualitative evaluation led by the therapist (fig. 1). There are some methods for evaluating the dexterity. For example, the method used today by the occupational therapist is based on the functional evaluation by a direct analysis of the other activity acting as operator (cinesiologic analysis):

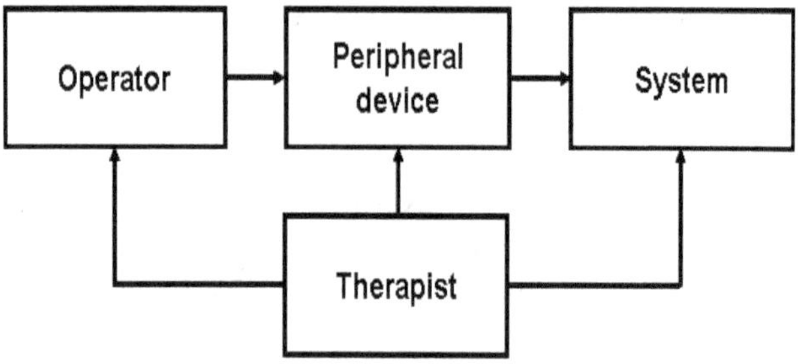

Fig. 1. Evaluation scheme for normal therapy session.

The therapist acts on the operator, the peripheral device and the system. This system can be a personal computer, an external system such as powered wheelchair or a toy. The feedback used by the therapist is qualitative. The therapist is able to adapt the device changing internal parameters (such as sensibility, position, as well as, the configuration of system). These corrected actions are done following the therapist expertise.

3. Objective

PLEIA (Peralta H., 2006) software can be integrated into the evaluation scheme (fig. 2) as assistive system for the therapist.

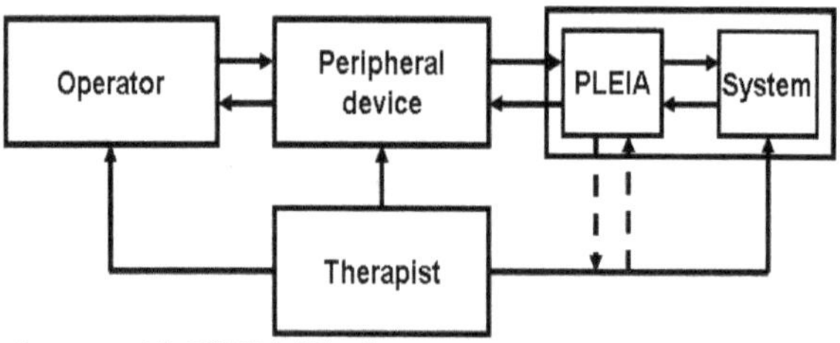

Fig. 2. Evaluation scheme with PLEIA Platform.

PLEIA gets information from the peripheral device. The therapist can access to these information. Then he can act on PLEIA, on the peripheral device or on the system. The evaluation of their capabilities by the interface capabilities is essential. Today in the scope of adaptation and quantitative measures of capacity, few evaluation standard methods exist. The evaluation are oriented to handicap, but the information measured just allow to determinate delay and trajectory by basic indicators. Therefore, it is necessary to find new methods to evaluate the peripheral devices by computers processing's mean. The monitoring of the user capability is useful for determining the diagnostic information. The plan for the rehabilitation could be also based on evaluation result (Dipietro, L. 2003). Thus, it is necessary to have a set of quantitative criteria, a therapy methodology and common tools to be applied by the occupational therapist.

The objective is then to define suitable exercises associated with quantitative criteria in order to evaluate the adaptation between the user and the peripheral (fig. 3). It includes performance but also handling evaluation at a time and on a period training.

4. Related Research

4.1 Evaluation studies

There are studies to determine analytical evaluation from the pointing devices with the user interaction. The first work about the hand movement is the Fitt's Law which is based on a model of human psychomotor behavior developed in 1954. It gets the measure of a Movement Time (MT) index. This is the result of the relationship between movement time, distance, and accuracy. Many works about the evaluation of movement and Human Computer Interaction (HCI) are based on this law.

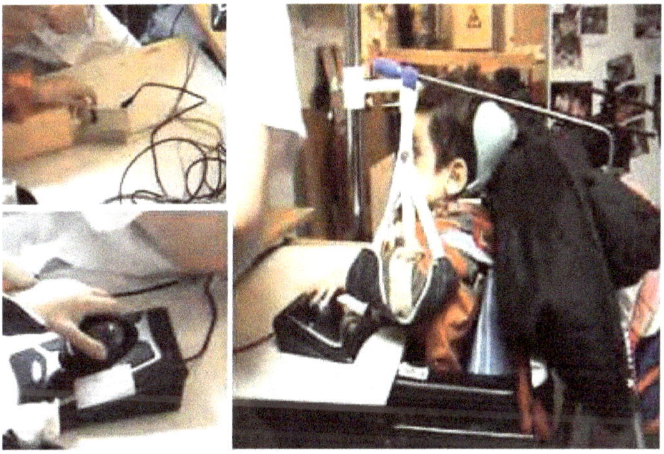

Fig. 3. Examples of peripheral device.

The main interest in this law is that it can be applied to pointing and dragging using a mouse, trackball, joystick, and touch screen (Keates, S., 2002) (Soukoreff, R. 2004). Mackenzie (MacKenzie, I., 2001) proposed seven new accuracy measures to evaluate computer pointing devices. The measures are intended to elicit subtle differences among devices through an analysis of the cursor movement along the cursor path. The ISO standard to assist evaluation of pointing devices is ISO 9241: "Ergonomic design for office work with visual display terminals (VDTs)." The part 9 is "Requirements for non-keyboard input devices". In (ISO 9241-9) are included mouse, joysticks, track ball, tablets and overlays, touchpad, touch sensible screens. The standard specifies the quality of the input devices in terms of performance criterion: "it is considered useable, if users can achieve a satisfactory level of performance on a given task and maintain an acceptable level of effort and satisfaction".

4.2 Methods to improve the mobility with pointing systems

If the interface is correctly adapted to the abilities of user, there are many solutions to improve it. Some solutions have been developed for accessibility and mobility. These solutions are based on command sensor adaptation processing. For example, "smart wheelchair", "adaptive interfaces" and "adaptive commands" (Thieffry, R., 2005) develop assistive methodology in order to reduce the physical, perceptual, or cognitive skills necessary to operate with safety a powered wheelchair or another system (walker or computer pointing system). Other works on assistive robotic wheelchair system improve the acting by the design of specific sensor interfaces like in the Wheelesley (Yanco, H., 2002). (Kang, S., 2004) shown one joystick for a system like an electric wheelchair. This system helps to drive easily and safety. Another system was experimented. (Jeong, H. 2004) proposed a new Human-Computer-Interaction (HCI) method for a quadriplegic, which is controlled by clenching teeth. Two clenching patterns, did seven instructions including rest, up, down, left and right as well as click and double click actions are made for the control of a pointing device. The control source is EMG1. An experimental system of voice interface is presented in (Tellex, S., 2005). It is an alternative controlled manner. The system "understands" natural language motion commands. The works show the possibility to compensate and improve the user mobility. The big parts of such systems use a pointing interface as command access. The questions are then: How could the users have the right peripheral device? It is convenient for his proper abilities? Can another interface improve his development on the control of his system? A step of evaluation with different interfaces is necessary.

4.3 Evaluation platforms

Platforms for improving the HCI acting based on exercises have been developed (Shimizu, H., 2006) for re-educational therapy. Today, the computer applications include graphical interfaces. Actions as "click", "displace", "drag and drop" are essential to handle a computer. There are many software, for handicapped persons that basically are centered on learning. For example, Judy Lynn Software, Inc. offers different categories of software for different patient (depending upon age and symptom), these work to improve certain activity as visual tracking, cause effect, hand - eye coordination, etc. We can find similar software of many companies as: Marblesoft, Simtech publication, Widget software. In conclusion, the exercises proposed by these softwares have an educational interest but they do not include a performance evaluation of user acting. Adeprio Diffusion proposes to save the results of patient acting. Efficasouris (Adameczek, A., 2005) is a software developed to evaluate the pointing capabilities of patient with the mouse, saving the performance. The designers have built four modules: 1) The game module, 2) The statistical module to save the performance data of patient, 3) Diagnostic or User identification and personal perception (this module is a questionnaire model, used to know qualitative the point of view on test and software) and the last one, 4) Virtual Keyboard, serves to design a virtual keyboard adapted to the patient from the analysis data. The last module is the objective of efficasouris. The medical team realizes subjective analysis (based on a questionnaire) and objective analysis which are made directly (observation of the interaction with the user during the test) and indirectly (using cameras and record data performance). The software has three indexes: task time, task error, and clicks number (accuracy). Another example is Catch Me™ by lifetool. It is evaluation software with interesting properties as creation of exercises, tuning of exercises and parameters configuration as mouse speed, colors, forms, wallpapers, volume. The analyzed results are: game time, right actions number, wrong actions number and average time by action. This does not include information on the user handling.

The following section explains the main idea for therapy methodology on PLEIA software.

---

[1] Electromyogram (EMG)

5. PLEIA

5.1 Description of Software Platform for Interface & Interface Evaluation (PLEIA)

The PLEIA software platform (by French acronymic) is our specialized evaluation platform. The PLEIA proposes an open methodology (fig.4) to evaluate the user's dexterity with the pointing devices using different peripheral computer devices at the end of the process. It allows to adapt these devices to characteristic of user using different feedback modes (light, sound, haptic, etc...) dedicated to occupational therapist. PLEIA tools allow to elaborate specific exercises based on functional systems: from computer interface to wheelchair command.

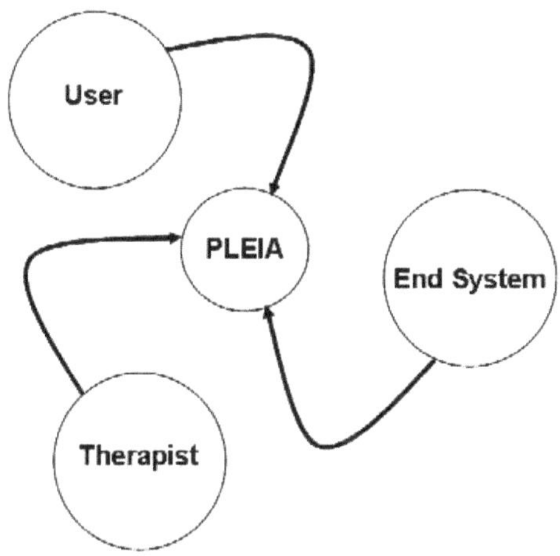

Fig.4. PLEIA as centre of the evaluation, assistance and compensation process.

The therapy session could be oriented on different goals: function learning (especially for the young children), evaluation of dexterity with different peripheral and generalization for other systems like wheelchair command. PLEIA is composed on three blocks with the same functionalities:

- **PLEIA evaluation**: This module was programmed to evaluate the dexterity through 5 main tests: 1) Reach Target, 2) Drag and drop, 3) Follow path, 4) Click Targets, 5) Exploration screen zones. This chapter is centered on this module.
- **PLEIA functional awaking**: This module allows user to act on real object (robots, toys, etc.). It is dedicated for the young children. The same evaluation could be done.
- **PLEIA functional**: This module is dedicated to evaluate handling of a powered wheelchair (often goal of the therapy).

PLEIA is a program that allows therapist to create specific exercises with scenarios. It could be connected to different peripheral interfaces (joystick, trackball, mouse, keyboard, etc.) and act on devices as robot (khepera™), toys and electric wheelchair. All information and performance data (time, errors, coordinates, etc ...) are analyzed. The patient tests different peripheral devices. The therapist evaluates which is more adequate for pointing systems. Different analytic indexes have been developed (see section 6). The therapist could create suitable configurations of exercise (named scenarios) with different tuning parameters such as cursor speed, sound, cursor and objects dimensions and appearance. This platform can be connected for remote experiment with other medical centers. Basically, PLEIA includes different exercises. The proposed test could include different elements, such as obstacles, objectives to reach, object to take, trajectories, cursor. These elements are shown in (fig. 5).

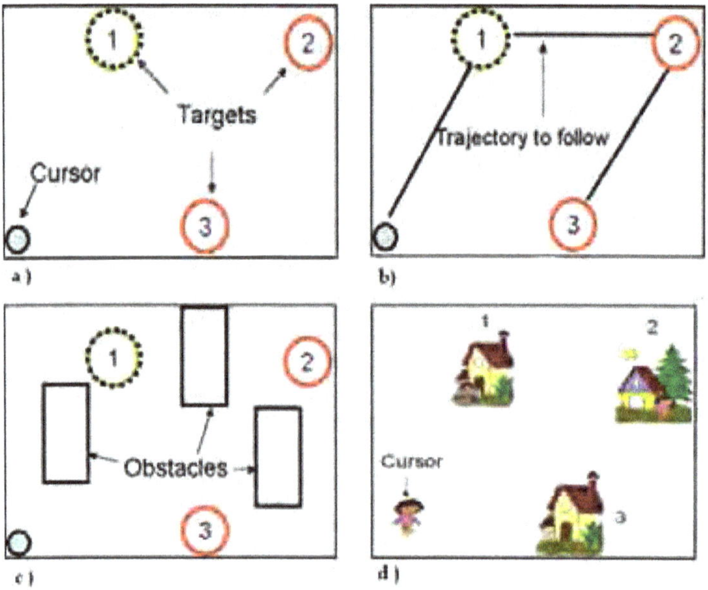

Fig. 5. Exercise models on PLEIA Software with the same scenario: a) Reach the targets, b) Follow path, c) Avoid the obstacles, d) Mode tuned.

Reach the targets (fig 5a), the aim of this test is to evaluate a displacement. The trajectory is shown by sequence of object. The dotted circle is the next objective to reach. The (fig. 5b) shows the same configuration of target, with path constraint. The next scenario (fig. 5c) is used when the patient present uncontrolled movements. The trajectory includes targets and obstacles to avoid. The (fig. 5d), shows the same test with different images. The therapist uses them to improve the attention of children. Fig. 9 present other example of PLEIA test.

5.2 PLEIA Functionalities

The functionalities that PLEIA offers are:

- Exercise configuration assistance:

The configuration of exercise is based on a wizard processing in order to be user friendly.
The medical team is able to choose the suitable exercise for evaluating the patient performance. We suggest five main model exercises: (1) Reach target: reaching certain objects on the computer screen. (2) Drag and drop: It refers to the capacity to hold a button and at the same time do the displacement. (3) Follow path: It evaluates the capacity of following a track. (4) Click on the targets: this test has been thought to measure the user accuracy, with different target sizes. (5) Exploration screen zones: this exercise evaluates work reachable space. It is very important to mention that the objects designed by the therapist on the scenario (trajectories, obstacles, wallpapers, etc) can be simple or complex depending upon the type of exercise. The decision is taken by the therapist.

- Patient test information:

PLEIA memorizes user actions (see section 6).

- Performance indexes as trajectory length, errors, clicks used in the exercise, accuracy, time delay, and command analysis.
- Assistance Mode:

To compensate the patient disability, We used feedback such as visual, audio, or vibration associated to test conditions (ex. Impact with the obstacle) to inform the user. Specific assistance like sensitive attraction could be used in the execution.

6. Method evaluation

6.1 Participants.

We present in this section, two children evaluations, Claudia and Robert. Each participant was identified as "child with disability" by the medical team. They can not use mouse, basic joystick or trackball because of their limitation in the mobility and muscular weakness. The fatigability is another factor to take into account. The test must take a few minutes (1 to 2 min), and the session has a 45 min duration at the worst case fro the good results.
Claudia is four years old child. She suffers from myopathy. She uses minitrack stick. She handles it with the left index finger. Special technical adaptations are required (fig. 6).
Robert is seven years old child. He suffers from myopathy, uses a mini joystick HMC™ with InfraRed connection. Robert uses the left thumb finger to handle his medical aid.
We have then introduced new indicators that could help the therapists to evaluate the performance of each patient.

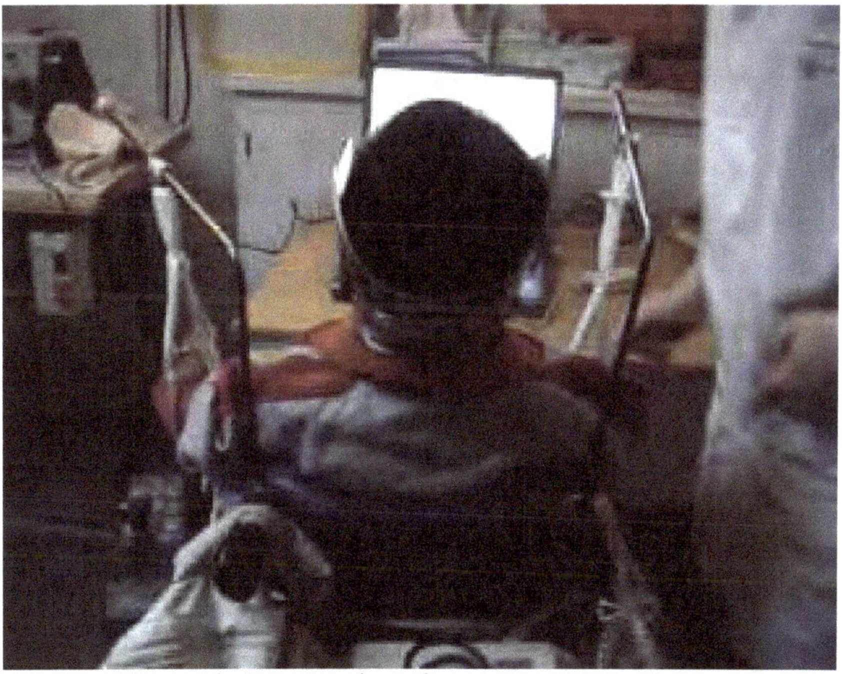

Fig. 6. Claudia with special adaptations for makes a test on PLEIA software.

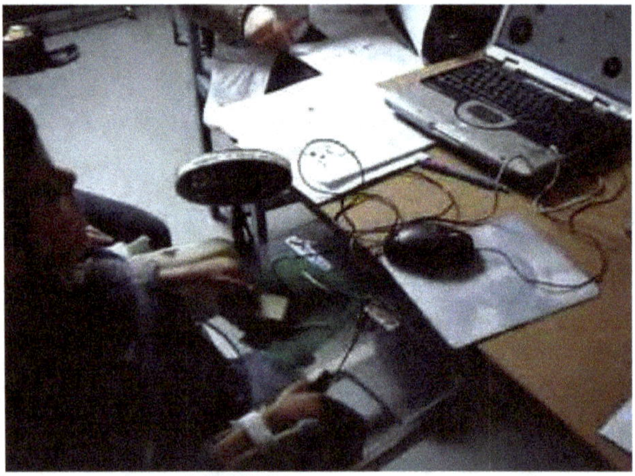

Fig. 7. Robert in therapy session with PLEIA.

These indicators have been implemented in a software platform (PLEIA). It is developed in collaboration with the Raymond Poincare Hospital and Saint Maurice Hospital (Paris Hospital).

PLEIA include user information. It includes the data of test, date, disabilities of patient, and other information of patient.

The patient is placed in front of monitor (between 0.60 m to 0.80 m). The computer's devices are installed in the best condition of comfort and functionality for the patient. This last condition depends upon the deficiency and the position of the patient (fig. 8).

6.2 Measurement and performance indexes

The indicator based on a set of performance focus the peripheral adaptation problem. In other words, they allow quantifying the realization of pointing tests and to appreciate the choice and the configuration of the peripheral device. They carry out comparisons to appreciate the evolution of the results of one user or relative to different classes of users.

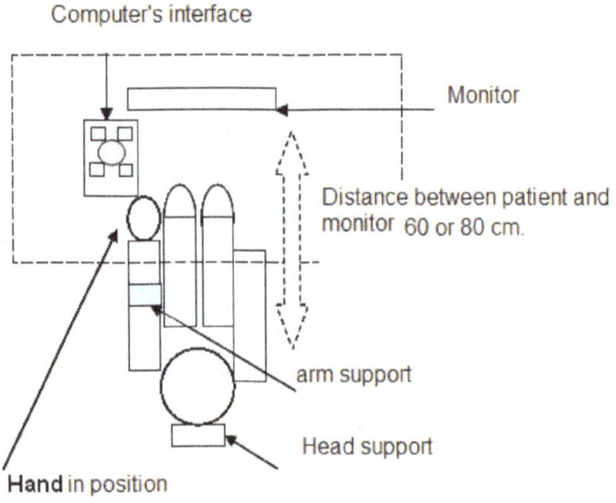

Fig. 8. Localization of patient.

We defined two groups of indicators: (a) task indicators which use direct results of the test execution, (b) comfort indicators which are centered on the behavior of the patient.

1) Task indicators: The indicators of tasks are the first order indicators which give a direct classification of the performances of the user. Based on tests, we retained three basic measurements:

- **Total time of exercise (TT)**: It is the time to finish the exercise.
- **The Covered Distance (CD):** It is the addition of all cursor displacement.
- **The collision (C) or Failure (F)** is a problem occurrence in the test: collision with obstacle, target unreachable.

2) Comfort indicators: The indicators of comfort have been introduced to evaluate user easiness in manipulating the device. The proposed indicators are:

- **Pause Rate (PR):** This indicator calculates the ratio of cursor stop delay in the exercise. This indicator expresses the "fatigue" of the user on a specification test with peripheral.

$$PR = \frac{PT}{TT} \quad (1)$$

PT: Pause time
TT: Test time.

- **User Action (UA).** This indicator estimates the number of user action on the peripheral interface.

$$UA = \sum_{i=0}^{TT} \left[(K_1 \Delta I_1)_i^2 + (K_2 \Delta I_2)_i^2 \right] \quad (2)$$

ΔI_1, ΔI_2: Peripheral inputs variation (between two sequential inputs).
TT : Test Time
i : Sample time in the test.
K_1,K_2: Normalization gains

- **Command Load (CL):** This indicator estimates the interface action number of the user versus a reference user.

$$CL_{user} = \frac{UA_{user}}{UA_{ref}} \quad (3)$$

UV_{ref} : User action variation (Valid person).
UV_{user}: User action variation (User)

- **Efficient Coefficient (EC).** It estimates the efficiency of user commands. An inefficiency is defined as the user actions that tend not to optimize the result of the test

$$EC = \sum_{i=0}^{TT} \left[\left((K_1 I_1)_i^2 + (K_2 I_2)_i^2 \right) * K_3 \Delta Gd_i \right] \quad (4)$$

ΔGd_i : Goal distance variation on the sample i

ΔI_1, ΔI_2: Peripheral inputs variation.
TT : Test Time
i : Sample time in the test.
K_3,K_1,K_2: Normalization gains

- **Efficient Load** (EL). This ratio estimates the user efficiency between the Reference Efficient Coefficient (EC) getting of valid user and the User Efficient Coefficient, multiplied by the Rate Time. This Ratio Time is defined as reference total time (time to finish the test by the Reference User) and the user total time.

$$EL_{user} = \frac{EC_{ref}}{EC_{user}} * \left(\frac{TT_{ref}}{TT_{user}} \right) \tag{5}$$

EC_{ref} : Efficient Coefficient (Valid user).
EC_{user} : Efficient Coefficient (user).
TT_{ref} : Test Time reference (Valid user)
TT_{user} : Test Time reference (user)

7. Experimentation

The exercise designed for the children by the occupational therapist (fig. 9) is a sequence of 12 targets.

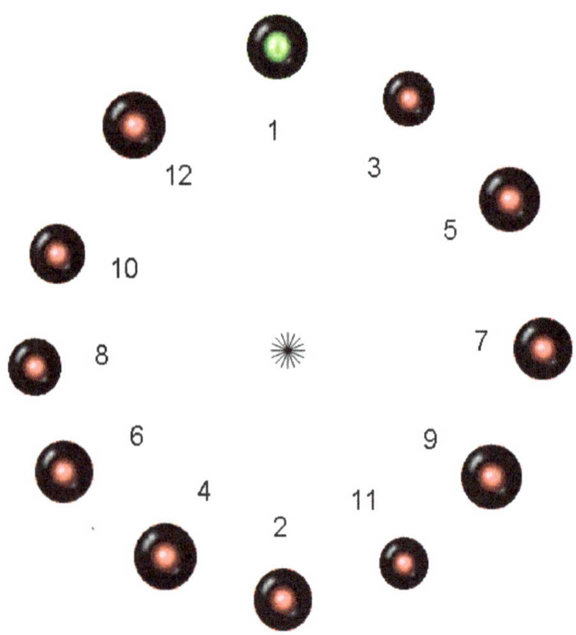

Fig. 9. Exercise designed for the Children

For a best understanding, PLEIA (configured by the therapist) displays sequentially only the next target, and hides the others. When the next target is reached, it is cleared and another appears. One sound can be also associated (feedback configuration, target reaching). This exercise does not have obstacles avoidance and the aim is the evaluation of dexterity.

- Experimentation with the abilities of Claudia.

Claudia knew PLEIA in November 2006. Her mobility and understanding were limited and difficult. This child had trouble with the test "follow path". This child could not avoid obstacles and the movements sometimes were without control. Then, the therapist proposed a test without obstacles and path. At first time it was only a simple test with one target. She practiced the test many times. After, the therapist proposed an exercise more complex. Test with 12 targets to reach. This article is based on two evaluations done in February 2007, November 2006 with the same 12 target test (fig.10 and 11) and the same technical aide and settings. Before , she practiced the model test proposed by the therapist without data saved. The therapist explained and practiced with her the activity and movements wanted. The therapist says when the patient has understood the activity, then, the data are saved.

The first session, Claudia made four practical test, the data were saved after (fifth test). The total test in the first session was eight. Trajectories at the beginning were sometimes uncontrolled.

The second session, the practical test number, was increased, because, the therapist saw that the patient did the test without difficulty, the test number in this session was nine. We can see that the movements in the second test are more optimized. The understanding about the aim of the exercise is better. She has a tactic to reach the target: when she goes to reach the next target, the displacement is very fast and exceeds the position of the target, then, she comes back to the target with circular and controlled slowly movement.

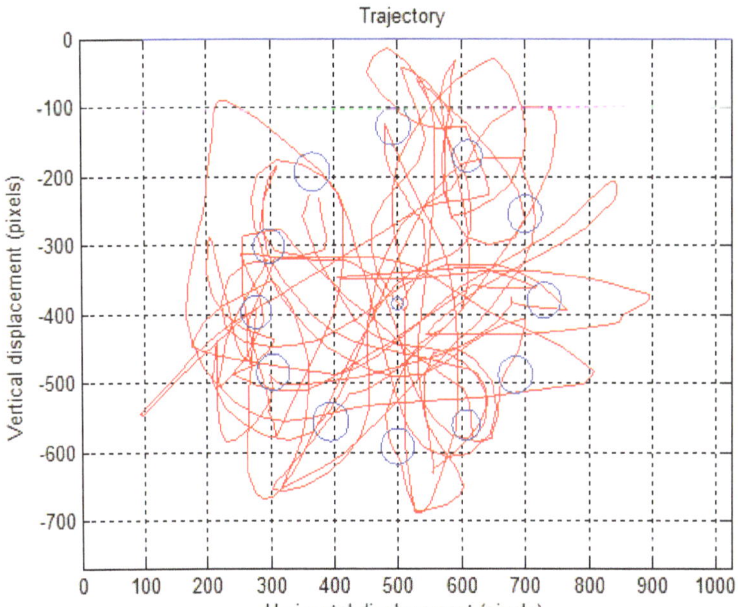

Fig.10. Trajectory of Claudia in November 2006.

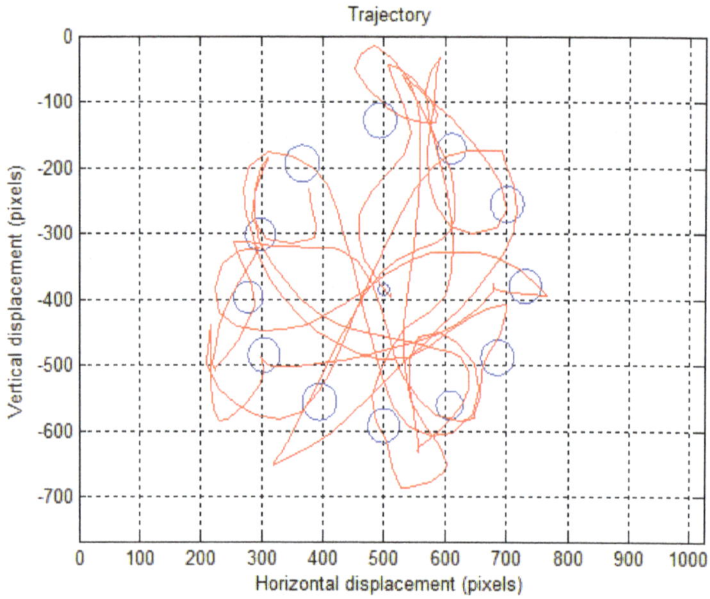

Fig.11. Trajectory of Claudia in February 2007.

The fig.12. Shows the evaluation phases distance in time (ms) for the two exercises. The scope of the first curves (noted (a)), is longer than the second (noted (b)). The displacement in the first exercise is slower than in the second test. The user action index (UA) represent user action on the peripheral device, this index is a function of the energy cost that the user must employ to realize the test. This index gives information to the adaptation between the user and his peripheral.

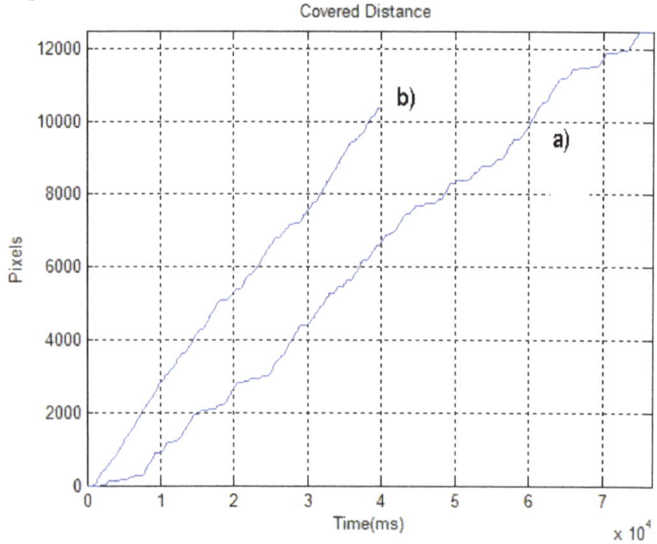

Fig. 12. Covered distance of two trajectories: a) November test, b) February test.

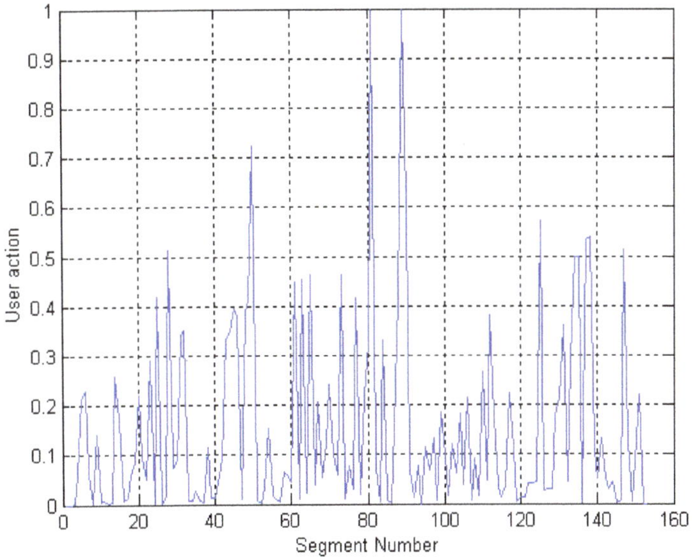

Fig. 13. User Action (UA) in November.

The Command Load (**CL**), shows the rate between the Action User versus a Reference User. Claudia acts more on the peripheral in the first test (2.43 on **CL)** . The efficiency Load (**EL**) is different (8 to 27 %). In fact Claudia had understood the test because the **RP** was lower (13.65 to 2.5). It is not an adaptation of peripheral but an adaptation of Claudia (a cause of training). She was more ready for the evaluation test (see table 1).

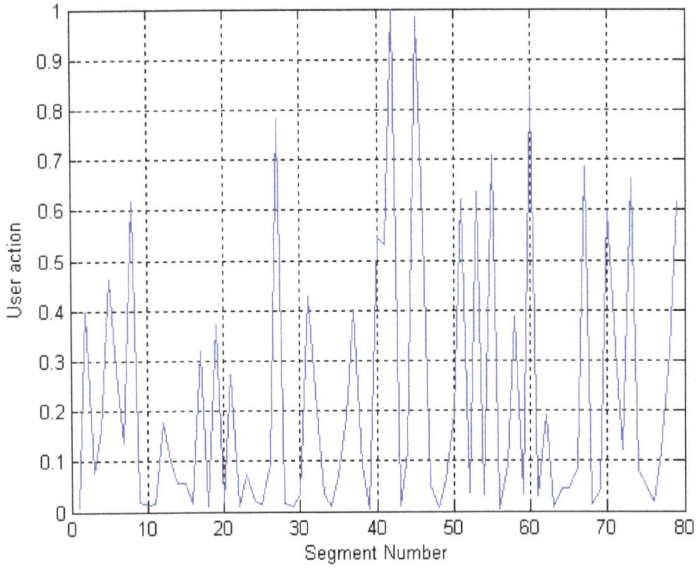

Fig. 14. User Action (UA) in February.

Sample	Test Time (TT) (ms)	Covered Distance (CD) (pixels)	Rate of Pause (RP) (%)	Command Load (CL)	Efficient Load (EL) (%)
Nov2006	76900	12500	13.65	2.43	8
Feb2007	39900	10500	2.5	0.89	27

Table 1. Claudia results.

- Experimentation with Robert

The first contact of Robert with PLEIA was in May 2006. The test shows, were made in November 2006. He has a good control on the technical aid but he acts slowly. The same exercise was used, in similar conditions.

Fig. 15 and 16 show two trajectories. We can notice that he has a good control on his technical aid. The trajectories are "cleaner" and very specific, He has a little problem with the diagonal trajectory, but the straight lines are good.

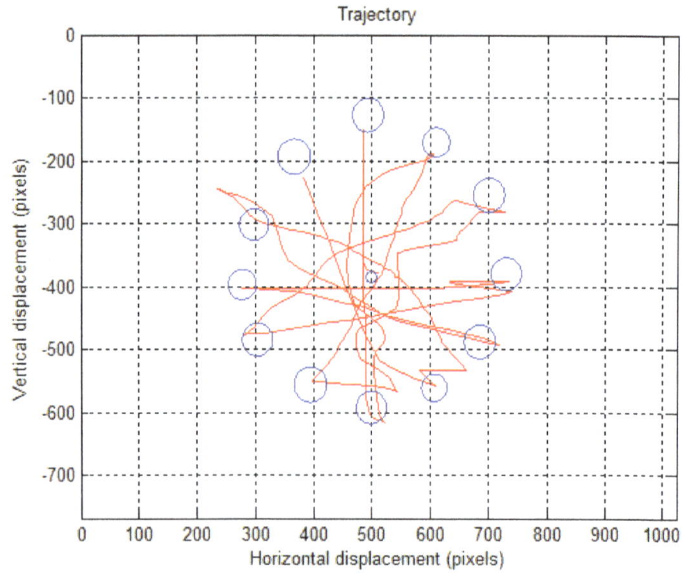

Fig. 15 Robert first trajectory

The occupational therapist observes that when Robert reaches the target, he makes a little pause. He is planning a few seconds the best trajectory to reach the next target. He has employed more time in the test 1 that the test 2 (10 %).

Between the two test, Robert has increase the number of actions (CL = 1.14 to 1.58 %) with some benefit (TT decrease of ~10%). However, he increases his efficiency (EL from 53 to 97%), see table 2.

In fact, in comparison with Claudia, the behavior is similar however he has a biggest pause rate (16.80). It means that Robert is more cerebral and he takes advantage from pause to stratify the next actions. Claudia is more reactive on peripheral. The result is that Robert acts more efficiently that Claudia.

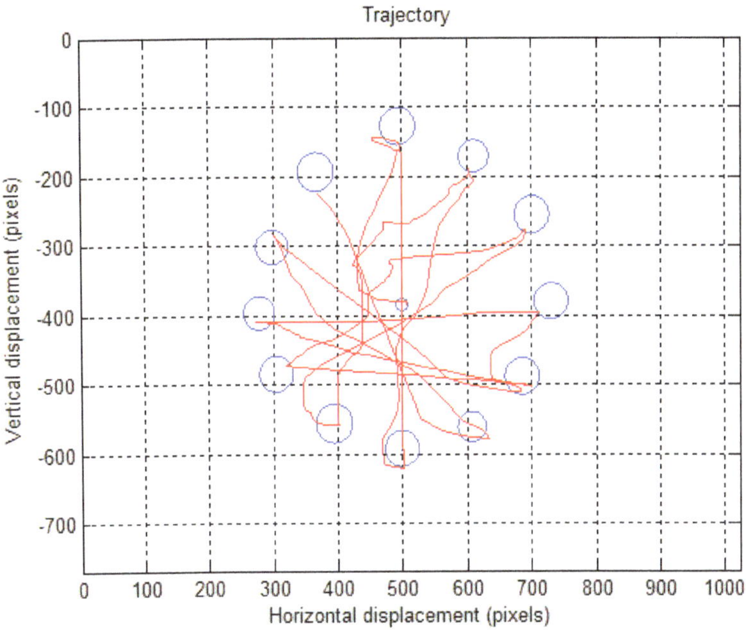

Fig. 16. Robert second trajectory.

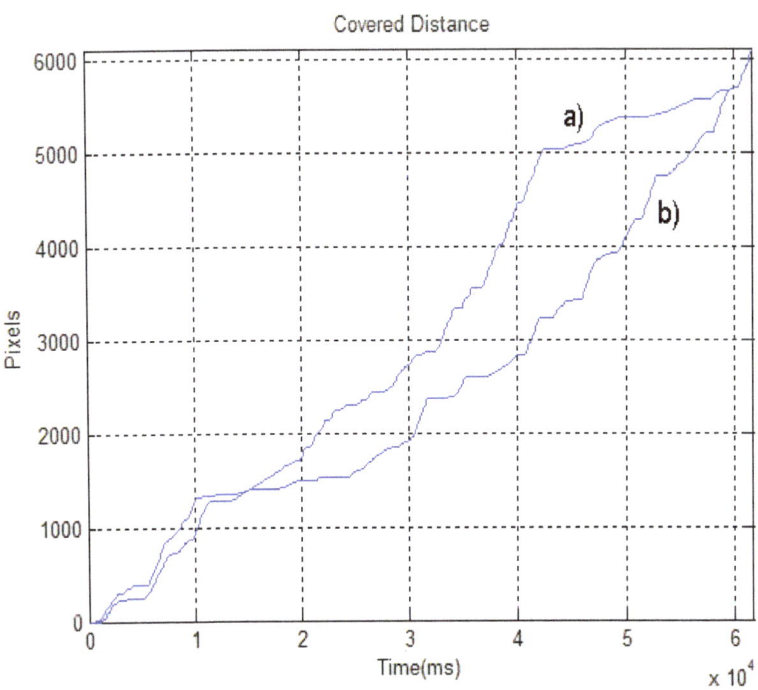

Fig. 17. Robert Covered Distance (first test (a) and the second test (b)).

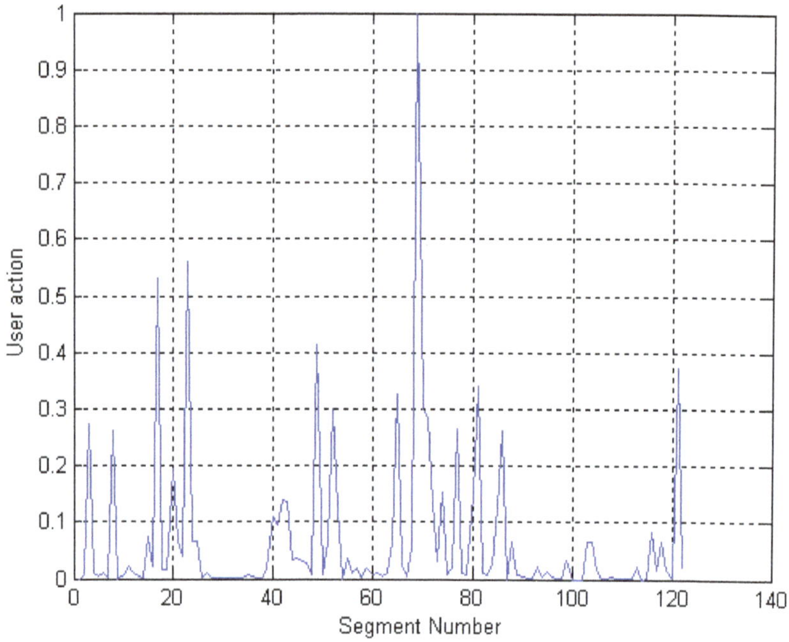

Fig. 18. User Action (UA) in the Robert first test.

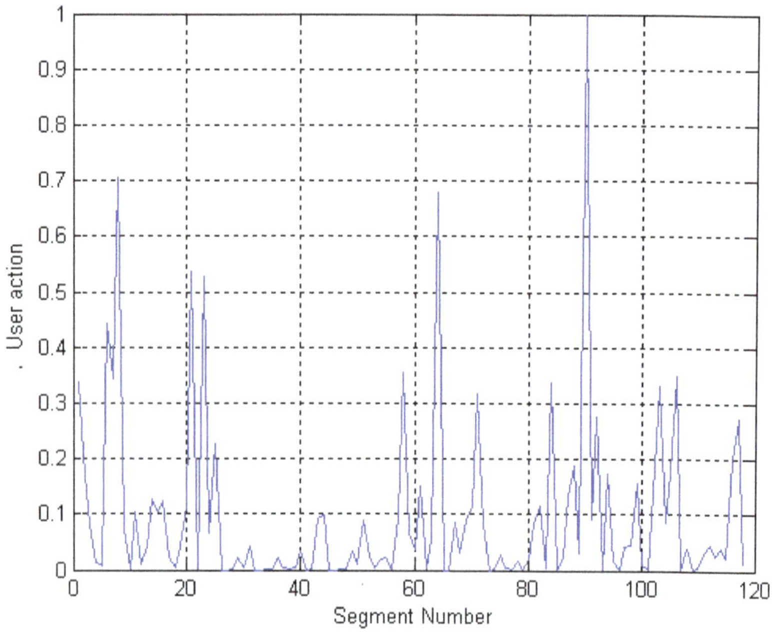

Fig.19. User Action (UA) in the Robert second test.

Sample	Test Time (TT) (ms)	Covered Distance (CD) (pixels)	Rate of Pause (PR) (%)	Command Load (CL)	Efficient Load (EL) (%)
Test1	61800	6125	14.56	1.14	53
Test2	59500	5690	16.80	1.58	97

Table 2. Robert results.

8. Conclusion

Today the methods used by the medical team and occupational therapist are often qualitative. PLEIA software can be employed as a tool to evaluate the pointing user's capabilities.
We proposed the new indexes to improve the classical evaluations methods that use the common factors as distance, time, errors and trajectory.
The index command load shows the energy that the user employs to act on his technical aid. This energy could be not to be in direct relation with the efficiency, when the user realizes a task.
PLEIA's capacities can be expanded as rehabilitation platform, telerehabilitation and experimentation platform for HCI systems with different haptic devices.
The experiments are based on the real evaluation cases.
In two cases, we evaluated the initial capabilities. The occupational therapist conclusions were: interface difficulties, some uncontrolled movements and the technical aid needs a best adaptation. The trajectories and indicators showed clearly this behavior. Claudia has a good interest with the exercises of PLEIA. The therapist detects that she has the same behavior as she rides her electric wheelchair.
We start test PLEIA with the other modules in order to evaluate children with robots and wheelchair. In these modules, all indicators are included. We will compare evaluation tools.

9. Acknowledgments

We thank Medical team and all occupational therapists of Raymond Poincare Hospital (Brezin unit 4), the Specialized Educational Center (Champigny France) and the Informatics' Unit of National Saint Maurice Hospital for his assistance in all experimentations in PLEIA.

10. References

Adameczek A. & Choquet T., & Huynh, Lefur .2005. Efficasouris: Outils pour les Ergothérapeutes et Clavier Virtuel. Report of project of studies, DESS HANDI, Nouvelles Technologies et Handicaps Sensori-moteurs, Paris ,France. March 2005.

Buaud, A., Roussel D.,. Truchot B,(2003). Evaluation process based on user's need: ergonomic evaluation of multimedia games for visually impaired children. AAATE 2003, Dublin, Ireland, September 2003. IOS Press, Craddock G., McCormack L., Reilly R., Knops H., Amsterdam, The Netherlands, pp. 237-241.

Dipietro,L. Sabatini, A. Paolo,D. (2003). Evaluation of an Instrumented gloved for hand movement acquisition. Journal of Rehabilitation Research and Development Vol. 40, No. 2 ,(March/April 2003),pp 179-190.

ISO/DIS 9241-9 Ergonomic requirements for office work with visual display terminals, non keyboard input device requirements. International Organisation for Standardisation, 1998.

Jeong, H. & Kim J. Choi, J. Lecture Notes in Computer Science (LNCS), Spring Berlin, ISBN 978-3-540-22312-2

Kadouche, R.,& Abdularazak B., Mokhtari, M .(2004). Designing an evaluation method for computer accessibility for people with severe disabilities. Proceding of 9th International Conference on Computers Helping People (ICCHP) with Special Needs, Springer, pp. 845-848, ISBN:3-540- 22334-7, Paris, France, July, 2004.

Kang, P. J. K. (2004). A Hand Gesture Controlled Semi-autonomous Wheelchair. Proceeding of 2004 IEEE/RSJ International Conference on Intelligent Robots and Systems, Vol.. 4 No. 2, pp.3565 - 3570, September 28 - October 2, 2004 , Sendai, Japan.

Keates, S., Hwang, F., Langdon, P., Clarkson, P.J., Robinson, P. (2002). Cursor Measures for Motion impaired Computer users. Proceedings of the ASSETS 2002 ACM Fifth ACM Conference on Assistive Technology-, New York, pp. 135-142, ISBN 1-58113-464-9, Edinburgh, Scotland

MacKenzie, I.S. & Kauppinen T., Silfverberg, M.(2001). Accuracy Measures for Evaluating Computer Pointing Devices. CHI '01: Proceedings of the SIGCHI conference on Human factors in computing systems, ACM Press, pp. 9-16.ISBN 1581133278, Seatle Washington, 31 march-5 april.

Peralta , H. & Riman, C., & Monacelli, E., A reconfigurable Evaluation and Assistance Platform for Handicapped People. Interational Conference on Intelligent Robots and Systems IROS 2006, IEEE, Beijing , Chine, October 9-15, 2006

Shimizu H, C. S. M. (2006). Programmed Instruction to teach pointing with a computer mouse in preschoolers with developmental disabilities. Research in Developmental Disabilities, Vol.27 ,No.(2), Mar-Apr 2006, pp. 175-189, PMID: 15970426.

Soukoreff R.W., Mackenzie I. S. (2004). "Towards a standard for pointing device evaluation, perspectives on 27 years of Fitts' law research in HCI." Int. J. Human-Computer Studies: 751–789.

Tellex, S., and Roy, D. (2006). Spatial routines for a simulated speech-controlled vehicle. Proceedings of the 1st ACM SIGCHI/SIGART conference on Human-robot interaction, 2006,pp. 156--163, ISBN: 1-59593-294-1, Salt Lake City, Utah, USA. March 02 - 03, 2006 ACM Press

Thieffry, R., Monacelli ,E. Laplace S. (2005). Adaptative Command and Generalization to Locomotion Aid Systems. Proceedings of the 2005 IEEE International Conference , ICRA, pp. 2643 - 2648, April 18-22, Barcelone, Spain.

Yanco, H. A. (2002). Evaluating the Performance of Assistive Robotic Systems. Performance Metrics for Intelligent Systems, NIST, Gaithersburg, MD, August 2002

Internets Sites

(Adeprio diffussion) http://www.adeprio.com

(Judy Lynn) http://www.judylynn.com/

(Marbesoft) http://www.marblesoft.com/

(Simtech publication) http://www.hsj.com/products.html

(Widgit software) http://www.widgit.com/

4

The Rehabilitation Robots FRIEND-I & II: Daily Life Independency through Semi-Autonomous Task-Execution

Christian Martens*, Oliver Prenzel** & Axel Gräser**
*University of Bremen, Institute of Automation***
*Rheinmetall Defence Electronics**
Germany

1. Introduction

The rehabilitation robotic systems FRIEND[1]-I (Martens et al., 2001) and its successor FRIEND-II have been developing at the Institute of Automation (IAT), University of Bremen, Germany, since 1997 and 2003 respectively. The systems belong to the category "intelligent wheelchair mounted manipulators". They focus on users with high spinal cord injury, or with similar handicaps, who are unable to control the manipulator by means of a keyboard or joystick. The systems offer support during daily life activities and at professional life. The strategic objective of the FRIEND as well as the succeeding AMaRob[2] project, which focuses on the usage of FRIEND-II within the context of an intelligent environment, is to research into new methods to control the robotic system in such a way that their users become independent for at least 1.5 hours without support by nursing staff. Beside the aspect that this is one of the main requirements expressed by potential users, the fulfillment of this objective would have a strong impact on the commercialization of the rehabilitation robotic system itself.
This article gives an overview of the FRIEND project and the robotic systems there from evolved. It is divided into a practical part, which presents the systems from a user oriented perspective, and into a theoretical part, which satisfies the system-engineer's point of view. The user oriented part outlines the different development steps, functional improvements, hardware setups and lessons learned since 1997. Here, the facilities of the FRIEND-I system as well as a description of the innovations of the FRIEND-II system, currently under development, are described with specific emphasis of the AMaRob project. The reader becomes aware of the functionalities and services offered by the FRIEND rehabilitation robot and of the challenging technical complexity with which the development has to deal. The theoretical part is focused on the concept of semi-autonomous task-execution as a means of reasonable complexity reduction. Due to the consequent application of this concept a technically manageable robotic system emerges, which is able to execute tasks on a high level of abstraction in a reliable and robust manner. Within this context semi-autonomous task-

---

[1] FRIEND - Functional robot arm with user-friendly interface for disabled people
[2] AMaRob - Autonomous manipulator control for rehabilitation robots

execution is used as a synonym for system initiated and controlled user involvement during task-execution. For the realization of this approach the control architecture MASSiVE[3] has been designed and implemented. It supports task-execution on the basis of a priori defined and formally verified task-knowledge. This task-knowledge contains all possible sequences of operations as well as the symbolic representation of objects required for the execution of a specific task. The seamless integration of user interactions into this task-knowledge, in combination with MASSiVE's user-adapted human-machine interface (HMI) layer, enables the system to deliberately interact with the user during run-time. It is shown how MASSiVE's application within the FRIEND-II system supports the future development of new services that increase autonomy of the users.

2. Evolution of Rehabilitation Robots

The development of rehabilitation robots started at the end of the 80ies in the last century. It was driven by the intention to support elderly and disabled people during daily life activities, making them more independent from care personnel or relatives. Additionally, the promising concept of an artificial assistant should be improved and technologically explored. This explains the chronological order of the appearance of different kinds of rehabilitation robots as they are presented in the following.

The first step in the evolution of rehabilitation robots was the development of fixed workstation systems that could execute pre-programmed tasks, like picking up paper from a printer or taking a book from a bookshelf. Quite popular systems of this category are DeVAR (Van der Loos, 1995; Mokhtari & Amni, 2001), ProVAR (Wagner et al., 1998; Van der Loos et al., 1999), RAID (Dallaway & Jackson , 1993; Eftring, 1994), MASTER-RAID II (Dallaway et al., 1995; Busnel et al., 1999; Mokhtari & Amni, 2001) or CAPDI (Casals et al., 1999). All these systems have in common that they consist of an industrial robot that is mounted at a workstation. Furthermore, they possess HMIs that are adapted to their users' special needs resulting from his or her disability.

Due to their structured and well known environment, fixed workstation systems could process complex task efficiently. Because this ability is limited to these predefined tasks, it turned out that these systems were too restrictive for a flexible use, e.g. in the domestic environment. This was the main motivation for the development of special purpose wheelchair mounted manipulators, like MANUS (Mokhtari & Amni, 2001), Wessex/Weston robot arm (Hillman et al., 1999) or RAPTOR (Mahoney, 2001). By means of different HMIs, e.g. joystick, keyboard or space-mouse, the user can control the gripper of the arm with respect to a Cartesian coordinate system or control each joint of the arm directly. In contradiction to industrial robots the main goal for the development of these manipulators was to create lightweight robot arms that satisfy special security requirements resulting from the direct human-machine interaction. This comes along with a loss of positioning accuracy, so that the pre-programming of complex action sequences, even in structured environments, was no longer possible. This is the reason why the control of these systems can only be performed on a low level of abstraction. For example, the user can command the direction for the arm movement or open and close the gripper. Even though this kind of control offers a great flexibility in use, it puts a high cognitive load on its users. Especially for complex tasks

---

[3] MASSiVE - Multilayer Control Architecture for Semi-autonomous Service Robots with Verified Task Execution

this is tiresome and comes along with a loss of concentration (Kawamura et al., 1995). Additionally, the kinds of HMIs which come along with these manipulators exclude tetraplegic (spinal cord injuries above vertebrae C5) or persons with a similar clinical picture.
A possible approach to encounter the above mentioned problems is to develop fully autonomous and mobile assistants, which are able to execute tasks on a high level of abstraction. Example systems of this category are MOVAR (Van der Loos, 1995), URMAD (Innocenti et al., 1994), MOVAID (Dallaway et al., 1995), WALKY (Bolmsjö & Neveryd, 1995) or Care-O-Bot (May & Schäffer, 1999). All these systems consist of a mobile platform with a manipulator mounted on it. In order to act in an unknown environment they are equipped with different kinds of sensors, like ultra-sonic or laser-beam distance sensor, cameras etc. All sensors as well as the platform and the manipulator itself are connected to a computer system that processes the user commands and controls all peripheral components.
At this point it has to be mentioned that, even though the above introduced idea of an autonomous robotic is as old as the history of robotics itself (Engelberger, 1989), its consequent realization has to be stated as unrealistic at the moment: Assuming that solutions for currently unsolved technical problems, like the real-time interpretation of camera images, are at hand, a fully autonomous system is cost-intensive and performs tasks with poor efficiency and reliability (Dario et al., 2004). This is because of its inherent high technical complexity. A manageable system with predictable behavior is required. With respect to the current state of science and technology, this requirement can be fulfilled only if the user's cognitive capabilities are taken into account, i.e. the robot executes the tasks semi-autonomously (Laschi et al., 2001; Martens et al., 2002; Colle et al., 2002).
Semi-autonomy takes the users' cognitive capabilities into account whenever a complex decision or environmental identification has to be made. Example systems of this category are the workstation mounted systems ISAC (Kawamura et al., 1995) and MUSIIC (Kazi, 1996; Kazi et al., 1997) as well as the wheelchair based systems KARES (Bien et al., 2001). The main principle is to offer simple but fully autonomous skills that can be activated by the user if necessary. Examples are the visually controlled grasping of objects (Lang et al., 2000), force-torque controlled drink serving (She et al., 2003b) or weight controlled pouring of a drink (She et al., 2003a). Because these skills are realized by sensor-based closed loop control processes, their execution becomes robust against dynamic environmental changes, even in unknown environments.
Even though offering autonomous executable skills reduces the amount of necessary user interactions during task-execution, a high cognitive load for the user still remains. He or she still has to remember the preconditions that have to be satisfied prior to the skill activation. For example, if a glass has to be grasped in a visually controlled manner, whereas the camera is mounted on top of the gripper (Lang et al., 2000), the user first has to move the gripper into the vicinity of the object to be grasped. Only if the underlying image processing system is able to extract significant features, the execution of the reactive grasping skill will be successful. Here, the approach of semi-autonomous task-execution, as it has been developed for the FRIEND-II robotic systems since 2003, will reduce the users' cognitive load. In the following, the rehabilitation robotic systems FRIEND-I & II are presented in general. Afterwards, the realization of the latter mentioned concept is described in detail.

3. Rehabilitation Robots FRIEND-I & II

This section gives an overview of the development steps of the FRIEND-I and FRIEND-II system as they have been undertaken since 1997. It is shown that the evolution of FRIEND-I closely correlates to the general evolution of rehabilitation robots as it has been described in the previous section. With the realization of an autonomously executed "serve-drink task" its full potential was tapped, so that the development of FRIEND-II started. FRIEND-II comes up of with a multitude of new hardware as well as software features that simplify the realization of flexible and robust task-execution. First, the new hardware setup is introduced in detail, before FRIEND-II's role as a subsystem embedded in an intelligent environment within the context of AMaRob is described.

3.1 FRIEND-I

FRIEND-I consists of an electric wheelchair and a MANUS (Exact Dynamics, Netherlands) robot arm. The robot arm is controlled by a PC, which is mounted on the backside of the wheelchair. For user interaction an LC-display is used. In order to execute different tasks autonomously, FRIEND-I is equipped with a stereo pan-tilt-zoom camera system, mounted on the back of the wheelchair, and a "smart tray". The tray is mounted at the front side of the wheelchair. It is characterized as "smart" due to its ability to locate object positions as well as to measure object weights, as described later in this section. A picture as well as a diagram of FRIEND-I is given in Fig. 1.
The first approach, to make the robot arm controllable for people with insufficient flexibility in their hands and arms for using a joystick or keyboard, was to equip the system with a speech control interface (Borgerding et al., 1999). By means of simple commands the robot can be operated with respect to different coordinate systems. The user can enter naturally spoken commands that are transformed into direct robot control actions. For example, if the user wants to pick up an object placed on the tray, a possible command sequence might be "Hand forward", "Hand down", "Stop", "Gripper open", "Hand forward", "Stop", "Gripper close". Because the user observes the actions of the robot arm continuously, he or she might interrupt the actions in erroneous situations.

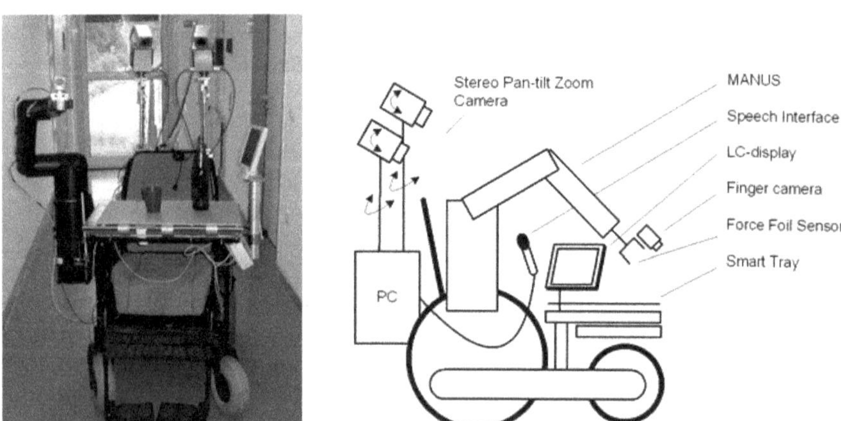

Fig. 1. Front view of FRIEND-I in summer 2003 (left) and schematic drawing (right).

By means of the speech interface it is possible even for a completely paralyzed user to command complicated tasks like grasping a bottle, pouring a drink in a glass and serve it to him- or herself. The drawback of this approach is that it requires high concentration over a long period of time. Therefore, in analogy to the robotic systems listed within the introduction, the succeeding approach in the FRIEND project was to pre-program often repeated tasks, like pouring and serving a drink or to put down objects on the tray. Even though it was convenient to activate the execution of these tasks by a single command, their application was too inflexible for the treatment of daily life activities.

A promising alternative was to increase the abstraction level of the commands by offering autonomously executable sensor-based skills[4]. The first implemented skill of this category was the camera controlled grasping of arbitrary objects. For its realization a finger camera was mounted on top of the robot gripper (Lang et al., 2000). If the user wants to grasp an object he or she moves the gripper into the neighborhood of the object to be grasped, until it can be seen by the finger camera. Starting from this position a visually controlled grasping action can be started with the command "grasp object". During the execution of the autonomous grasping action an underlying visual servoing algorithm continuously interprets image features that are assigned to natural or artificial markers on the objects.

The implemented grasping skill turned out to be robust during execution. Even under changing illumination conditions or with changes in the position of the target object the grasping tasks could be finished successfully without human intervention. It was possible to grasp an object placed in the workspace of the robot arm by means of three to five simple commands in comparison with 15-20 commands as necessary with direct voice control. Besides the reduction of necessary commands the whole execution time was reduced up to three times in average. This was the motivation to enhance the level of abstraction for task-execution again. The representative task of filling a glass with a drink and serve it to the user, short: the "serve-drink task" was chosen. The realization of this task unveils a number of challenging technical problems to be solved, which are also representative for further tasks. Therefore, the investigation and realization of the "serve-drink task" has the potential to develop a general method for robust high-level task-execution in rehabilitation robotic systems.

The underlying scenario of the task can be described as follows: A glass and an open bottle, filled with an unknown amount of drink, are arbitrarily placed on FRIEND-I's tray. After the user has entered the command "serve drink", the system has to fill the glass with the drink and move it to the mouth of the user. After the user finished drinking, the glass has to be put back on the tray. At the first sight the "serve drink task" seems to be trivial and restricted, but it deserves closer attention. First, the system has to locate the glass and bottle on the tray, grasp the bottle and move it close to the glass. Afterwards, the glass has to be filled and the bottle has to be placed back on the tray. Then the glass has to be grasped and moved close to the user's mouth. Finally, the glass has to be put back on the tray, ready for a succeeding pouring action. The execution of this scenario solely on the basis of image processing and visual servoing is very ambitious, especially if a robust behavior under all possible environmental conditions is requested. Additionally, unreliable behavior may cause dangerous situations for the user. To prevent such situations and to increase the system's reliability a "smart tray" was developed that is used in combination with the vision sensors (Volosyak et al., 2003).

The tray can be divided into two subsystems: A scale for the measurement of weight changes of objects placed on the tray and a touchpad for the detection of their positions. The

---

[4] These operations are characterized as skills, since they represent indivisible atomic functionalities of the system that execute autonomously sub-tasks by means of continuously processing sensor information. Examples are grasping an object or pouring a drink.

scale consists of an off-the-shelf digital scale with a measuring precision of ±1g that is connected to the main system PC. The position detection is realized by a touchpad sensor that was developed at the IAT. The touchpad consists of a 48x30 matrix, where each matrix element has binary output. Binary 1 denotes the presence of a weight greater then 3g per element, 0 indicates that there is no load on the corresponding matrix element. Hence, the result can be treated as a binary image and known image processing methods can be used for object localization. Fig. 2 (right) depicts the raw binary touchpad image resulting from a cup and a bottle that are placed on the tray. The outputs of the touchpad are processed by a microcontroller and send to the main PC. It is obvious that the positions of object segments can be easily determined on the basis of the binary touchpad image. But it is also evident that the amount of information from these images is insufficient for object identification. Here, additional sensor data is required that is fused with the touchpad information. By means of the information coming from the smart tray in combination with image processing results provided by the stereo-camera system, an autonomously executable "serve-drink task" was realized (Radchenko et al., 2004). The objective was to demonstrate that care personnel could place the involved objects, i.e. the glass and the bottle, on arbitrary positions on the tray and the system is able to execute the rest of the task autonomously. Even though this approach was independent of calibration, as it was for the pre-programmed tasks described before, the realization was fixed in the manner that the system could not be used for the processing of varying task scenarios. With the introduction of a flexible software-architecture this problem is solved within FRIEND-II, as described in the following.

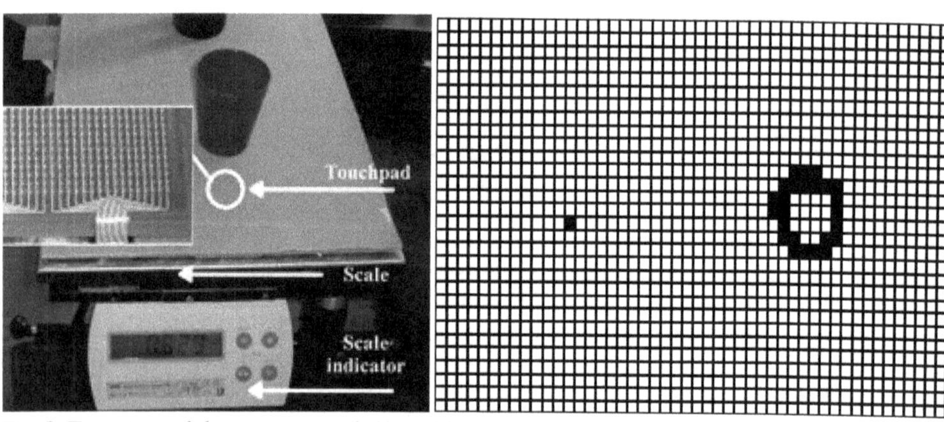

Fig. 2. Top view of the smart tray (left) and binary image of the sensor matrix (right).

3.2 FRIEND-II

The development of the FRIEND-II system started in 2003 with the objective to improve the FRIEND-I system and to benefit from the lessons learned so far. On the one hand, there were different shortcomings in FRIEND-I's hardware setup. On the other hand the flexibility of the control concept and the software-architecture in FRIEND-I was a rather basic approach that aimed to demonstrate the feasibility of rehabilitation robotic support scenarios. This section discusses the different extensions of FRIEND-II with respect to the hardware configuration, whereas the control concept MASSiVE is discussed in detail in the succeeding section.

Hardware Setup for Dexterous Manipulation in Clustered Environments

The MANUS robotic arm, which has been used in FRIEND-I, corresponds with its 6-joints kinematical structure to industrial robots. Such a structure turned out not to be suitable for dexterous manipulations. The ability to master manipulations with obstacle avoidance in clustered and mainly non-structured home environments is mandatory for the application in rehabilitation robotic scenarios.

Within FRIEND-II a dexterous 7 degrees-of-freedom robotic arm, which has been developed by Amtec Robotics (Berlin, Germany) under functional specifications by IAT, is used. It has a humanlike kinematical structure: The arm is composed of a series of turn- and pan-joints with perpendicular axes respectively. The arm is mounted on a linear axis which allows it to drive in a specific home position and reduce visibility if not in use (Fig. 3). At the wrist a multi-axis force/torque sensor, model Gamma, from ATI-Industrial Automation (NC, USA) is integrated. This compact, light and robust monolithic transducer uses silicon strain gauges, providing high noise immunity, to sense forces and torques from all three directions of the tool frame. To process the strain gauge information into CAN-Bus information a compact wrist mounted electronics unit has been developed. The robot arm is equipped with an Otto Bock SensorHand[5] as a gripper. The necessary mechanical as well as electrical adaptations were made in agreement with Otto Bock Health Care (Duderstadt, Germany). A gripper force and a slip control mode, which will be activated from the FRIEND-II system, are integrated in the SensorHand. As it has proven to be a benefit for the realization of robust operations, FRIEND-II is, like its predecessor, equipped with a smart tray for determination of object positions and weight changes. The camera Sony EVI-D70P was selected for the FRIEND-II image acquisition system. The selection was made on the basis of requirements for minimal lighting of the scene and particularly on the basis of a cost-effective connection of the camera with a pan-tilt head. The chosen pan-tilt zoom video camera system is mounted on the frame-rack behind the user.

With the help of the described improved hardware setup and the implementation of the new software control concept MASSiVE, the first successfully implemented scenario was an extended drink serving scenario, since this could serve as reference scenario for comparison with FRIEND-I. This scenario was presented at the Hannover-Fair 2005 and it turned out that during the whole week a robust execution, in the sense of the following explanation, took place. Independent of the initial configuration of bottle and glass (sometimes placed by fair visitors) the pouring action was executed as pre-determined. Beside the statement that a stable accuracy from different initial conditions is related to the improved manipulative capabilities of the new robotic arm, two other hardware components contributed also to the enhanced overall performance: The Otto-Bock gripper with its integrated intelligent force-control guaranteed a firm grip even on a slightly wet bottle. Furthermore, the force-torque-sensor enabled to implement a more flexible placing of objects even on non-tactile surfaces like an ordinary table. All in all the improved hardware setup of FRIEND-II is the basis for currently ongoing implementation of further scenarios. The well focused development of different representative and complete rehabilitation robotic scenarios on the basis of the experiences gathered with the FRIEND systems is the objective of the AMaRob project, which will be discussed in the following.

---

[5] http://www.ottobockus.com/products/upper_limb_prosthetics/myoelectric_hands_sensorhand.asp

AMaRob Project: Support Scenarios for Daily Life Autonomy

The project AMaRob is funded within the BMBF[6]-program "Leitinnovation Servicerobotik" (IAT, 2007; DLR, 2007). The overall objective is to demonstrate that 1.5 hours of complete autonomy from care personnel or nursing staff can be realized for tetraplegic people, solely supported by a rehabilitation robot. The suitability for daily use as well as efficiency from the economical viewpoint in one ADL (activities of daily living) and two working scenarios is to be examined. An important aspect with respect to the successful project process is the interdisciplinary cooperation. From the beginning on, therapists (Neurological Rehabilitation Center Friedehorst, Bremen, Germany), designers (i/i/d - Institute of Integrated Design, Bremen, Germany) and various experts for the different technological components (Meyra, Kalletal-Kalldorf; Otto-Bock, Duderstadt; Amtec Robotics, Berlin; IGEL GmbH, Bremen; all from Germany) are cooperation partners in the AMaRob project.

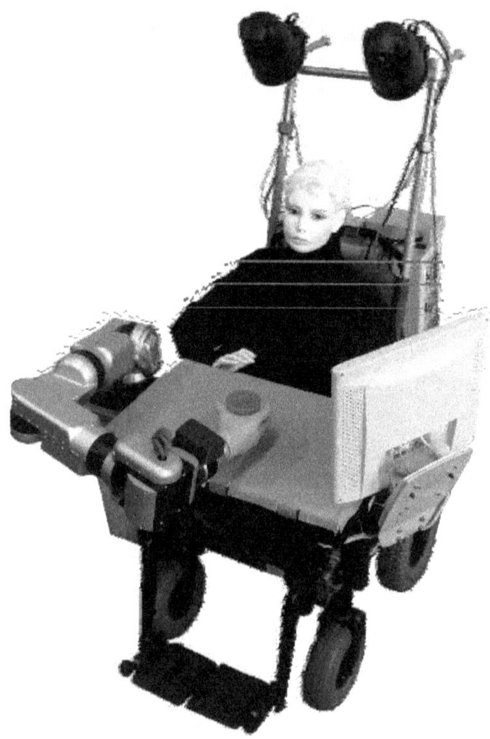

Fig. 3. Rehabilitation robotic system FRIEND-II.

The main development goal in the ADL scenario is the complete process of preparing and eating a meal. This starts with the retrieval of the desired meal from the storage, the proper heating procedure with respect to the contents of the meal, the eating and drinking procedure and finally the clearance of the dishes. In the first working scenario different electronic

[6] BMBF - German Federal Ministry of Education and Research ("Bundesministerium für Bildung und Forschung")

components are tested on the basis of manual inspection as well as functional tests. These tests are common tasks that are often accomplished by disabled people with remaining manual capabilities in the workshops at Friedehorst. The second working scenario deals with a service desk in a library, where books are rented or returned, and dues are paid, reservations are handled, etc.

During the AMaRob project, a redesign of FRIEND-II will take place. Development goals are an improved design for daily use, a smoother integration of sensors and actuators, including the new generation of Amtec Robotics manipulators. Another aspect that is valid for the development of all three scenarios is the investigation of methods to integrate distributed smart components, also known as ambient intelligence or ubiquitous computing (Korondi & Hashimoto, 2003). Its objective is to support the process of task-execution and to lower the technical complexity of the rehabilitation robotic system itself. Based on the experiences gathered with the smart tray within the FRIEND projects, it will be considered to place tactile skins on certain platforms that are in the center of manipulation, e.g. parts of the worktop in the kitchen or the desk in the workshop or library. Furthermore, RFID[7]-tags attached to objects will enable the decentralized storage of object relevant information, e.g. cooking instructions for a meal placed in a smart fridge that is equipped with RFID antenna. Fig. 4 illustrates an exemplary setup of an "intelligent" kitchen environment. With such an intelligent environment, a distributed system evolves with hardware that is distributed physically and that is managed by different processors. In Fig. 4 on the right side, a prototypic installation of an intelligent kitchen environment is depicted. Instead of using a real fridge, the first setup includes a cupboard, representing the fridge. This cupboard is equipped with two tactile layers, which consist of the same tactile skins as that one used for the smart tray component of the FRIEND-II system. Thus, less technical complexity of the rehabilitation robot itself is necessary with respect to required sensors and algorithms to retrieve location information about the meals in the smart fridge. Under the upper cupboard layer an RFID antenna is installed which covers the space above the two layers. The meal to be prepared for the disabled user is arranged on a special meal tray, which fulfils the following conditions:

- It is graspable by the robotic gripper
- The material is suitable for the heating in a microwave oven, is food safe and can be easily cleaned after usage
- The lid is equipped with RFID tags. This lid is also manageable by the robot and can be removed before heating to avoid damage of the RFID tag in the microwave oven.

Once care personnel inserts a meal in this kind of smart fridge, meal specific information will be stored on the RFID tag. This includes a description of the meal, cooking instructions and minimum durability. During the process of meal preparation, the locally stored meal information directly drives the heating procedure in the microwave oven. This oven is also part of the intelligent environment, since it is directly controllable from the system without manipulative interaction and consequently also reduces the technical complexity of FRIEND-II.

Besides the ongoing improvements on the hardware level and the application and enhancement of an overall software control concept, other key developments will be undertaken within AMaRob. This includes fast motion planning for collision free, intelligent and

[7] RFID – radio frequency identification

smooth manipulation in clustered environments (Ojdanic et al., 2006) or the realization of improved machine vision concepts respectively.

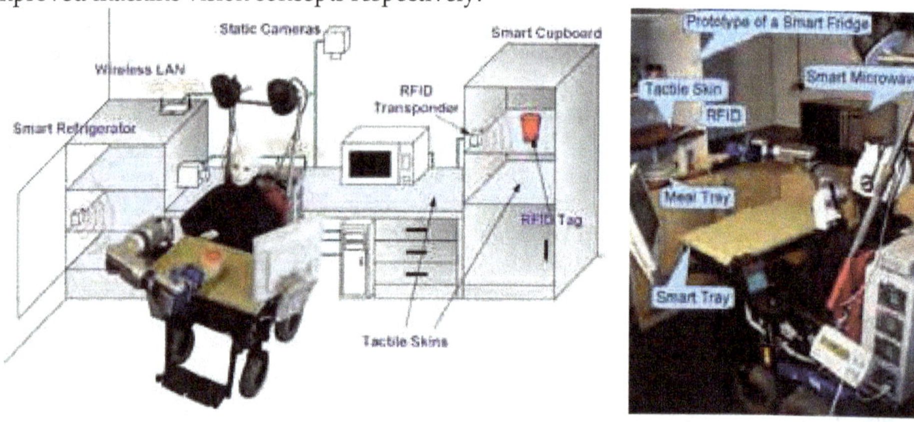

Fig. 4. FRIEND-II in intelligent environment, schematic version (left), first prototypic installation (right).

4. Semi-Autonomous Task-Execution

The preceding sections concentrated on the functional aspects of the FRIEND systems. This section is focused on the application of software-technical methods that help to cope with the inherent complexity of the robotic system and its environment. First, the design and implementation of an appropriate software-architecture is described. Afterwards, within the context of this architecture, task-knowledge data-structures, suitable for the inclusion of the user, as required for semi-autonomous task-execution, are introduced. It is shown how the consequent application of these concepts leads to a robotic system, which is able to execute tasks robustly on a high level of abstraction.

4.1 The Software-Architecture MASSiVE

From the software-technical point of view the realization of a service robot comes up with a multitude of challenging tasks to be solved within the context of an architecture: Distributed calculation, reactions to environmental changes and control of electro-mechanical devices under hard real-time requirements, processing of complex algorithms, adaptation to heterogeneous hardware interfaces, ergonomic human-machine interaction and autonomous planning of action sequences. The preceding enumeration doesn't claim to be exhaustive.

It turned out that hybrid multi-layer architectures, like TCA (Coste-Maniere & Simmons, 2000) or 3T (Bonasso et al., 1998), are predominating in the field of fully autonomous systems, since they provide a combination of deliberative and reactive behavior. A deliberative component is necessary for the creation of a high-level plan, i.e. for having a system that is able to receive task requests and to define a mission goal. The inclusion of reactivity has proven to be a suitable mean to achieve robustness with respect to environmental disturbances, comparable to the reflex system of living organisms. Therefore, a typical hybrid multi-layer architecture consists of three layers:

- Deliberator: Plans operations on a high level of abstraction, i.e. with the help of a symbolic planning strategy.

- Reactive Layer: Has access to the actuators and sensors of the system and offers reactive operations in the form of closed control-loops (i.e. coupling of sensors and actuators).
- Sequencer: Is responsible for the activation and deactivation of operations in the reactive layer according to the plan generated by the deliberator. Therefore, it plays the role of a mediator between deliberator and reactive layer.

Besides these layers a world model is included that contains the current system's perspective on the world according to the task to be executed. Due to the hybrid approach a separation of world-model data into two categories is mandatory: The deliberator operates with symbolic object representations (e.g. *C* for the representation of a cup), while the reactive layer deals with the sensor data taken from these objects, so-called sub-symbolic information. Examples are the color, size, shape, location or weight of an object.

To fulfill the requirements in the field of rehabilitation robotics, the software control architecture MASSiVE has been developed at the IAT. This control architecture is derived from the generally successfully applied architectures of autonomous systems as introduced before. However, in the field of rehabilitation, the user can be included in to the process of task execution, which leads to modifications towards a semi-autonomous system. Furthermore, the analysis of typical rehabilitation robotic support scenarios revealed the fact that these scenarios are mostly composed of a finite set of reusable basic operations (Martens, 2003b).

Fig. 5 depicts the emerging scheme of the modified control architecture. With respect to the semi-autonomous task-execution, the deliberator component of traditional hybrid control architectures has been replaced by an HMI, whereas symbolic planning is performed within the sequencer. The evident role of the HMI is the translation of high abstraction level task requests from the user (e.g. "Fetch cup", "Pour in a drink", etc.) into commands that are forwarded to the sequencer for further processing. Additionally, the HMI provides a complete infrastructure for task related user interactions. This includes the direct control of actuators within context-based constraints given by the sequencer. Within MASSiVE, the role of the sequencer is to act as a global control unit that coordinates the cooperation between all levels of the architecture (Martens et al., 2002). It is designed as a discrete-event-controller that operates on the basis of predefined task-knowledge, so-called process-structures, and generates task related action sequences.

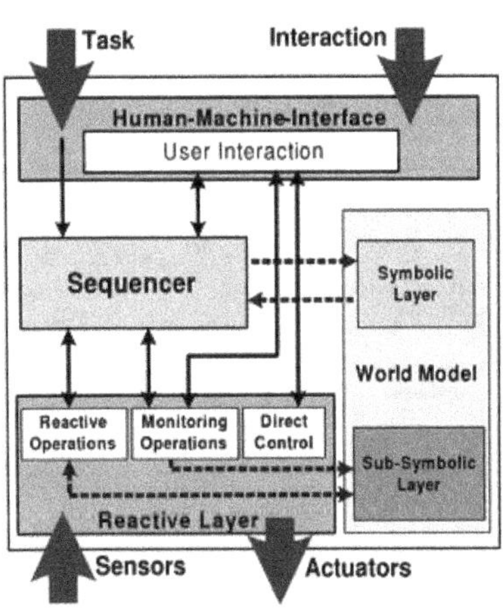

Fig. 5. Schematic overview of the control-architecture MASSiVE.

These process-structures are the basis of the principle to pre-structure the support scenarios. Despite their a-priori definition, they are still flexible enough to process a requested task under varying initial conditions, i.e. they can handle different initial situations and varying kinds of task participating objects. Due to the implicit restriction to task relevant information, this approach guarantees, in contradiction to classical AI-based task planning, a finite and, in the meaning of real-time suitability, reasonable size of the planning search space. Additionally, the formal verification of the task-knowledge with respect to reachability of situations or the correctness of its execution becomes possible. Even though this has no impact on the offered functionality of the robotic system, it is evident that the latter aspect plays a vital role for the commercialization of rehabilitation robots in general.

A planned action sequence consists of operations that are elementary from the sequencer's viewpoint. This motivates the term elementary executable operations (*EEOPs*). *EEOPs* include user interactions (e.g. identification of an object), direct control of actuators (e.g. movement of the camera system), monitoring operations (e.g. visual feature extraction of already identified object) and reactive operations (e.g. visually controlled object grasping). Thus, the basic operations already implemented for the FRIEND-I system are realized within this context as *EEOPs*. Due to the uniform software interface of *EEOPs*, the sequencer can generate action sequences independently of the kind of operation that has to be taken into account. After the generation of an *EEOP*-sequence is finished, the sequencer maps the *EEOPs* to skills that are executed asynchronously on distributed software-servers. These servers are part of the reactive layer or the HMI, respectively. In the reactive layer, a network of servers offers basic system skills that are grouped within the servers according to functional cohesion, as described in the following.

Infrastructure for Semi-Autonomous Task-Execution within Distributed Systems

The sequencer of the MASSiVE architecture (Fig. 6) consists of two modules that are designed as active objects: The *Task Planner* and the *Task Executer*. Active objects are a software design pattern to separate the execution of a method from its calling context with the help of threads, whereas the method's implementation is independent of any threading details (Gamma et al., 1995). Thus, the planner and executer are able to act independently. This enables the control of skill execution in the reactive layer as well as reactions in the planning layer like interruption of ongoing task execution or re-planning of required operation sequences.

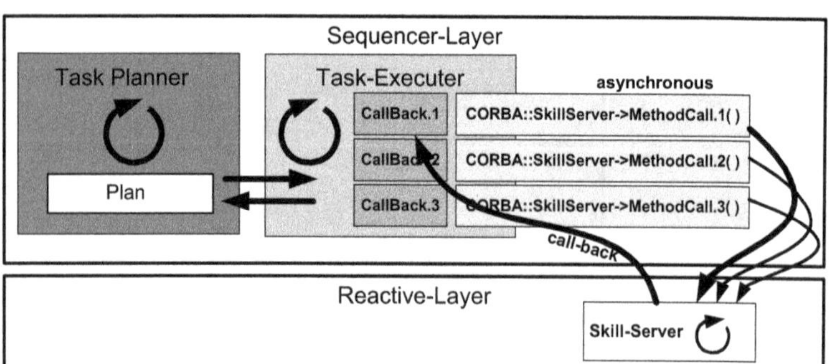

Fig. 6. Communication from sequencer layer.

To be able to execute several operations simultaneously, asynchronous calls of skill-methods are necessary. Furthermore, the operations may run on different processors, e.g. because of system-hardware that is distributed physically as it is the case for remote smart devices. The distribution of skill execution capabilities should be adaptable in a flexible manner, i.e. without changing the system structure or extensive re-implementations, to have the opportunity at hand to scale the computing power available for a single skill. All these demands are fulfilled entirely with the help of standardized and platform-independent communication infrastructures based on CORBA (Common Object Request Broker Architecture, (Gamma et al., 1995)). The following section describes the design and realization of the CORBA based reactive layer.

Reactive Layer

The name reactive layer resides from its purpose to provide reactive behavior. This means to directly couple sensorial input with the control of an actuator (i.e. to design a control loop) to establish autonomous behavior that is robust against dynamic environmental changes. As depicted in Fig. 5 the reactive layer is furthermore responsible for offering monitoring operations (based on input from the sensors) as well as direct control of the actuator (manipulative skills). The latter aspect is important for example when user interaction in the form of direct actuator-control becomes necessary. Due to this, several skill servers provide the necessary basic operations, i.e. skills, of the robotic system by accessing the sensors and actuators of the system or remote smart devices. This means, a skill layer has access to a hardware layer, whereas different hardware servers encapsulate basic hardware functionalities.

Skills have to operate on the already mentioned sub-symbolic environmental information. As shown in Fig. 5, the sequencer including the symbolic planning engine accesses the symbolic layer of the world model. Thus, the sequencer (on the basis of high-level process-structures and symbolic descriptions) is responsible for the correct abstract modeling of that segment of the environment that is relevant to the current task-execution. To administrate all sub-symbolic information in a structured manner, a sub-symbolic world model server is introduced within the reactive layer. Here, sub-symbolic information is stored with reference to symbolic information from the upper layer of the world model and consequently a connection between both layers of the world model (and therefore also between these both information layers) is established.

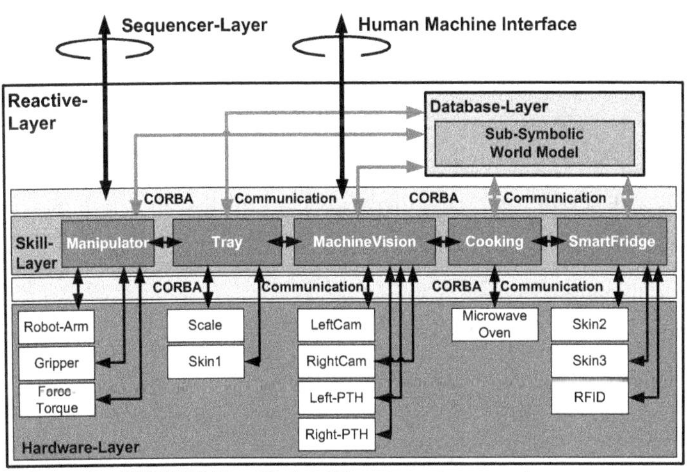

Fig. 7. Reactive layer for FRIEND-II with intelligent environment.

Skill Server

The criterion for separation into several skill servers is derived from the functional entities of the system. That means, one skill server offers all the system operations that have to be assigned basically to one certain entity. In case of scenarios that take place in an intelligent environment as introduced in Chapter 3.2, the necessary skill-servers are the *Manipulator-*, *Tray-*, *MachineVision-*, *Cooking-* and *SmartFridge-Skill-Server*, with their assigned hardware-servers as depicted in Fig. 7. Here, for instance, the Cooking-Skill-Server provides skills to access the hardware-server *MicrowaveOven* and thus to control this remote device or to extract data from it.

From the software-technical point of view, skills are methods of a skill server that are executed asynchronously. This means skill-methods are non-blocking and will return immediately after their activation. The problem of asynchronous execution is that no values or parameters can be returned. Therefore, sub-symbolic data that is generated during skill execution is stored within the world model. The information on the status of skill execution (e.g. successful execution) has to be transmitted via another communication way. For this issue call-back objects are introduced, which can be accessed by the skill caller and the skill method itself. Call-backs are also used for sending information from the skill caller to the skill while it is executing. This could be for example the command to stop the skill or to re-parameterize it. Fig. 6 already showed how the task executer within the sequencer maps call-back objects to asynchronously invoked methods and Fig. 8 demonstrates the communication mechanisms between sequencer- and skill-layer in more detail.

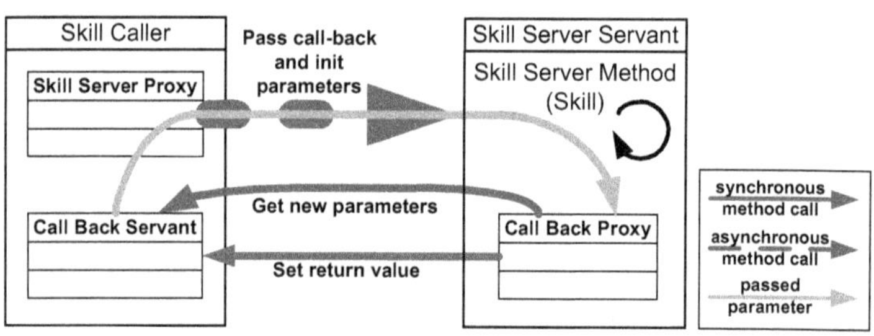

Fig. 8. CORBA-based asynchronous communication.

Hardware Server

For each hardware component, like the robot arm, a hardware server is implemented (see Fig. 7), which itself is connected to a certain skill server. The design principle is that only methods of this skill server can access the hardware directly. This decouples the upper layers of the software structure from the hardware. In case a hardware component is replaced, only the implementations of the hardware server methods have to be adapted, whereas the parameters of each method remain.

If for a hardware-component/-server a fast communication is required, i.e. the communication offset of CORBA cannot be accepted, a local instance of the hardware server implementation class can be used and the communication can be carried out via shared memory. Also the combination of client and servant in one process is possible. All three possibilities of using a hardware server are fully exchangeable and no re-design or new implementation is necessary.

Human-Machine-Interface

For the realization of the user involvement, which is initiated and controlled by the system, the HMI offers an interface that enables the sequencing layer to initiate user assistance via user interaction skills. From the user-centered viewpoint, the overall objective is to offer an intuitively controllable interaction skill, which hides all technical details, like the selection of necessary hardware resources or the control of the data flow. The connection between the HMI and MASSiVE is established by a software component that uses the interface of the sequencer to start and stop system tasks and offers a software-server to enable the sequencer initiating user interactions. From the sequencer perspective, the invocation of a user interaction is thus handled exactly like a skill activation within the reactive layer.

So far, the architectural concept designed for semi-autonomous task-execution has been discussed. In the following, process-structures as a substantial aspect for the control of user interactions and autonomous system operations within MASSiVE are presented.

4.2 Task-Knowledge Driven User-Interaction

According to the structure of the control architecture, process-structures come in two levels of abstraction: Abstract process-structures (PS_A) are associated with the abstract (symbolic) layer of task-knowledge representation and describe tasks in a user-oriented and non-technical way. This level of abstraction is suitable for task-oriented programming purposes (Martens, 2005). Elementary process-structures (PS_E) represent the part of the task-knowledge that is required within the environmental-related (sub-symbolic) level. The information on this level of abstraction subsumes necessary hardware resources, like sensors and actuators, as well as *EEOPs*. In the following, the different steps of task processing on the basis of abstract as well as elementary process-structures will be discussed. The activity diagram depicted in Fig. 9 gives a conceptual overview on the steps that are undertaken to process a task request in MASSiVE.

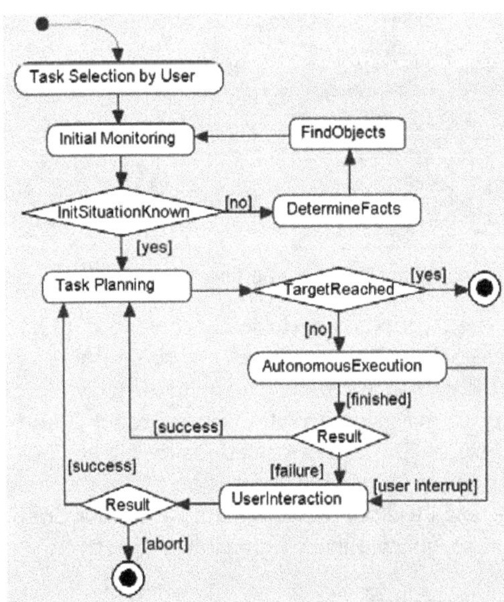

Fig. 9. Overview on task processing within MASSiVE.

Task Request

First, with respect to the task request from the HMI, the sequencer selects and loads an abstract process-structure. Abstract process-structures are derived from data-structures typically used in assembly planning, namely AND-OR-nets (Cao & Sanderson, 1998). Within the context of MASSiVE they have been enhanced with first-order predicate logic facts that assign, in a STRIPS[8]-like manner, pre- and post-conditions to the operations contained in the net. Aditionally, facts are used for the description of object states and relationships.
Fig. 10 depicts an iconic model of a possible PS_A that is assigned to the task request "Fetch cup". The iconic PS_A contains all object-constellations (*OC*s), i.e. objects in physical contact, which might appear during the execution of this task, as well as all possible operations performed by the system. Within this context *all* has to be interpreted as from an application programmer's viewpoint. The operations are called composed operators (*COP*), since they represent a composition of *EEOP*s and their decomposition takes place on the level of PS_E. They interconnect the different *OCs* of the PS_A, meaning that the system transforms the constellations of objects by executing a sub-task. Due to their derivation of AND-OR-nets, there are three different kinds of *COP*s: Assembly and disassembly operations as well as internal state transitions. The semantics of the first two types is self explaining, whereas the latter version is used to represent internal changes within a single *OC* without changing the components being in physical contact (e.g. moving a book on a table).

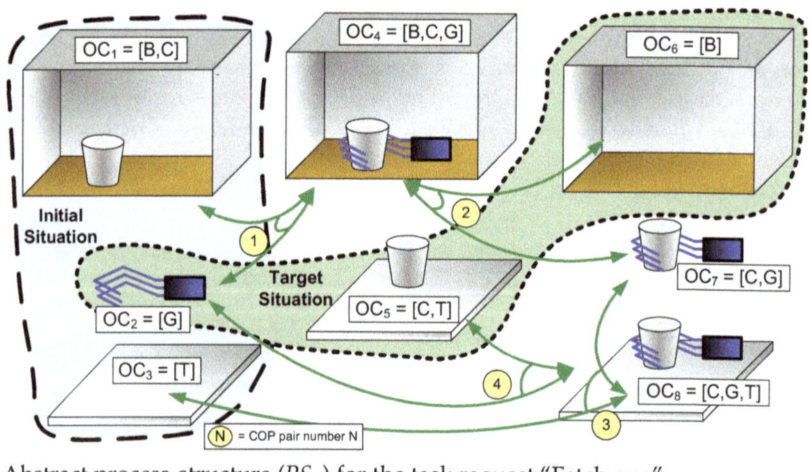

Fig. 10. Abstract process-structure (PS_A) for the task request "Fetch cup".

As listed in Table 1, the "Fetch cup" scenario solely consists of *COP*s of the first two categories. The numbers of each pair of operations refer to the numbers given in Fig. 10. The objects involved in the task scenario are a box *B* (e.g. an abstract representation of an already opened cupboard), a cup *C*, the gripper of the service robot *G* and a table *T*. Some exemplary *OC*s of Fig. 10 are: OC_1 = "the cup is located inside the box", OC_4 = "the grasped cup is located inside the box" or OC_5 = "the cup is located on top of the table". Beside the enumeration of contained objects, each *OC* possesses a set of first order predicate logics facts, which represent the object states as well as their relationship respectively.

[8] STRIPS: Stanford Research Institute Problem Solver (Fikes, 1971)

No.	**List of COPs used in Fig. 10:** (AOP - assembly operation, DOP - disassembly operation)
1	AOP: GraspObjectInContainer(G, C, B) DOP: DepartFromContainer(G, C, B)
2	AOP: PlaceObjectInside(G, C, B) DOP: GetObjectOutside(G, C, B)
3	AOP: PutDownObject(G, C, T, FreePlacePos) DOP: MoveObject(G, C, T, FreePlacePos)
4	AOP: GraspObject(G, C, T) DOP: Depart(G, C, T)

Table 1. Composed operators of the "Fetch Cup" scenario.

On the basis of *OC*s a situation S_k is described as follows: S_k is a set of *OC*s that contains all objects of the PS_A exactly once and is part of the situation-graph (Prenzel, 2005), which interconnects all valid situations via the operations defined within the PS_A. Assuming the correctness of the PS_A, which is verified automatically off-line, a target situation S_T can be reached from any situation S of the situation-graph via the application of a finite number of operations. This circumstance is the basis of the planning concept applied in MASSiVE, which is explained in more detail below. S_T has a fix association with the task to be solved according to the given task request. For the example task depicted in Fig. 10 the target state is defined as: $S_T = \{OC_2, OC_5, OC_6\}$, i.e. the task request "Fetch cup" is associated with the target situation where the cup has finally been placed on the table and the empty gripper as well as the empty cupboard remain.

So far, the explanations concentrated on the design of a PS_A. Its information is used to drive the planning process of a task request. Here, according to the conceptual sequence of activities depicted in Fig. 9, the task related PS_A is loaded first. Afterwards, the so-called process of initial monitoring is started. This process determines the initial situation S_I of the chosen PS_A that corresponds to the current environmental situation. From out this situation a path to the target situation can be processed.

Initial Monitoring

The situation monitoring process is controlled by the information contained within the set of situations associated with a PS_A and is executed in a semi-autonomous manner also (Prenzel, 2005). As illustrated in Fig. 9, the monitoring process consists of the determination of the first order logic facts that are assigned to the different *OC*s. Within the given process-structure, the set of facts listed in Table 2 has to be determined during initial monitoring.

To give an illustration of the monitoring approach in MASSiVE, the example of finding the cup to be retrieved from the cupboard will be taken into account. Fig. 11 shows a respective setup of a user interaction that will occur in this case. Here, the FRIEND-II system has been moved in front of a cupboard in which several cups are placed. During this user interaction the user is requested by the system to control the pan-tilt head devices (and thus move the cameras), so that the object of interest is in their sight (the left camera image is displayed to the user). During the movement of the cameras, the image processing system segments objects positioned in the middle of the camera image in real-time. The segmentation result is overlaid to the image, so that the user is able to decide whether the desired object is highlighted or not.

Fact	Description
HoldsNothing(G)	The gripper G holds nothing.
IsInFreePos(G)	The gripper G is in a free position.
IsInsideContainer(C, B)	The cup C in inside the container B (box).
HasFreeStoringSpace(B, C)	The box B has enough free space for the cup C.
IsGripped(G, C)	The cup C is gripped by the gripper G.
IsPlacedOn(C, T)	The cup C in place on top of the table T.

Table 2. Set of facts in "Fetch Cup" scenario.

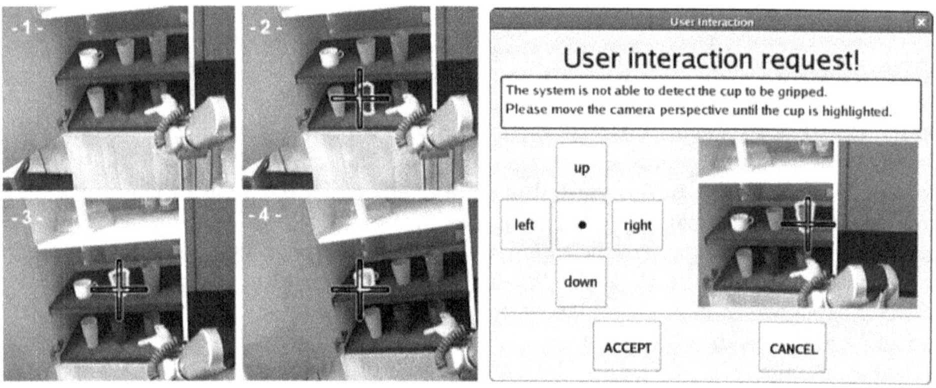

Fig. 11. Experimental setup for finding a cup in a cupboard.

With respect to finish the initial monitoring, the determination of other task relevant objects is performed analogously within a user interaction in case the autonomous object detection fails (or is not unique). After the initial object detection is completed, additional object specific sub-symbolic information is extracted according to the concept of object-anchoring (Prenzel, 2005). This information is stored in the sub-symbolic layer of the system's world model (Fig. 5), to be accessible for all skills that are executed within the reactive layer. Thus, during further task processing steps the degree of the system's autonomy increases with the increasing amount of acquired environmental information.

Task Planning and Execution

According to Fig. 9 task planning and execution takes place, after the initial situation S_I is monitored successfully. Planning is necessary in order to determine a sequence of operations that is adapted to the current environmental situation. The applied planning method is equivalent on both levels of process-structures, i.e. PS_A and PS_E, as exemplified in the following: In the scenario of Fig. 10 with its assigned PS_A it shall be assumed that the initial situation has been determined during initial monitoring. Thus, the task planning objective is to transform this initial situation $S_I = \{OC_1, OC_2, OC_3\}$ into the target situation $S_T = \{OC_2, OC_5, OC_6\}$. Since the transformation of situations is realized by means of the execution of operations, the generation of action sequences is reduced to a graph search problem. Here, the search is realized by means of the Dijkstra algorithm (Martens, 2003a). According to the assumed initial situation S_I, the first *COP* in the sequence of planned *COPs* is *GraspObjectInContainer*. Because this *COP* cannot be executed directly within the architecture, it has to be decomposed to a level of abstraction that deals with *EEOPs*.

The result of the *COP* decomposition, i.e. its assigned elementary process-structure (PS_E), is depicted in Fig. 12. Here, to reduce the complexity of the illustration, only a segment of the complete PS_E is shown – the upper part, as indicated by the dashed box, has been left out. However, the principle of a PS_E can be clarified as follows: The flow of control is modeled on the basis of a Petri-net. As depicted, transitions of this Petri-net are arranged in pairs (or tuples), which represent the execution of an *EEOP*. Each transition of a pair (or tuple) represents the execution of an *EEOP* with different execution results. This is denoted by the different return values. The different nature of *EEOPs*, as introduced in Chapter 4.1, is specified with the help of the prefix in the transition name: *DC* stands for "direct control" of an actuator, *USER* for "user interaction and *REAC* for "reactive operation", i.e. an *EEOP*, which is in fact a closed control loop that couples sensors and actuators. *EEOPs* of the fourth category, the "monitoring operations", with the prefix *MON*, are not part of the depicted segment of PS_E.

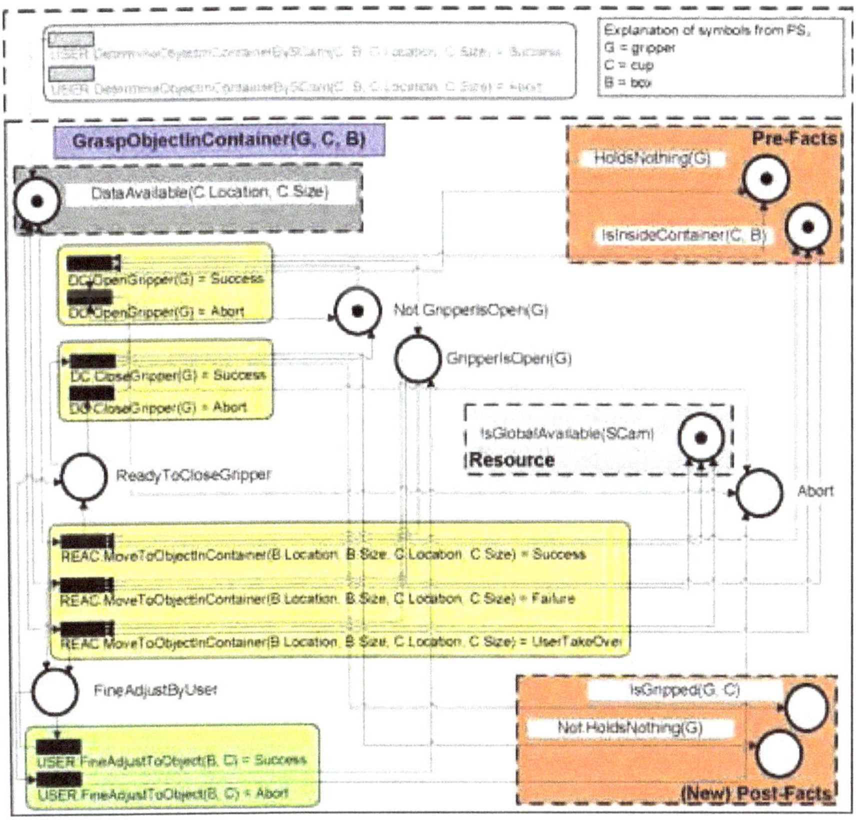

Fig. 12. Section of elementary process-structure (PS_E) representing the *COP* "*GraspObjectInContainer*" (upper part is left out).

Task planning on the basis of the Petri-net is equivalent to the planning process performed on the basis of the PS_A. Starting from an initial situation (initial marking with tokens in the Petri-net) the shortest sequence of operations (fired transitions) is calculated by means of the

Dijkstra algorithm. During task execution, a single transition from out a pair (or tuple respectively) is fired according to the actual return value of the respective *EEOP*. If the return value fits to the pre-planned one, the next *EEOP* of the plan is chosen. Otherwise, a re-planning step has to be performed. Because decomposition has the meaning of replacing the formal parameters of a PS_E with the actual parameters determined by the PS_A, the resulting sequence of *EEOP*s considers the objects that have been localized during the initial monitoring process.

The elementary process-structures in the form of a Petri-net include different modeling aspects and represent the following:

- Control flow (e.g. controlled involvement of the user into data monitoring or direct actuator control)
- Resource usage (e.g. *IsGlobalAvailable(SCam*[9]*)*)
- Data flow and data availability (e.g. *DataAvailable(C.Location, C.Size)*)
- Interconnection to abstract layer and to the world model via facts (e.g. *HoldsNothing(G)*)

The advantage of using Petri-nets as a modeling tool is the availability of mathematical methods for the structural analysis of PS_E. Due to the illustrated stringent and application specific syntax within a PS_E, offline verification becomes possible. This includes the verification with respect to dead-locks, resource-conflicts, modeling errors, state-reachability, availability of sub-symbolic data and the direction of data flow (Martens, 2003b).

During runtime, the initial marking in a PS_E is set according to the current status of task execution. For the example depicted in Fig. 12, since the task participating object *B* (box) and *C* (cup) have already been identified during the initial monitoring process, a new acquisition of the data is not required. Thus, the token in the place "*DataAvailable(C.Location, C.Size)*" will be part of the initial marking. In any other case, where this information which is required for the subsequent manipulative operation *REAC.MoveToObjectInContainer* is not yet available, it will be generated within the upper part (not depicted) of the PS_E via monitoring *EEOP*s or user interactions respectively. The target marking in a PS_E, which is required to apply planning by graph search, is specified during the definition of a PS_E. One rule with respect to the target marking specification is that it has to include the post-facts associated with the *COP* assigned to a certain PS_E. Post facts in Fig. 12 are *IsInsideContainer(C, B)* (also pre-fact), *IsGripped(C, G)* and *Not.HoldsNothing(G)*. With the help of post- and pre-facts, the connection and consistency between the sub-symbolic control level (PS_E) and the abstract level (PS_A) are guaranteed.

Here, according to the given state of the Petri-net, the manipulative *EEOP*s *DC.OpenGripper, REAC.MoveToObjectInContainer* and *DC.CloseGripper* will be executed. Within the reactive manipulation *EEOP*, a motion planning algorithm is started, which retrieves and operates on the previously (during initial monitoring) generated environmental information from the world model (Prenzel et al., 2006; Ojdanic et al., 2006). Due to the structure of the task-knowledge contained within the PS_E and the usage of the Dijkstra algorithm, the result of the planning process is that autonomous *EEOP*s are executed first and user interaction *EEOP*s follow in case the system fails (this general idea is also illustrated in Fig. 9). Furthermore, manipulative *EEOP*s can be interrupted by the user, e.g. in case he can already foresee a possible collision. This is indicated by the "[user interrupt]" transition in Fig. 9 or the third

---

[9] SCam = Stereo-camera system

transition of the reactive *EEOP* in Fig. 12 respectively. The concrete and more detailed description of this kind of interaction enforced by the user is discussed in (Lüth et al., 2007). The complete planning and execution cycle is continued until the given task is completed or has been aborted, e.g. according to the user's intention or due to a critical and irresolvable system status.

The described approach leads to a system that is able to operate robustly, even if it is not able to execute all steps fully autonomously. Moreover, it supports the evolutionary development of the system with increasing autonomy. This means, it is possible to initially realize a rehabilitation robotic support scenario with a low level of autonomy and to replace missing autonomous functionality with user interactions. Subsequently and in an evolutionary manner, more and more user interactions are replaced by autonomous operations by developing more intelligent skill algorithms or using additional sensors and actuators.

For recapitulating this section it is referred to Fig. 9. After the user's initial task selection, the first system controlled user interaction takes places within the initial monitoring. Initial identification tasks that cannot be solved fully autonomously without unreasonable increase of technical complexity are given back to the user to be solved by him. The same approach is taken into account within the ongoing process of task-execution.

5. Conclusion

This paper gives an overview of the functional capabilities of the rehabilitation robotics systems FRIEND-I and FRIEND-II as well as an introspective view of the used underlying control principles and applied software techniques. It is shown that during the different development steps of FRIEND-I the control of the system evolved from out direct speech control of the manipulator up the fully autonomous execution of a "serve-drink task". It turned out that the control of a rehabilitation robot like FRIEND-I becomes possible for a person without manipulative capabilities in his or her arms and hands. But there is still the need for more robustness and reliability in execution, flexibility in usage and relief for its users, if the overall objective of 1.5 hours of autonomy for daily life activities has to be reached. The most important lesson learned within the FRIEND-I project is the application of the semi-autonomous task execution principle. The motivation is that the involvement of the user's cognitive capabilities has the potential of reducing the system's complexity dramatically, so that a technical manageable system emerges.

The consequent implementation of this principle has been realized within the successor system FRIEND-II. On the one hand FRIEND-II comes up with new sophisticated hardware components like a 7 DOF manipulator or a force-torque controlled gripper. It is evident that the usage of these hardware components leads to more robustness in execution. On the other hand FRIEND-II has been software-technically designed for its application within an intelligent environment, where different daily life as well as working scenarios, as specified within the AMaRob project, will be managed. It is shown that the beforehand mentioned requirements of user involvement and distributed execution, as necessary for its application within the intelligent environment, are satisfied by the multi-layer architecture MASSiVE. For user involvement, MASSiVE offers an infrastructure for task-knowledge driven task planning, whereas the user interaction is an integral part within this knowledge. During task execution the system requests the user whenever it has to come to a decision on a cognitive level and the algorithmic realization of this process it too complex and error prone. But even though the user is requested, he or she is relived from tiresome and complicated tasks like remembering the necessary sequence of actions that have to be fulfilled before the execution of the next steps becomes possible. Within MASSiVE's HMI-level the current task context is known, so that a specific and efficient request limited to the current context can be initiated. This has been demonstrated by the detection of a certain cup in a cupboard full of cups, where the application of a well known image segmentation algorithm leads to the same results, from the user's point of view, as a complex image analysis.

The requirement for reactive and distributed execution is satisfied by MASSiVE's reactive layer, which is controlled by the intermediating sequencer. From the sequencer's point of view the reactive layer is as a pool of skills, from which some have to be selected and combined according to a task plan in order to reach the goal of a requested task. Within this context the reactive layer encapsulates the underlying hardware and offers environmental information on a pre-processed symbolic level. Because each hardware component is managed by a separate software server, which itself is managed within the reactive layer according to a well defined server interface concept, the inclusion of new components, like the smart devices within the intelligent environment, has no design consequences for the superior levels like the HMI-layer or the sequencer respectively.

The first task scenario which has been managed with FRIEND-II on basis of MASSiVE is the "serve-drink task" also. Even though the functional improvement with respect to FRIEND-I is not evident, its execution is more flexible from the viewpoint of software technique. Within FRIEND-I subtasks of the "serve-drink task", like grasping, replacing or putting down objects, were programmed in a pre-determined sequence. Within FRIEND-II these subtasks evolve from out a planning process performed on basis of task-knowledge. Due to this flexibility the next development steps concentrate on the implementation of new subtasks, i.e. skills that will be integrated into the already existing task-knowledge data-basis. On the basis of this extended task-knowledge new tasks, as specified within the AMaRob project, will be managed within the next two years.

Another area of active research, which is also important with respect to further improvements of rehabilitation robots, is the system control via non-invasive brain-computer interfaces (BCIs). In (Lüth et al., 2007) first results are presented that show the feasibility of user interactions in MASSiVE solely on the basis of brain signal interpretation. The applied principle is the detection of either the characteristic P300 waveform or steady state visual evoked potentials (SSVEP) in the visual cortex of the user, who is concentrating on a continuously blinking light source. The bandwidth of this kind of input media is still very low and also it is currently not yet possible to realize user interactions with fast reaction times. However, due to ongoing improvements of this technique, a very promising opportunity to command a robotic system arises for highly handicapped users.

6. References

Bien, Z. Z.; Song, W.-K; Kwon, D.-S.; Chung, M.-J.; Park, H.-S.; Kim, D.-J.; Kim, J.-H. & Lee, K. (2001). A Wheelchair Robot System and its Various Interface Methods for the Disabled Persons, *Proceedings of the 1st Workshop on Technical Challenge for Dependable Robots in Human Environments,* Seoul, Korea, May 21-22, 2001

Bolmsjö, G. & Neveryd, H. (1995). WALKY, an Ultrasonic Navigating Mobile Robot for the Disabled, *Proceedings of the 2nd TIDE Congress*, pp. 366-370, ISBN 978-90-5199-220-5, Paris, France, April 1995, IOS Press, Amsterdam

Bonasso, R.; Kortenkamp, D.; Schreckenghost, D. & Ryan, D. (1998). Three tier architecture for controlling space life support systems, *Proceedings of IEEE International Joint Symposium on Intelligence and Systems (SIS) 1998*, pp. 195-201, ISBN 0-8186-8548-4, Rockville, MD, USA, May 1998

Borgerding, B.; Ivlev, O.; Martens, C.; Ruchel, N. & Gräser, A. (1999). FRIEND - Functional Robot Arm with User Friendly Interface for Disabled People, In:, *Assistive Technology on the Threshold of the New Millennium: AAATE'99, Proceedings of the 5th European Conference for the Advancement of Assistive Technology*, C. Bühler, H. Knops (Ed.), pp. 286-290, , IOS Press, ISBN 1-58603-001-9, 1st-4th November 1999, Amsterdam

Busnel, M.; Coulon-Lauture, F.; Détriché, J.-M.; Le Claire, G. & Lesigne, B. (1999). The robotized workstation -MASTER- for users with tetraplegia: Description and evaluation. *Journal of Rehabilitation Research and Development*, Vol. 36, No. 3, July 1999, pp. 217-229, ISSN 0748-7711

Cao, T. & Sanderson, A. C. (1998). AND/OR net representation for robotic task sequence planning, *IEEE Transactions on Systems, Man and Cybernetics*, Vol. 28, Issue 2, May 1998, pp. 204–218, ISSN 1094-6977

Casals, A.; Merchan, R.; Portell, E.; Cufi; X. & Contijoch, J. (1999). CAPDI: A Robotized Kitchen for the Disabled and Elderly, *Proceedings of the 5th European Conference for the Advancement of Assistive Technology (AAATE)*, pp. 346-351, ISBN 1-58603-001-9, Düsseldorf, Germany, November 1-4, 1999, IOS Press, Amsterdam

Colle, E.; Rybawzyk, Y. & Hoppenot, P. (2002). Arph: an assistant robot for disabled people, *Proceedings of IEEE International Conference on Systems, Man and Cybernetics*, pp. 176–181, ISBN 0-7803-7437-1, Yasmine Hammamet, Tunisia., 6-9 October 2002unKhoc cho nho thuong voi trong long, khoc cho noi sau nhe nhu khong. Bao nhieu yeu thuong nhung ngay qua da tan theo khoi may bay that xa... http://nhatquanglan1.0catch.com

Coste-Maniere, E. & Simmons, R. (2000). Architecture, the backbone of robotic systems, *Proceedings of International Conference on Robotics and Automation*, pp. 67–72, ISBN 0-7803-5886-4, San Francisco, CA, USA, April 2000

Dallaway, J.L. & Jackson, R.D. (1993). CURL - today and tomorrow, *Proceedings of the 2nd Nordic Workshop on Rehabilitation Robotics*, Orup Rehab Center, Sweden (HADAR, Malmö),, September 1993

Dallaway, J. L.; Jackson, R. D. & Timmer, P.H.A. (1995). Rehabilitation Robotics in Europe. *IEEE Transactions on Rehabilitation Engineering 1995*, Vol. 3, No. 1, March, 1995 pp. 33-45, ISSN 1063-6528

Dario, P.; Dillman, R. & Christensen, H. I. (2004). EURON research roadmaps, *Key Area 1 on Research Coordination*, http://www.euron.org

DLR. (2007). Key research program "Leitinnovation Servicereobotik", *www.service-robotik.de*, DLR - Project executing organization for German Federal Ministry of Education and Research ("Bundesministerium für Bildung und Forschung")

Eftring, H. (1994). Robot control methods and results from user trials on the RAID workstation, *Proceedings of the 4th International Conference on Rehabilitation Robotics (ICORR)*, pp. 97-101, Wilmington, Delaware, USA, June 1994

Engelberger, J. F. (1989). *Robotics in Service*, MIT Press, ISBN 0-2620-5042-0, Cambridge, MA, USA

Fikes, R. & Nilsson, N. (1971). STRIPS: A new approach to the application of theorem proving to problem solving, *Artificial Intelligence, Vol. 2*, pp. 189-208. Reprinted in Readings in Planning, J. Allen, J. Hendler, and A. Tate (Ed.), 1990, Morgan Kaufmann Publishers, San Mateo, California

Gamma, E.; Helm, R.; Johnson, R. & Vlissides, J. (1995). *Design Patterns: Elements of Reusable Object-Oriented Software,* Addison-Wesley Professional, 1st edition ed., 1995, ISBN 0-2016-3361-2

Hillman, M. R. et al. (1999). Design of a Wheelchair Mounted Robot, *Proceedings of the 5th European Conference for the Advancement of Assistive Technology (AAATE)*, pp. 316-321, ISBN 1-58603-001-9, Düsseldorf, Germany, November 1-4, 1999, IOS Press, Amsterdam

IAT. (2007). AMaRob - Autonomous Manipulator Control for Rehabilitation Robots, *Project-webpage, www.amarob.de*

Innocenti, C.; Mondino, G.; Regis, P. & Sandini, G. (1994). Trajectory Planning and Real-time Control of an Autonomous Mobile Robot Equipped with Vision and Ultrasonic Sensors, *Proceedings of the International Conference on Intelligent Robots and Systems (IROS) 1994,* pp. 1861-1866, ISBN 0-7803-1933-8, Munich, Germany, September 12th-16th, 1994

Kawamura, K.; Bagchi, S.; Iskarous, M. & Bishay, M. (1995). Intelligent robotic systems in service of the disabled, *IEEE Transactions on Rehabilitation Engineering,* Vol. 3, No. 1 , Mar 1995, pp. 14 -21

Kazi, Z. (1996). Multimodally Controlled Intelligent Assistive Robot, *Proceedings of 16th Annual RESNA Conference*, pp. 348-350 Salt Palace Convention Center, Salt Lake City, Utah, USA, June 1996

Kazi, Z.; Chen, S.; Beitler, M.; Chester, D. & Foulds, R. (1997). Grasping at Straws: An Intelligent Multimodal Assistive Robot, *Proceedings of the 5th ICORR'97,* pp. 87-90, Bath Institute of Medical Engineering, University of Bath, UK, April 1997

Korondi, P. & Hashimoto, H. (2003). Intelligent Space as an Integrated Intelligent System, *Keynote Paper in Proceedings of the International Conference on Electrical Drives and Power Electronics,* pp. 24-31, 2003

Lang, O.; Martens, C & Gräser, A. (2000). Realisation of a Semiautonomous Grippingskill for the Support of Disabled People, *Proceedings of Robotik 2000,* pp. 273-278, ISBN 3-18-091552-8, Berlin, 29./30. June 2000, VDI Berichte 1552, VDI Verlag GmbH, Düsseldorf

Laschi, C.; Teti, G.; Tamburrini, G.; Datteri, E. & Dario, P. (2001). Adaptable semi-autonomy in personal robots, *Proceedings of IEEE International Workshop on Robot and Human Interactive Communication,* pp. 152–157, ISBN 0-7803-7222-0, Bordeaux, Paris, France, September 2001

Lüth, T.; Ojdanić, D.; Friman, O.; Prenzel, O. & Gräser, A. (2007). Direct control in a rehabilitation robotic system via a Brain-Computer Interface, Proceedings of the International Conference on Rehabilitation Robotics ICORR, Noordwijk, Netherlands, 13-15 June 2007

Mahoney, R. M. (2001). The Raptor Wheelchair Robot System, *Proceedings of the 7th International Conference on Rehabilitation Robotics (ICORR) 2001,* Mokhtari, M. (Ed.) Integration of Assistive Technology in the Information Age, pp. 135-141, ISBN 1-58603-171-6, Evry, France, IOS Press, Amsterdam

Martens, C.; Lang, O.; Ruchel, N.; Ivlev, O. & Gräser, A. (2001). A FRIEND for Assisting Handicapped People. *IEEE Robotics and Automation Magazine,* Vol. 7, No. 1, March 2001, pp. 57-65, ISSN 1070-9932

Martens, C.; Kim, D.-J.; Han, J.-S.; Gräser, A. & Bien, Z. Z. (2002). Concept for a modified hybrid multi-layer control-architecture for rehabilitation robots, *Proceedings of the*

3rd *International Workshop on Human-friendly Robotic Systems,* pp. 49-54 Daejeon, Korea , January 21-22, 2002

Martens, C. (2003a). Generation of parallel executable control sequences for rehabilitation robotic systems on the basis of hierachical petri-net based task representation, In: *Methods and Applications in Automation,* B. Lohmann, A. Gräser, (Ed.), pp. 73–85, Shaker Verlag, ISBN 3-8322-4502-2, Aachen

Martens, C. (2003b). *Teilautonome Aufgabenbearbeitung bei Rehabilitationsrobotern mit Manipulator,* Ph.D. thesis University of Bremen, Shaker-Verlag, ISBN 3-8322-2400-9, Aachen

Martens, C. (2005). Task oriented programming of service-robots on the basis of process-structures, In: *Methods and Applications in Automation,* B. Lohmann, A. Gräser, (Ed.), pp. 45–56, Shaker Verlag, ISBN 3-8322-4502-2, Aachen

May, T. & Schäffer, C. (1999). Care-O-bot: A System for Assisting Elderly and Disabled Persons in Home Environments, *Proceedings of the 5th European Conference for the Advancement of Assistive Technology (AAATE),* pp. 340-345, ISBN 1-58603-001-9, Düsseldorf, Germany, November 1-4, 1999, IOS Press, Amsterdam

Mokhtari, M. & Amni, C. (2001). Assistive Technology for the Disabled People: Should it Work? The French Approach, *Proceedings of the 2nd International Workshop on Human-friendly Welfare Robotic Systems,* pp. 134-136, KAIST, Daejeon, Korea January 2001, HWRS-ERC, Daejeon

Ojdanic, D.; Ivlev, O. & Gräser, A. (2006). A new fast motion planning approach for dexterous manipulators in 3D-Cartesian space, *Proceedings of ISR-Robotik Joint Conference on Robotics,* p. 49, ISBN 3-18-091956-6, International Congress Centre Munich, Germany, May 15-17 2006, VDI Wissensforum IWB GmbH, Düsseldorf, Germany

Prenzel, O. (2005). Semi-autonomous object anchoring for service-robots, In: *Methods and Applications in Automation,* B. Lohmann, A. Gräser, (Ed.), pp. 57–68, Shaker Verlag, ISBN 3-8322-4502-2, Aachen

Prenzel, O.; Ojdanic, D. & Gräser, A. (2006). Manipulative Robotic Tasks in Smart Home Environments, *Proceedings of 4th International Conference On Smart Homes and Health Telematics (ICOST),* pp. 172-179, ISBN 1-58603-623-8, ISSN 1383-813X, Belfast, Northern-Ireland, UK, June 26-28, 2006, Series: Assistive Techology Research Series, IOS Press, (Ed.) C. Nugent, J.C. Augusto, Vol. 19

Radchenko, O.; Martens, C.; Pape, A.; She, H.; Volosyak, I. & Gräser, A. (2004). FRIEND – An Intelligent Assistant in Daily Life, In: *Advances in Rehabilitation Robotics: Human-friendly Technologies on Movement Assistance and Restoration for People with Disabilities - Part II Rehabilitation Robots for Assistance of Human Movements, II.1 Conceptions and Experimental Design,* Ed.: Z. Zenn Bien, Dimitar Stefanov, pp. 95–126, Springer-Verlag, ISBN 3-540-21986-2, Heidelberg, Germany

She, H.; Martens, C. & Gräser, A. (2003a). Application of Programming by Demonstration in the Rehabilitation Robotic System FRIEND, *Proceedings of the 8th International Conference on Rehabilitation Robotics (ICORR) 2003,* pp. 39-42, ISBN 89-88366-09-3, Daejeon, Korea, 23-25 April 2003, HWRS-ERC

She, H.; Martens, C.; Gräser, A.; Kim, D.-J.; Lee, H.-E. & Bien, Z. Z. (2003b). Soft Computing-based Robust Contact/Non-contact Detection during Serving a Beverage Task, *Proceedings of the IEEE International Conference on Fuzzy Systems (FUZZ-IEEE 2003),* pp. 613-617, Marriott Pavilion Downtown Hotel, St. Louis, MO, May 25-28, 2003

Van der Loos, H.F.M. (1995). Lessons Learned in the Application of Robotics Technology to Field of Rehabilitation. *IEEE Transactions on Rehabilitation Engineering*, Vol. 3, No. 1, March 1995, pp. 46-55, ISSN 1063-6528

Van der Loos, H.F.M.; Wagner, J.J.; Smaby, N.; Chang, K.-S.; Madrigal, O.; Leifer, L.J.; Khatib, O. (1999). ProVAR assistive robot system architecture, *Proceedings of International Conference on Robotics and Automation (ICRA) 1999*, pp. 741-746, ISBN 0-7803-5180-0, Marriott Hotel, Renaissance Center, Detroit, Michigan, May 10-15, 1999, IEEE Robotics and Automation Society

Volosyak, I.; Radchenko, O.; Pape, A., Martens, C.; She, H.; Wendland, E. & Gräser, A. (2003). Smart tray for the support of a wheelchair mounted manipulator, *Proceedings of the International Conference on Economic, Engineering and Manufacturing Systems ICEEMS 2003*, ISBN 973-635-215-3, Brasov, Romania, 23-24 October, 2003

Wagner, J.J; Van der Loos, H.F.M; Leifer, L.J. (1998). Dual-Agent User Interface for an Assistive Robot, *Proceedings of the 21st Annual RESNA Conference*, pp. 286-288, ISSN 0883-4741, ISBN 0-932101-4-2, Minneapolis, MN. Washington DC, June 1998, RESNA Press

5

Applications of a Fluidic Artificial Hand in the Field of Rehabilitation

Artem Kargov[1], Oleg Ivlev[2], Christian Pylatiuk[1], Tamim Asfour[3], Stefan Schulz[1], Axel Gräser[2], Rüdiger Dillmann[3] and Georg Bretthauer[1]
[1]Institute for Applied Computer Science, Forschungszentrum Karlsruhe, Germany
[2]Institute of Automation, University of Bremen, Germany
[3]Institute of Computer Science and Engineering, University of Karlsruhe, Germany

1. Introduction

Since the early middle of last century, use of artificial robotic hands in the field of rehabilitation has been associated with prosthetic devices used for the therapy of upper limb deficiency. Artificial manipulators of the last century were used in general for industrial applications or for service tasks of telemanipulation.
In the last three decades, service robotics developed very rapidly. In recent years, robotic systems which are able to complete service tasks in direct cooperation with humans became popular [Yuta at al., (2006)].

Modern robotic rehabilitation devices are intelligent systems used for movement assistance, physical support and indoor navigation, physical rehabilitation, vocational rehabilitation, and interactive entertainment [Bien, Stefanov (2004)].
Dextrous manipulation has become the subject of research for many scientists around the world and artificial hands are used in a wide area of applications [Venkataraman, Iberall (1990)].
Investigations of hand construction, artificial design, and manipulation abilities resulted in the development of different hand prototypes for service robotics, prosthetics, and rehabilitation [Muzumdar (2004); DeLaurentis et al., (2000); Pons et al., (1998); Pons et al., (2000); Lee et al., (2000); Light, Chappell, (2000); Weir *ff* et al., (2001); Kyberd et al., (2003); Walker (2003); Boblan et al., (1999); Plettenburg (2002); Hirzinger et al., (2004); Jacobsen et al. (1986); Townsend (2000)].

In view of the dexterity of natural hands, it may be assumed that there are problems in the development of dextrous artificial hands, including controllability, hand geometry, hand functionality, development and placement of sensors; sensory fusion, and the need for better actuators [Subramanian T. Venkataraman, Thea Iberall (1990)].
As regards the different criteria related to artificial manipulators, which were discussed in research literature, we share the opinion that acceptance of robotic devices by the user plays a very important role in the development of manipulator constructions. Safety and simplicity of usage are no less important aspects of device architectures. Universality of components, their modularity and changeability should be taken into account and can allow for reducing the energy consumption and production costs of

This chapter will highlight applications of an artificial robotic hand actuated by flexible fluidic actuators developed at the Forschungszentrum Karlsruhe (Karlsruhe Research Centre, Germany) [Kargov et al., 2006].

Flexible fluidic actuators were developed as an alternative to other actuation principles of today, such as electromotors, shape memory alloys, or McKibben muscles.

Up to date, fluidic actuators have impeded the design of artificial actuation systems due to their relatively high weight and low power. Modern fluidic actuators have already been identified as being particularly suitable for macrorobotics, compared to other actuator technologies and considering several criteria, including stress improvements, bandwidth, intrinsic compliance, packaging, good power to weight ratio, and high dynamics [Hollerbach et al., 1992].

2. Fluidic artificial hand

2.1 System components and mechatronic design

Since 1999, a multifunctional artificial hand has been developed at the Karlsruhe Research Centre that meets modern technical standards. This development was based on the invention of new flexible fluidic actuators [Schulz at al, 1999]. The construction of first actuators was easy. They were built of thin plastic films in a very compact manner as a two-layered body with two separated chambers which contained a small pipe for fluid supply. The elastic chambers were expanded when the pressure was applied to the actuator. This expansion behaviour was taken into account by a new concept of an artificial finger joint, which was presented in 2000. The functional principle of such artificial joints consists in converting the energy of chamber inflation into a rotational movement between two thin plates that are connected to each other (Fig. 1a,b). Different prototypes of fluid actuators based on this principle have been built by the Institute of Applied Computer Science up to date [Schulz at al, 1999].

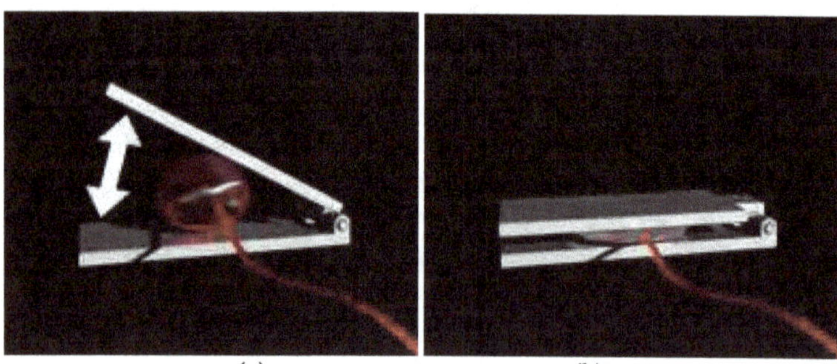

(a) (b)

Fig. 1a,b. Functional principle of flexible fluidic actuators.

The current model of an artificial finger joint consists of a flexible fluidic actuator made of a reinforced flexible bellow. Both fronts of the actuator are attached to solid fittings mounted on the joint, which transmit the pulling force of axial expansion to the joint (Fig. 2.). A special tissue covers the bellow and reduces the radial expansion of the actuator under pressure.

Two major advantages of these actuators are their low weight and inherent compliance. Each actuator weighs only 2.6 grams and is built of lightweight materials. In comparison with fluid cylinders, flexible fluidic actuators can transmit energy in the same manner, but have a higher power-to-weight ratio at the same pressure and volume. Small dimensions of actuators of 12 mm in diameter and 12 mm in length allow for an integration directly in the artificial finger joint. A torque of up to 0.8 Nm can be achieved for such joint at 6 bar pressure.

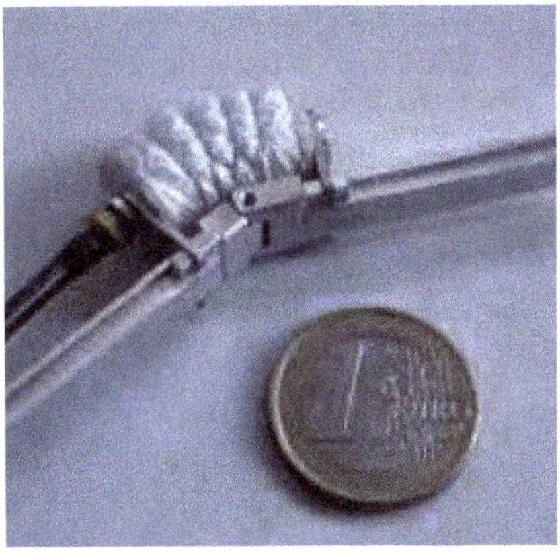

Fig. 2. Flexible fluidic actuator with artificial joint.

The development of artificial joints led to the design of a multi-articulated artificial hand (Fig. 3.). Biometric data of a natural hand were used to design the prototype of this robot hand. Made of lightweight aluminium with high tensile strength properties, the basic construction consists of the 5-fingered durable and stable mechanical framework with a natural appearance. The artificial metacarpus with the fingers is made up of artificial bones and joints. The number of joints can be varied for other prototypes and optimised for special applications without almost any losses of the anthropomorphic appearance of the hand, its dexterity, functioning, and high dynamics.

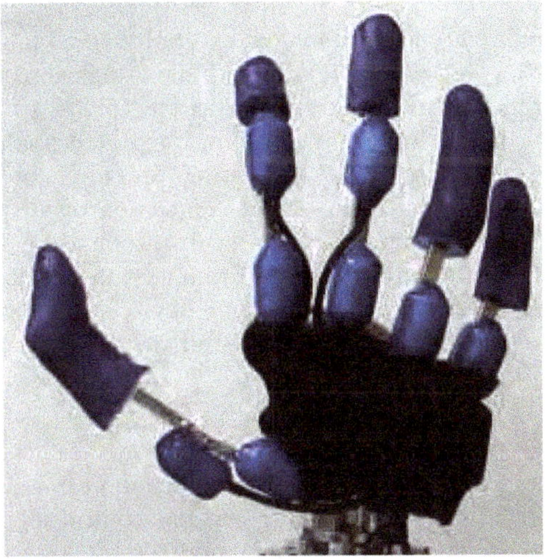

Fig. 3. Current prototype of a fluid hand

All joints and actuators in the hand are constructed identically. This makes the hand construction modular, actuators can be interchanged with each other, and the number of degrees of freedom can be changed. Consequently, redesigning of the end manipulator and the whole reconstruction of the system are not necessary.
Current prototypes of a fluid hand have 8 active actuated joints and 3 passive joints which are not actuated. The index and middle fingers have four active joints. The ring and small fingers have one actuated joint and one passive joint each. The thumb is actuated by two joints. The base joint of the thumb is placed perpendicular to the middle joint to achieve an opposite movement.
Other important components of the fluid hand are electronic valves and the control unit (Fig. 4.), which are integrated in the artificial metacarpus. Valves and electronics are custom-made, as suitable commercially available devices are lacking.

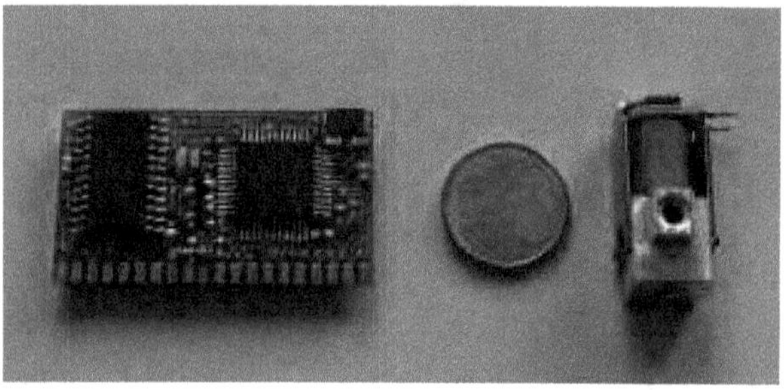

Fig. 4. Electric valve and control unit.

Valves are operated according to the mono-stable principle. They supply the fluid for fluidic actuators and keep the fluid pipeline closed, if no current is applied. In this way, the position of fingers can be saved during grasping. Small dimensions of valves of 23x11x13 mm allow for their integration in the hand. Low power consumption of the valves of 1 Watt saves energy and a flow rate of 14 l/min (by air) ensures a high dynamics of hand movements.
The electronic unit is built by SMD technology, except for some few discrete components, and arranged on a four-layered circuit board. With the dimensions of 51 mm / 40 mm / 9 mm, it consists of a programmable microcontroller PIC16F877 by Microchip (Microchip Technology Inc., USA), drivers for the valves, an integrated analogue-digital converter which can digitize 8 signals collected by positioning, pressure, and tactile sensors as well as mini connectors which allow for the direct connection of all periphery units to the electronics. Sensors can be integrated optionally in the hand and use analogue/digital ports to communicate with the control unit. Additionally, the electronics offers I2C, CAN, and SPI interfaces to interact with external robotic devices, such as the robot arm and an RS232 interface for programming the control unit and diagnosing the whole control system from a PC.

2.2 Control architecture and functioning

Communication and data transfer between the controller and external devices take place via serial CAN, SPI, I2C or RS232 interfaces. In general, control signals, such as the joint number, angles for positioning the joints or a number of programmed grip types are transmitted from the external control system to the fluid hand in this way.

A fluid hand works as follows: the controller collects external control signals and operates four mono-stable valves via the respective driver modules. Microvalves provide the corresponding flexible fluidic actuators with external air pressure. The actuators are inflated under pressure, forces of expansion are generated, and the flexion movement of hand digits is achieved. The extension movement is performed by a spring element.

2.3 Performance and functionality

Due to the use of fluidic actuators and the possibility of controlling each joint separately, a large operating range of hand motion is achieved. Every digit of the hand with an active base joint can be flexed by up to 90°. All actuators can be flexed independently of each other.

The possibility of moving each finger joint or joint group separately during grasping is a very important advantage of artificial hands with an anthropomorphic appearance and functionality. Using this benefit, artificial manipulators can perform in general all basic grasping patterns of human hands.

Different tasks of daily life, such as grasping and manipulating differently sized household objects, can be performed using a large number of combinations of movable joints. A cylindrical power grasp, precision grasp, tripod grasp, hook grasp, and spherical grasp can be performed. (Fig. 5.). The important functions of the index finger, such as pressing a key or operating a switch, can be implemented as well.

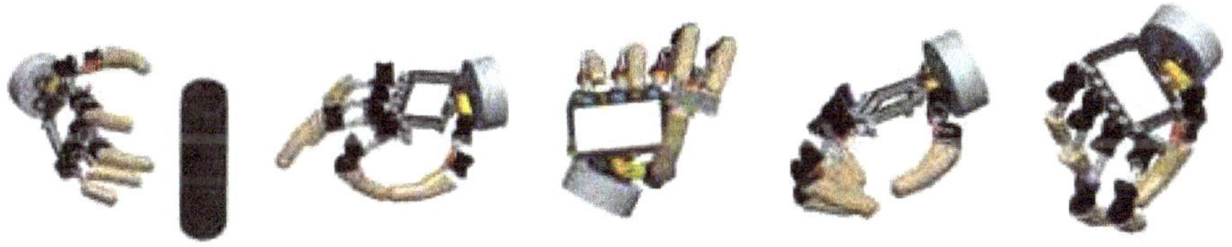

a b c d e

Fig. 5. Grip types which can be performed by the fluid hand. a - cylindrical power grasp, b - precision grasp, c - tripod grasp, d - hook grasp, and e - spherical grasp.

A multiple number of degrees of freedom (DOF) and compliance of the fluidic actuators and elastic finger pads give rise to a fluid hand with the specific feature of adaptive grasping. Artificial fingers conform to the shape of an object when grasping it. Additionally, the self-adapting properties of the hand provide for a correct distribution of contact force when grasping and manipulating objects, which is similar to that of natural hands.

2.4 Technical characteristics

The technical characteristics of the hand are presented in Table I. Small-sized and low-weight components were used for the mechanical construction of the hand, resulting in a low total weight of 350 g. The weight of the skeletal framework is 245 g, including 8 fluidic actuators and the elastic finger pads.

Prehension forces are distributed over a large contact area during grasping and stable holding with low grip forces is possible. Hence, a cylindrical object simulating the handle of a suitcase can be held with a maximum of 110 N in a hook grasp.

Using the custom-made valves, the hand can be closed within two seconds.

The fluid hand has different interfaces and can be integrated in different systems for service robotics and rehabilitation, which use different control interfaces.

The fluid hand requires an external power supply of 7.5V up to 12 V and air pressure supply of 6 bar.

3. Applications of a fluidic artificial hand

3.1 Humanoid robot for the household environment

3.1.1 System overview

The humanoid robot ARMAR-III [Asfour et al., 2006] has been developed within the German Humanoid Project (SFB 588: Collaborative Research Center on Humanoid Robots). The goal of this project is the development of humanoid robots which safely coexist with humans, interactively communicate with humans, and usefully manipulate objects in built-for-human environments. In particular, it is focussed on the integration of motor, perception, and cognition components, such as multimodal human-humanoid interaction and human-humanoid co-operation in order to be able to demonstrate robot tasks in a kitchen environment. Designing the robot is aimed at obtaining a humanoid that closely mimics the sensory and sensory-motor capabilities of the human being. The robot should be able to deal with a household environment and the wide variety of objects and activities encountered in it. Therefore, the robot must be designed in a comprehensive manner, such that a wide range of tasks (and not only a particular task) can be performed.

The humanoid robot ARMAR-III (Fig. 6) has 43 mechanical degrees of freedom (DoF): the head has a total number of 7 DoFs, the waist has 3 DoFs, each arm has 7 DoFs, each hand has 8 DoFs. The mobile platform has 3 DoFs. In addition, the hands consist of 16 DoFs. From the kinematics control point of view, the robot consists of seven sub-systems: head, left arm, right arm, left hand, right hand, torso, and a mobile platform. The upper body has been designed to be modular and light-weight while retaining a size and proportion similar to those of an average person. For locomotion, a mobile platform is used, which allows for holonomic movability in the application area. The head has seven DoFs and is equipped with two eyes. The eyes have a common tilt and can sway independently. The visual system is mounted on a four-DoF neck mechanism. Each eye is equipped with two digital colour cameras (wide and narrow angle) to allow for simple visual-motor behaviours, such as tracking and saccadic motions towards salient regions as well as for more complex visual tasks, such as hand-eye co-ordination.

The head features human-like characteristics in motion and response, that is, the neck and the eyes have a human-like speed and range of motion. Furthermore, the head is equipped with a microphone array, consisting of six microphones (two in the ears, two in the front, and two in back of the head). This is necessary for 3D acoustic localisation.

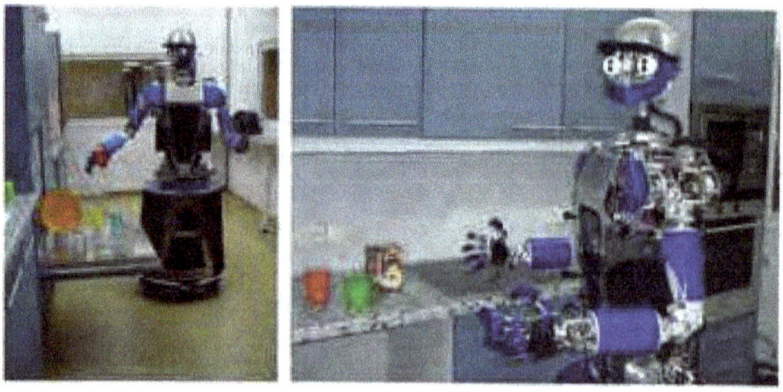

Fig. 6. The humanoid robot ARMAR-III in the demonstration environment (kitchen). The robot consists of seven sub-systems: head, left arm, right arm, left hand, right hand, torso, and a mobile platform.

The main goal of our research is to build humanoid robots which support people in their daily life. The main component of such a robot for handling objects is its manipulation system. The design of the arms is based on the observation of the motion range of a human arm. From the mechanical point of view, the human arm can be modelled by a first-order approximation as a mechanical manipulator with seven DoFs.
The sections of the arm are linked by one-DoF rotational joints, each specifying a selective motion. Consequently, the arms have been designed in an anthropomorphic way: three DoFs in the shoulder, two DoFs in the elbow, and two DoFs in the wrist. Each arm is equipped with a five-fingered hand with eight DoFs ([Schulz et al., 2004]). The goal of performing tasks in human-centred environments results in a number of requirements on the sensor system, especially on that of the manipulation system. To achieve different control modalities, different sensors are integrated in the arm. Each joint is equipped with motor encoders, axis sensors, and joint torque sensors to allow for position, velocity, and torque control. Due to space restrictions and mechanical limitations, the sensor configuration differs. For example, a sensor fitting into the elbow will most likely be too large for the wrist. In the current version of the arms, motor revolution speed, position of axis, and axis torque are monitored in each joint. In the wrists 6D force/torque sensors (ATI Industrial Automation, www.ati-ia.com) are used for position and force control. Four planar skin pads (see [Kerpa et al., 2003]) are mounted to the front and back side of each shoulder, thus also serving as a protective cover for the shoulder joints. Similarly, cylindrical skin pads are mounted to the upper and lower arms, respectively.

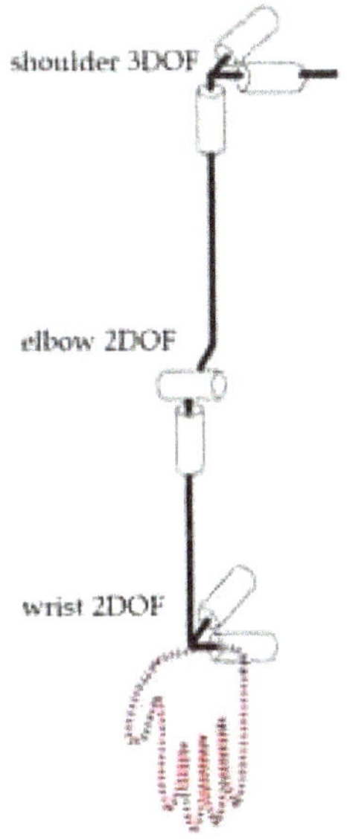

Fig. 7. Kinematics of the arm with 7 DOFs.

3.1.2 Control architecture

The control architecture comprises the following three levels: task planning level, synchronisation and coordination level, and sensor-actor level [Asfour et al., 2005]. A given task is decomposed into several sub-tasks. These represent sequences of actions the sub-systems of the humanoid robot must carry out to accomplish the task goal. The co-ordinated execution of a task requires the scheduling of the sub-tasks and their synchronisation with logical conditions, external and internal events.

Fig. 8 shows the block diagram of the control architecture with three levels, global and active models, and a multi-modal user interface [Asfour et al., 2005]:

- The task planning level specifies the sub-tasks for the multiple sub-systems of the robot. This level represents the highest level with functions of task representation and is responsible for the scheduling of tasks and management of resources and skills. It generates the sub-tasks for the different sub-systems of the robot autonomously or interactively by a human operator. The sub-tasks generated for the lower level contain the information necessary for the task execution, e.g. parameters of objects to be manipulated in the task or the 3D information about the environment. According to the task description, the sub-system's controllers are selected here and activated to achieve the given task goal.

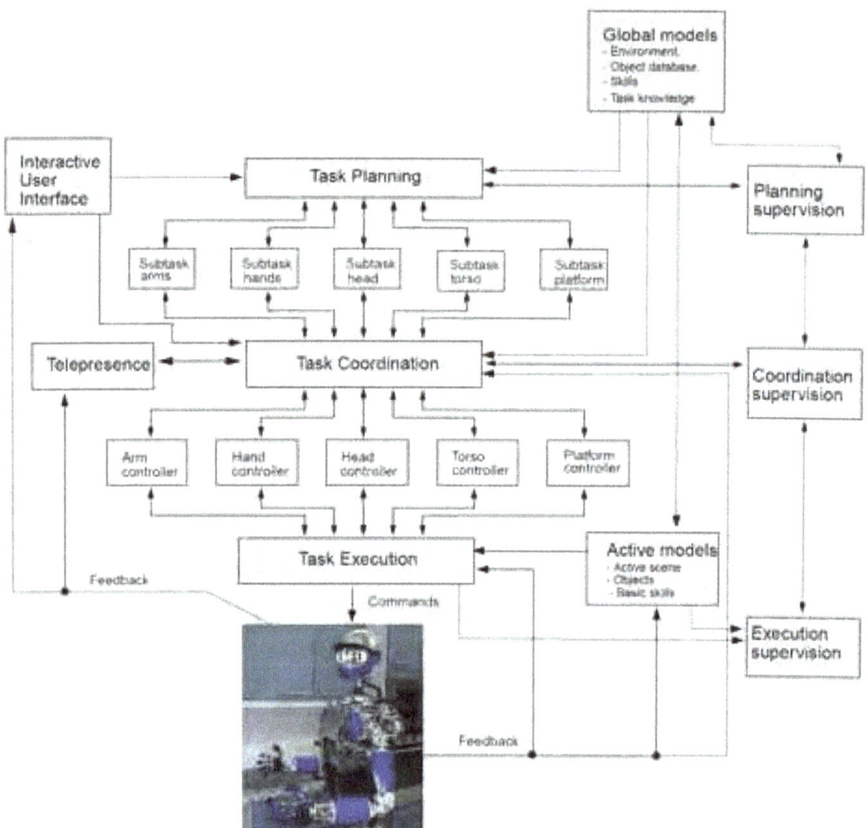

Fig. 8. Hierarchical control architecture for co-ordinated task execution in humanoid robots: planning, co-ordination, and execution level.

The task co-ordination level activates sequential/parallel actions for the execution level in order to achieve the given task goal. The sub-tasks are provided by the task planning level. As on the planning level, the execution of the sub-tasks in an appropriate schedule can be modified/reorganised by a tele-operator or user via an interactive user interface.

- The task execution level is characterised by control theory to execute specified sensor-motor control commands. This level uses task-specific local models of the environment and objects. Hereinafter, these models shall be referred to as *active models*.
- The active models (*short-term memory*) play a central role in this architecture. They are first initialised by the global models (*long-term memory*) and can be updated mainly by the perception system. The novel idea of the active models, as they are suggested here, is their independent actualisation and reorganisation. An active model consists of the internal knowledge representation, interfaces, inputs and outputs for information extraction, and optionally active parts for actualisation/reorganisation (update strategies, correlation with other active models or global models, learning procedure, logical reasoning, etc.).
- Internal system events and execution errors are detected among local sensor data. These events/errors are used as feedback to the task co-ordination level in order to take appropriate measures. For example, a new alternative execution plan can be generated to react to internal events of the robot sub-systems or to environmental stimuli.

In addition to graphical user interfaces (GUIs), the user interface provides the possibility for an interaction using natural language. Telepresence techniques enable the operator to supervise and tele-operate the robot and, thus, to solve exceptions which can arise for various reasons.

3.1.3 Integrated grasp planning and visual object localisation

As a first step towards a complete humanoid grasping system, an integrated approach to grasp planning has been developed [Morales et al., 2006]. The central idea of this system is the existence of a database with the models of all the objects present in the robot workspace. Based on this central fact, two necessary modules are developed: a visual system able to locate and recognise the objects and an offline grasp analyser that provides the most feasible grasp configurations for each object. The results provided by these modules are stored and used by the control system of the humanoid to decide and execute the grasp of a particular object. Fig. 9 gives an overview of the grasp planning system.

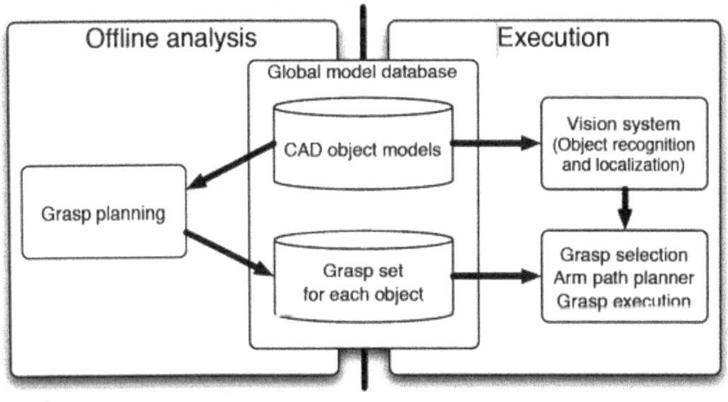

Fig. 9. An overview of the grasp planning system.

The grasp planning system consists of three components (see [Morales et al., 2006]):

- The **global model database**. It is the core of our approach. It does not only contain the CAD models of all the objects, but also stores a set of feasible grasps for each object. Moreover, this database is the interface between the different modules of the system.
- The offline **grasp analyser** that uses the model of the objects and of the hand to compute in a simulation environment a set of stable grasps. The results produced by this analysis are stored in the grasps database to be used by the other modules.
- A **online visual procedure to identify objects in stereo images** by matching the features of a pair of images with the 3D pre-built models of such objects. After recognising the target object, it determines its location and pose. This information is necessary to reach the object (see [Azad et al., 2006].

Once an object has been localised in the work scene, a grasp for that object is selected from the set of pre-computed stable grasps. This is instanced to a particular arm/hand configuration that takes into account the particular pose and reachability conditions of the object. This results in an approaching position and orientation. A path planner reaches that specified grasp location and orientation. Finally, the grasp is executed. These modules are not described in this paper, since they are still under development.

3.1.4 Outlook

The robot represents a highly integrated system suitable not only for research on manipulation, sensor-motor co-ordination, and human-robot interaction, but also for real applications in human-centred environments that make higher requirements on perception and action abilities of the robot. These are different scientific and technical problems, such as navigation, humanoid manipulation and grasping with a 5-finger hand, object recognition and localisation, task co-ordination as well as multi-modal interaction. The term multi-modality includes the communication modalities intuitive for the user, such as speech, gesture, and haptics (physical contact between the human and the robot), which will be used to command or instruct the robot system directly. Concerning the co-operation between the user and the robot - for example in the joint manipulation of objects - it is important for the robot to recognise the human's intention, to remember the acts that have already been carried out together, and to apply this knowledge correctly in the individual case. Great effort is spent on safety, as this is a very important aspect of the man-machine co-operation.

An outstanding property of the system is its ability to learn. As a result, the system can be led to new, formerly unknown problems, for example to new terms and new objects. Even new motions will be learned with the aid of the human and they can be corrected in an interactive way by the user.

3.2 Rehabilitation wheelchair system / Rehabilitation robot FRIEND-II equipped with the FZK hand: dexterous and safe manipulation

3.2.1. System description

The rehabilitation robotics system FRIEND developed by the Institute of Automation of the University of Bremen (IAT) can be used by disabled people, for instance, with upper limb impairments, to act more autonomously in daily life as well as in the working environment. For the detailed description of this robotics system, its main components, and envisaged functionalities see another chapter in this book about FRIEND I+II.

Service robots in general and rehabilitation robots in particular have to act in the real world and not in a specially installed working cell, i.e. an artificial world, as common industrial robots. To act safely and effectively in a real unstructured environment, this kind of robots requires dexterous manipulators with at least 7 joints (degrees of freedom or DoF) like a human arm. The effects of the limited motion repertoire of "Manus"-ARM, the 6-joint kinematic structure of which corresponds to that of an ordinary industrial robot, were demonstrated during the experiments with FRIEND-I [Martens et al., 2001]. The next generation of this rehabilitation robotics system, FRIEND-II (Fig. 10), therefore is equipped with a dexterous lightweight robot arm with 7 joints [Ivlev et al., 2005]. This electrically driven robot arm was developed by *amtec robotics*, Berlin (www.amtec-robotics.com) with the functional specification given by the IAT. To implement humanlike kinematics, the arm is composed of a series of turn and pan joints with perpendicular axes. The combination of a turn-pan-turn-joint is kinematically equivalent to a spherical joint like the human shoulder or the wrist joint. The middle (4th) pan joint corresponds to the elbow (Fig. 11). At the wrist, a multi-axis force/torque sensor of the type Gamma by ATI-Industrial Automation (NC, USA) is integrated. To increase the grasping capabilities, the arm may be equipped optionally with a 5-finger artificial fluid hand instead of a conventional two-finger gripper. In this way, the range of objects which can be grasped is extended and manipulation safety is improved thanks to the hand compliancy. Although it operates very closely to the user, this "soft" hand is safe and cannot harm a human or objects in the workspace. FRIEND-II also is equipped with a stereo pan-tilt-zoom camera system and a "smart tray" which is able to detect objects. The rack shown in Fig. 10, on which the cameras are mounted, was chosen to determine the optimal location of the cameras and will later be exchanged for a more ergonomic rack. The multi-processor control PC is mounted at the rear of the wheelchair.

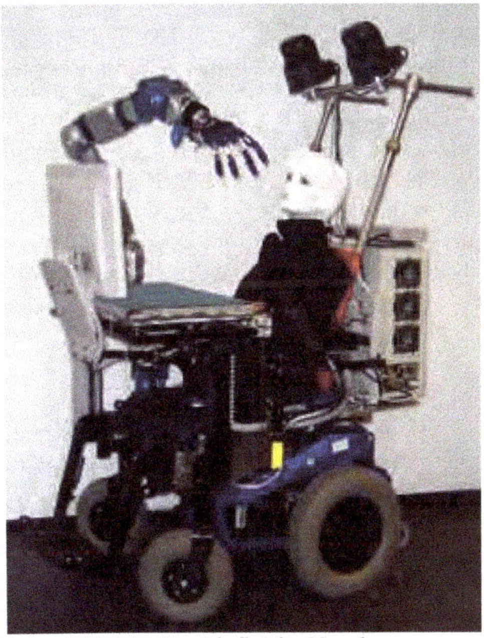

Fig. 10. Rehabilitation Robot FRIEND-II with fluidic Hand.

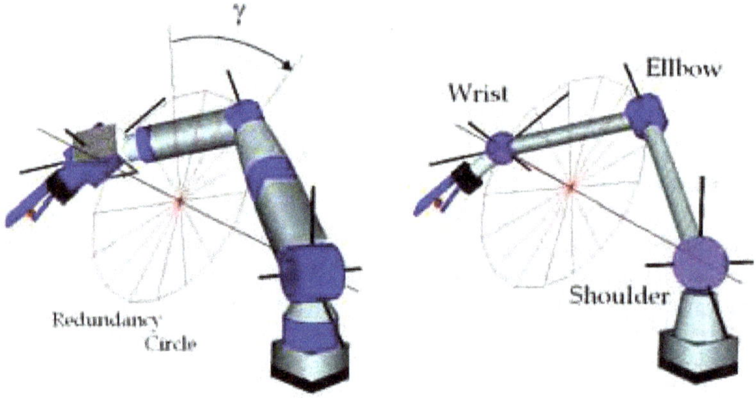

Fig. 11. Kinematic structure of a 7-joint manipulator and its self-motion manifold.

3.2.2. Grasping cases and dexterous arm control

Similar to a human arm, a dexterous manipulator with humanlike 7-joint kinematics allows for changes of the Cartesian elbow position in space without influencing the hand location. This feature is called *self-motion* and characterises in general the manipulative manifold of dexterous robots. In a 7-joint robot arm a manipulative manifold is a circle – the so-called redundancy circle, with the centre on the line connecting the intersection points of the shoulder and wrist joints (Fig. 11). The elbow position on the redundancy circle usually is determined by the redundancy angle γ. By varying γ, the arm configuration is changed without changing the hand location. This feature is utilised by the configuration control of dexterous 7-joint manipulators [Seraji, 1989]. Compared to conventional 6-joint kinematics, however, kinematic dexterity causes significant control problems, because dexterous kinematic structures with more than 6 DoFs are described by an underdetermined systems of non-linear algebraic equations.

For the successful and practically useable control of dexterous manipulators, a new control concept, called Kinematic Configuration Control (*KCC*), has been developed [Ivlev et al., 2000]. The concept combines the advantages of the kinematic control paradigm, enabling exact regulation of tool motion and typically used by conventional robots with 6 DoFs, with the possibility of precisely controllable changes of the robot configuration.

The standard algorithm of kinematic control is based on the following vector equation:

$$_{(s)}g = f(_{(n)}q), \tag{1}$$

which describes the relationship between the n-dimensional joint variables vector $_{(n)}q$ and the s-dimensional vector $_{(s)}g$ representing the location of the end effector (hand) in the workspace. The non-linear vector function f consists of s scalar functions specifying the kinematic structure of the robot as an open kinematic chain.

For non-redundant robots with n=s, the equation system (1) can be solved in a closed form: $_{(s)}q = f^{-1}(_{(s)}g)$. For each end effector location $_{(s)}g$ within the robot workspace $W \in \Re^s$, this solution yields a finite number of possible configurations. In the case of redundant kinematics n>s, the equation system (1) is underdetermined and can be solved in a so-called functionally closed form, when the inverse functions $f^{-1}(_{(s)}g, {}_{(r)}q)$ contain $r = n - s$ joint variables as parameters. In order to fully specify the equation system (1), r additional conditions (scalar equations) are needed.

In the case of 7 DoF kinematics n=7. The dimension s of the vector $_{(s)}g$ depends on the manipulation and/or grasping task. If the manipulation task follows a fully defined trajectory in the 3D Cartesian working space $W \in \Re^3$, the three Cartesian coordinates as well as the hand orientation angles are specified unambiguously and the vector is $_{(6)}g = [X, Y, Z, Yaw, Pitch, Roll]$ with s=6. The same condition results when grasping objects of parallelepiped shape, as for example a book (Fig. 12a). The hand location here may also be considered as having been determined completely, because the object may be gripped in the middle for equilibrium reasons. In this case, s=6 as well. Therefore, just one additional condition to resolve the redundancy will be needed for such kind of manipulation and grasping tasks.

However, such a fully defined specification of the hand location is encountered rather rarely in service and rehabilitation robotics. Figures 12b and 12c show two other typical grasping cases. If a cylinder (e.g. a glass or a bottle) must be grasped, the orientation angle *Yaw* cannot be defined precisely: in general, it may have an arbitrary value between 0° and ±180°. In this case, $_{(5)}g = [X, Y, Z, Pitch, Roll]$ with s = 5 and for redundancy, two additional conditions are required. When grasping a ball-shaped object, such as an apple or an egg, all three orientation angles are free, $_{(3)}g$ = [X, Y, Z], s = 3 and three additional conditions already will be needed to resolve the redundancy.

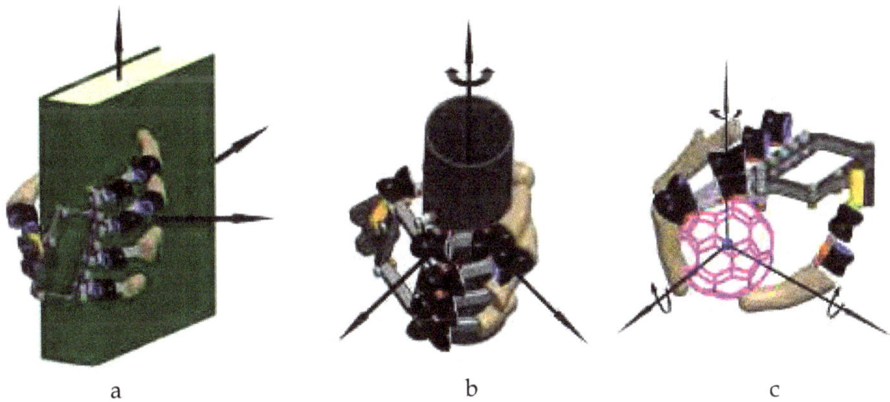

Fig. 12. a - completely defined hand location when grasping a book (s=6), b - Partly defined hand orientation when grasping a glass (s=5), c - Undefined hand orientation when grasping a ball (s=3).

The main idea of resolving redundancy in *KCC* in contrast to other concepts of closed solutions for 7-joint kinematics [Dahm 1997, Asfour 1999] is to control the robot arm relative to the actual robot pose (spatial posture) instead of the actual configuration, as it is typical of other control methods. The difference between a robot configuration and a robot pose is defined as follows: a pose is the placement of robot links and joints in the 3D Cartesian working space, while a configuration is a set of joint angles - i.e. a point in the 7D configuration space for a robot arm with 7 joints.

To control the robot arm relative to the current pose, the kinematic chain with a number of additional virtual (imaginary) links [Ivlev et al.,1997, Ivlev et al., 1999] is applied, such that the constrained kinematic structure becomes non-redundant - this means that the number of degrees of freedom becomes equal to the working space dimension. For the case of ${}_{(6)}g$ = [*X, Y, Z, Yaw, Pitch, Roll*], just one imaginary link will be needed. In the case of 7-joint kinematics, it connects the robot elbow with the Cartesian point, where the elbow was placed by the previous control cycle (Fig. 13). For this kinematic structure, the kinematic equations can be solved analytically - like for conventional robots with 6 joints, and the desired hand position can be achieved with high accuracy.

The optimised KCC algorithm described in [Ivlev et al., 2000] allows to calculate exactly the elbow position E_{min} on the redundancy circle with the minimal distance to the previous elbow position E' - say, with minimal length of the imaginary link. The implemented routine contains only 21 multiplications, 11 additions as well as 1 square root and, hence, is very fast: the calculation requires only 40 µs on a PC with a 1 GHz Intel processor [Ivlev et al., 2004]. Within a typical robot control cycle of 16 ms, enough time remains to simulate the variation of the elbow position on the redundant circle and to generate other valid robot configurations. After this, the best robot pose considering the current spatial situation can be selected.

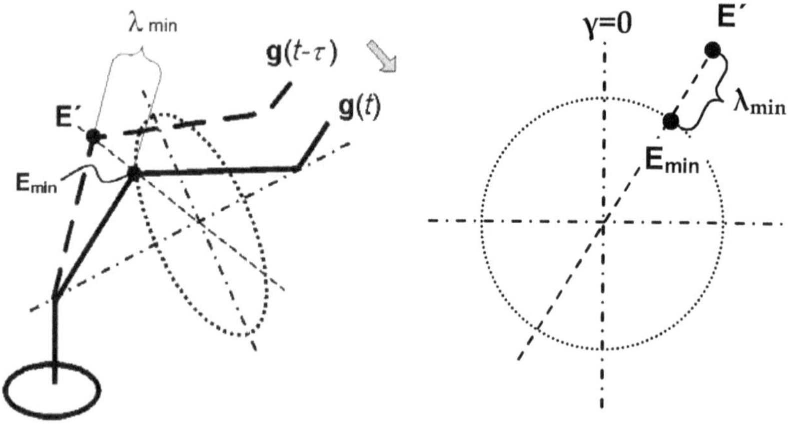

Fig. 13. Method of redundancy resolving in KCC.

In the grasping cases with s=5 and s=3, the new kinematic structures with two and four imaginary links, respectively, have to be assembled and the new inverse functions generated. In these functions, one or three parameters (lengths of imaginary links), respectively, must be chosen according to the current spatial situation. Alternatively, the inverse functions for the case s=6 (i.e. the fast optimised KCC algorithm) can be used. In this case, one (*Yaw*) or all three hand orientation angles *Yaw, Pitch,* and *Roll* (Fig. 12b and Fig. 12c) have to be varied in the hand location vector ${}_{(6)}g$ = [*X, Y, Z, Yaw, Pitch, Roll*] in addition to variations of the elbow position on the redundancy circle.

To simulate these variations and to choose a suitable hand orientation as well as an elbow position, the working environment, including the grasping object as well as the relevant obstacles, has to be mapped. To select a collision-free hand location and arm pose during the simulation process, the distances between obstacles and robot arm, including hand, have to be calculated permanently. In FRIEND, this problem has been solved by the so-called Mapped Virtual Reality (MVR) which models the spatial situation in an extremely simplified form and, at the same time, reflects the main spatial correlations [Feuser et al.,

2005]. The objects from the real world – obstacles, objects to be grasped as well as robot arm and hand - are mapped into this virtual reality as simple shapes covering the real objects. Only three simple 3D bodies are used in the MVR: cuboid, cylinder, and sphere. By combining these basic bodies, nearly any complex structure can be assembled. For object-oriented design, a base-class body is introduced, which provides the attributes all 3D bodies have. These are the position and the rotation. For the three simple 3D bodies, three classes are introduced, which all inherit from the base-class body: Cuboid, Cylinder, and Sphere. These classes add attributes which are needed for the description of the corresponding 3D body. For the cuboid, these are height, depth, and width, for the cylinder, height and radius, and for the sphere, only the radius.

For modelling robot links, a class CLink is used, which holds information about the transformation with respect to the previous link. This transformation is described by conventional DH parameters. To model the body structure of a link, a list is used, which holds objects of the three simple 3D bodies introduced before. Generally, a virtual robot consists of a certain number of links, where the number of links specifies the robot DoF. Therefore, the virtual robot is modelled by a list of CLink objects, where the order in the list describes the order of the links and their transformations, i.e. the kinematics of the virtual robot. The list and all needed methods are combined in the class CRobotModel.

The virtual obstacles are also modelled by the three simple 3D bodies and their class representatives and are stored in a list. The needed functionality is combined in the class CRobotWorld which inherits from CRobotModel. The result is a class which offers methods and attributes for modelling a robot and its environment.

The information in the class CRobotWorld can be used to calculate distances between the virtual robot and virtual obstacles. For this task, the GJK algorithm [Gilbert et al., 1988] is used. It provides information about the minimal distance between two convex polyhedrons and the minimal distance vector. The GJK algorithm only works with points (vertices) that describe the polyhedrons. For this purpose, a class Distance is introduced, which encapsulates the GJK algorithm and provides for a conversion of the classes describing the simple 3D bodies in a set of points. A cuboid can be described simply by eight vertices points, a cylinder has to be approximated by a set of points. To describe a sphere, it is not needed to approximate its surface by a polyhedron: its centre point and radius are sufficient. After computation by the GJK algorithm, the distance up to the sphere surface can be calculated by subtraction of the radius.

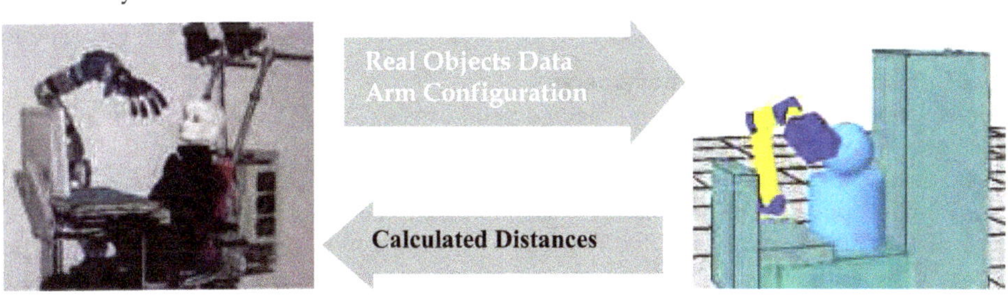

Fig. 14. Concept of Mapped Virtual reality (MVR).

The minimal distance to an obstacle can be obtained by calculating the distance between the obstacle and all body elements of each link of the robot and then choosing the smallest distance.

The classes CRobotModel and CRobotWorld both to render the virtual scene via OpenGL, but the main task of the MVR is to approximate a robot and its environment exactly enough to calculate the distances to obstacles. Therefore, very detailed graphical representation is not desired and not necessary.

In contrast to common VR, the task of which is to reflect the real world as exactly as possible and usually without influencing a situation in the real world, MVR interacts with the real world (Fig. 14). The robot configuration is transferred from the real robot and permanently updated. So, the virtual world reflects the real macro-situation and the distance can be calculated now without any difficulty instead of being measured. The task of external sensors (e.g. cameras) can be reduced to the detection of new objects which have to be mapped into the MVR instead of observing all obstacles in the workspace and measuring distances. Such task distribution increases the safety of manipulation by reduction of technical complexity.

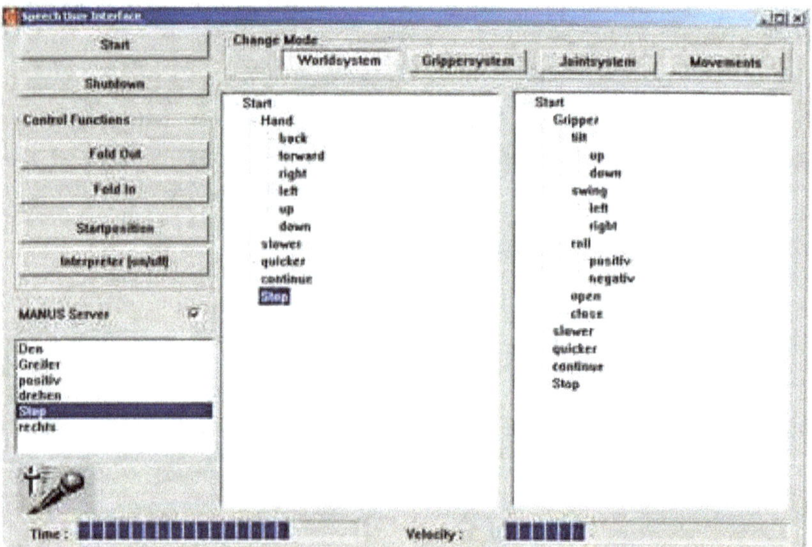

Fig. 15. Man-machine-interface with a speech command tree for the control of hand movements.

3.2.3. User–controlled hand movements

Many specific interfaces adapted to specific handicaps exist to control devices, e.g. devices which are controlled by the chin, tongue, eye position, etc. Speech recognition also is among these devices. An important requirement for the selection of the user interface is the general control philosophy "shared autonomy" which will be used in FRIEND-II [Volosyak et al., 2005]. Shared autonomy means that the robot acts autonomously at any possible time. But to restrict the complexity of the automation system and to enhance the overall robustness, a fall-back level is introduced. If the system detects a situation which cannot be resolved within the system's autonomy, it asks the user actively for support. This means that the system then relies on the mental capabilities of the user. The user can also actively take control of the robot and suspend the automation system. Speech recognition fulfils the requirement of a user interface for shared control. This is the reason why FRIEND-II is

equipped with a speech control interface shown in Fig. 15, which was also used in FRIEND-I [Martens et al., 2001].
The speech processing system translates naturally spoken words into commands. It consists of the two modules of speech recogniser and command interpreter. The speech recogniser consists of the speech recognition software ViaVoice Gold™ by IBM® , which translates naturally spoken commands entered via a microphone into specific words using pre-determined grammar. The recognised words are transmitted to the command interpreter which translates the words or text sequences received into system commands.
For safety reasons, the set of commands is organised in a hierarchical command tree. To suppress the misinterpretation of commands, such as interpreted noise or misspelled words, a path in the tree must be completed to cause a system action. This minimises the possibility of erroneous interpretations. If the system is in the user command mode and the command interpreter does not receive a permissible command within a fixed period of time, the system automatically returns to a safe state. The entire tree and the current state of the command are represented graphically on the flat screen, because the user can easily recognise the state of the system, if it is presented in the form of pictograms (Fig. 15).
Speech input allows for the control of the robot on different levels of complexity. Low-level commands which control directly a single robot joint or the robot tool (like "gripper up") are as possible as high-level commands like "pour in a drink". If the system is not able to recognise objects in the environment or if inconsistent data are retrieved from object recognition, the system may ask the user for support. In this case, the user may control e.g. the pan-tilt heads of the cameras.

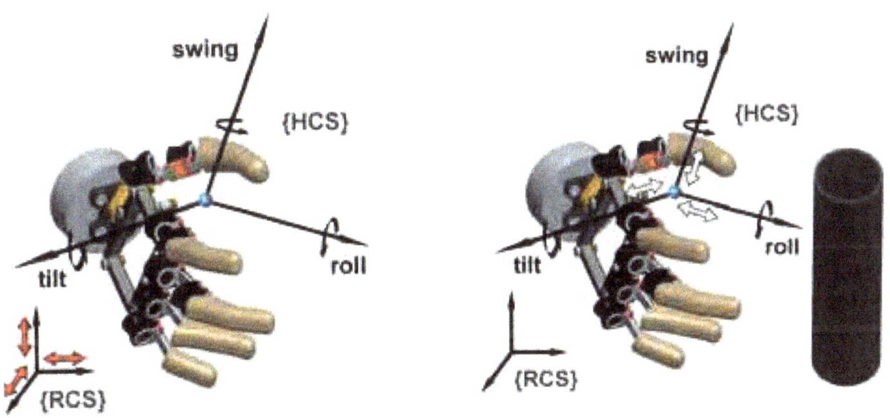

Fig. 16. Different reference coordinate systems during user-controlled hand movements: "mixed" motion directions (left), hand-fixed approaching movements (right).

By means of simple speech commands, the robot may be operated as usual by tele-operation of robot arms with respect to different coordinate systems: a reference coordinate system fixed to the robot arm base (RCS) as well as a coordinate system fixed at the hand (HCS). As shown in [Ivlev et al., 2004], the accuracy and stability of the end effector movements in the tele-operation mode increase due to the use of KCC compared to the so-called resolved-rate control which is used by default for the dexterous manipulator. The individual control of all joints is an alternative control variant and very useful, if complete arm reconfiguration through the manipulation is required. Such a situation may occur for example during manipulation in a cluster environment, while avoiding obstacles. The pre-condition is that the hand orientation can be changed freely. This means, for example, no filled glass has been grasped before.

In the manual control of some rehabilitation robots, for example "Manus"-ARM (www.exactdynamics.nl), translational Cartesian movement defaults occur relative to the RCS, the rotary ones occur for the HCS. These "mixed" motion directions are shown in Fig. 16, left. If the approaching movement of the hand to an object is commanded, however, the HCS system is significantly more comfortable for the user than the RCS coordinate system, as was found out in the first experiments with FRIEND. Figure 16 (right) shows the directions of the approaching motion to the object.

With the help of the speech control interface, the complete control sequences can be carried out. For example, if the user wants to pick up an object placed on the tray, a possible command sequence might be *Hand right – Hand left - Hand down – Stop - Hand open - Hand forward – Stop - Hand close*. With the last command, the power hook grip can be activated to grasp, for example, cylindrical objects, such as a bottle or a glass (Fig. 12b). To activate other kinds of grips of the dexterous fluidic hand, for example a "precision grip" or a "spherical grip", special commands can be programmed. Due to the general compliancy of the fluidic hand, however, the majority of relevant objects, such as a book or a ball (Fig. 12a and Fig. 12c), handled by FRIEND can be grasped safely with the power hook grip.

The elbow position on the redundancy circle can be commanded in the same way. Possible commands for this action may be "Elbow left"–"Elbow right" or "Elbow up"–"Elbow down" depending on the current position of the elbow. The first command set corresponds to the situation when the elbow is located close to the upper point of the redundancy circle (i.e. the position with redundancy angle $\gamma \approx 0°$, s. Fig. 17), where the "down" direction is not unique. In all other elbow placements, the second two commands are more convenient from the user's point of view and can be used for controlling the elbow without loss of safety. Since the user observes the actions of the robot arm continuously, he or she can interrupt its actions in erroneous situations at any moment. As the user is supported by MVR which observes the current spatial situation and anyway stops the arm movement when a collision with the user or the environment may occur, safety of the manipulation processes increases significantly and can be classified as dependable.

The extended manipulatory facility of the dexterous robotic system FRIEND-II in comparison with conventional 6-joint kinematics is illustrated in Fig. 17. In the spatial situation shown, it is possible to grasp the glass without colliding with the bottle only by a skillful use of all 7 joints.

3.2.4. Outlook

FRIEND II is intended to increase the usability of service robots designed for paralysed people with quadriplegia or similar disabilities (paralysis down from the neck due to spinal cord injuries above vertebra C6 and movement of arms, hands, and fingers is impossible). FRIEND II helps to be independent of nursing staff for several uninterrupted hours in professional and private life. To achieve this goal, a range of new technical solutions is introduced. Keywords for the new technology are: manipulative as well as sensory redundancy, shared autonomy, smart devices, and ambient intelligence [Volosyak et al., 2005]. Figure 18 presents the concept of an "intelligent kitchen". A large number of different action sequences like "pour in and serve a drink", "take, prepare, and serve a frozen meal", "support eating", "open a drawer", "fetch and handle a book", "fetch and handle some tool" are necessary to fulfill the user's demands, to overcome the complaints about the existing systems, and to give the user a minimum of independence of the nursing staff for several uninterrupted hours. As additional requirements, FRIEND II will have a human-like robustness and flexibility for the autonomous control of unforeseen variations in the environment. Use of the dexterous 7-joint arm with human-like kinematic configuration control and a compliant fluidic 5-finger hand will help at least to solve the problems of manipulative robustness, flexibility in handling objects, and safety.

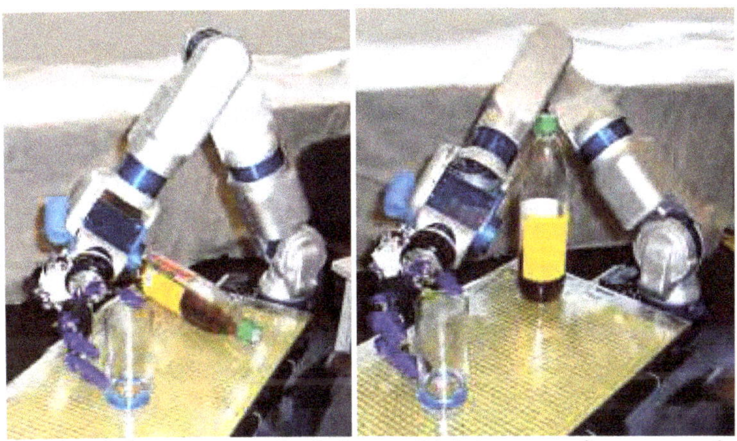

Fig. 17. Example of dexterous manipulation: a 6-joint arm can't grasp a glass without collision with a bottle (left); by controllable movement of elbow it will be possible (right).

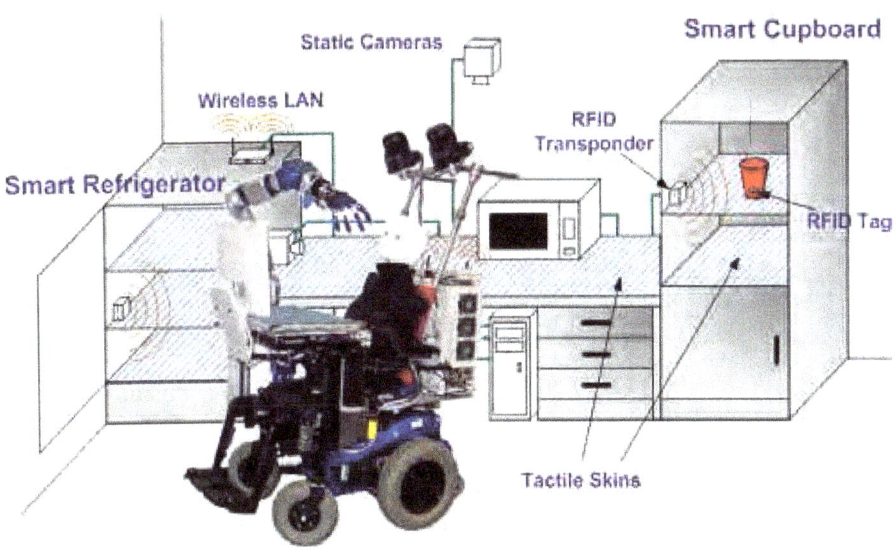

Fig. 18. FRIEND II in intelligent home environment.

3.3 Upper limb prosthesis

The loss of an upper limb implies a significant restriction of function and the individual has to cope with the stigma of being perceived as incomplete. Currently, upper limb-deficient individuals can either be fitted with a hook-type terminal device that provides good functionality and grasping force feedback, but poor cosmetics that are not accepted by most potential users in Europe. Therefore, most persons are fitted with a purely cosmetic hand or with an electrically driven hand that provides at least some cosmetic, but limited functionality. Since externally driven prostheses have been introduced to the market in the early 1970s an increasing number of patients have been fitted with these hands. However; approximately one third of all limb-deficient persons do not use their prosthesis at all [Atkins 1996]. In the last two decades, some of the achievements in the development of new materials and technologies were integrated in the design of artificial robot hands, resulting in higher dexterity. Artificial hands that are used in prosthetics have only very little in common with robot hands, which will be demonstrated in this chapter.

The following constraints should be considered when designing a prosthetic hand. They are based on the experience of different projects dealing with prosthetic hand design [Keller 1947, Peizer 1969, Weir 2003, Kyberd 2004, Pylatiuk 2007).

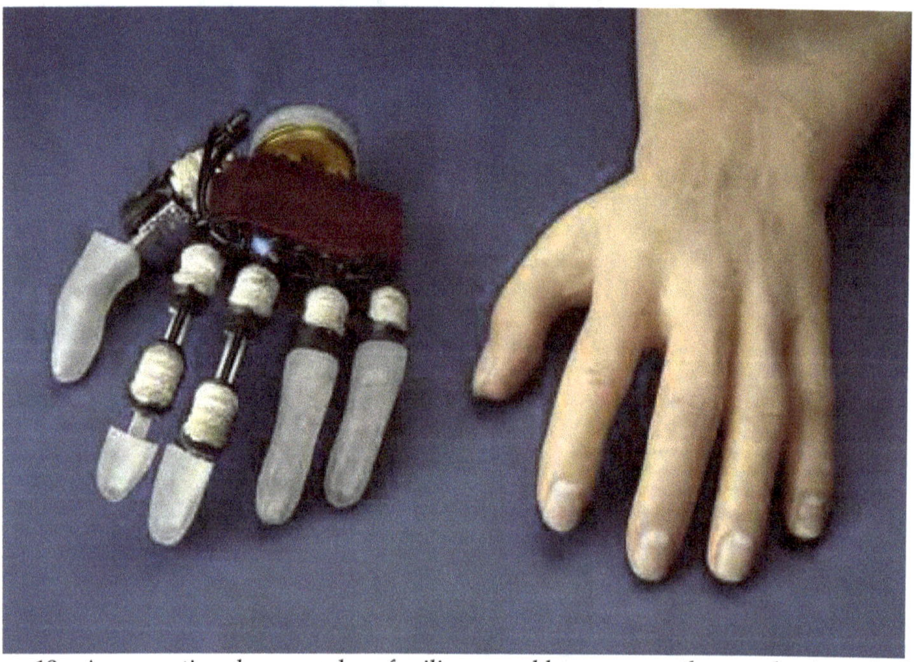

Fig. 19. A cosmetic glove made of silicone rubber covers the mechanics of the multifunctional prosthesis [Schulz 2005]. The thumb can be moved in a plane transverse to the index and middle finger.

- *Weight:* The mass of a prosthetic hand has to be below 500 grams. Otherwise, most users would not accept the technical aid. Every gram is perceived as an external load that must be carried, so the lighter a prosthetic hand is, the better accepted it will be. Although a lightweight design of robot grippers is also wanted in order to reduce the moments in the joints of the robot arm needed to move the terminal device, most commercial robot hands have a mass that considerably exceeds 500 g.

- *Compact design:* In prosthetic hands a very compact design is needed to allow for the fitting of a maximum number of upper limb-deficient persons. If not all requisite components were within the artificial hand, the large number of individuals with a transradial amputation could not be fitted. By contrast, many robot hands use the space at the forelimb to actuate the hand.
- *Appearance*: As most users of prosthetic hands, especially female users, do not want to attract attention to themselves, the design of a prosthetic hand should mimic a natural hand as closely as possible (Fig. 19). This includes different colours used to match the cosmetic glove to that of the user's skin. The design of robot hands usually is very technical. Additionally, the position of the thumb has a large impact on the appearance of the hand. In most commercial prostheses, the thumb's plane of motion is in direct opposition to the index and middle finger instead of a more natural transverse plane of motion.
- *Sound:* Any sound that originates from a prosthesis may annoy the user and should therefore be avoided. The noise level of commercial prosthetic hands is less than 45 dB at 1 m distance, which is almost imperceptible in surroundings with background noise, like an office.
- *Price*: The resources in most national health care systems are increasingly limited and in clinical practice, health insurance judges the therapeutic effects against the costs of a compensatory aid individually for every patient. In terms of economic efficiency, a prosthetic hand has to be a simple, but functional device, whereas robot hands typically are much more complex and, as a consequence, the expenses may be up to 20 times those of a prosthetic hand.
- *Power consumption*: The energy to process control signals and move the fingers of a prosthetic hand is typically supplied by rechargeable batteries of limited capacity. Therefore, efficient use of the battery energy is required and can be achieved by turning the controller to a stand-by mode when not used as well as by using actuators that do not require energy as soon as an object is grasped.
- *Sensors*: Robot hands need information from sensors about the flexion angle of each joint of the hand and about the occurring grasping forces, whereas commercial prosthetic hands do not have sensors, as the hand position is controlled visually by the user.
- *Grasping patterns:* The human hand is capable of grasping an object reliably with a vast number of different prehension patterns due to its versatility and ability to conform to the shape of an object. Commercial prosthetic hands only have one degree of freedom and, hence, can grasp only with a cylindrical power grasp or with the tip of the thumb, index, and middle finger. Multifunctional hands as described in detail in [Schulz 2005] offer additional prehension patterns (Fig. 20).
- *Grasping force:* A minimum pinch force of 67 N was proposed to enable the users to perform all activities with their artificial hands. If the fingers of a prosthetic hand have more than 1 DOF and, thus, can conform to the shape of an object, the requisite grasping force is significantly lower [Kargov 2004].

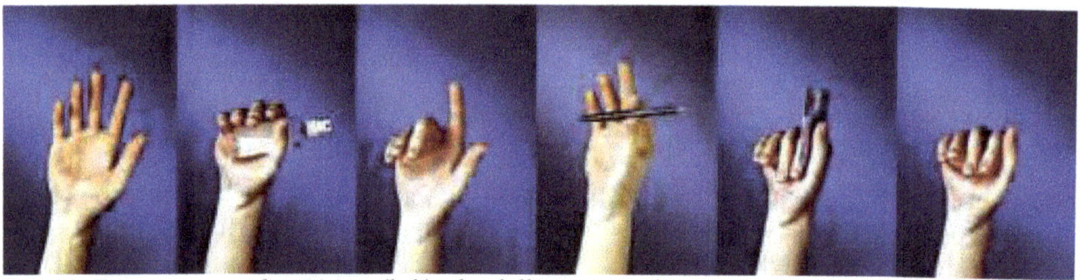

Fig. 20. From a neutral position (left), the following prehension patterns can be performed: cylindrical power grasp, index position, tip grasp, lateral grasp, and hook grasp.

- *Grasping speed:* Since their introduction in the 1970s, commercial prostheses have closed the fingers within one second, which can be taken as a benchmark. Just recently, prosthetic hands were introduced, which allow for much more speedy grasping.
- *Sensory feedback:* The lack of sensory information in electrically driven prosthetic hands is one of the main reasons for prosthesis rejection. The user has to estimate the force exerted by the prosthesis while grasping and the posture of the fingers has to be controlled visually.
- *Control:* Prosthetic upper limbs are typically controlled by switches, pressure sensors or myoelectric surface electrodes that are operated by the residual limb in the socket. The control of several independent DOFs has been a challenge, but with the introduction of microprocessors and new methods of biosignal analysis, future control systems will be easier for the patient to be learned and operation of the prosthetic aid will be more intuitive [Reischl 2004, Englehart 2003].
- *Reliability: Both* prosthetic and robotic hand users usually favour a reliable, but simple technical aid to a more sophisticated, independent device that malfunctions regularly. Especially users with a bilateral upper limb loss depend on their prosthetic hands.

Just recently, new prosthetic hands with increased functionality were presented [Schulz 2005, www.touchbionics.com]. For example the multifunctional prosthesis from the Forschungszentrum Karlsruhe, Germany allows for different prehension patterns and also includes sensory feedback [Schulz 2005, Pylatiuk 2006]. It is based on the same actuators described in 2.1 (Fig. 2), but it is driven by a micro hydraulic system (Fig. 4, 21), that is housed within the metacarpus of the hand.

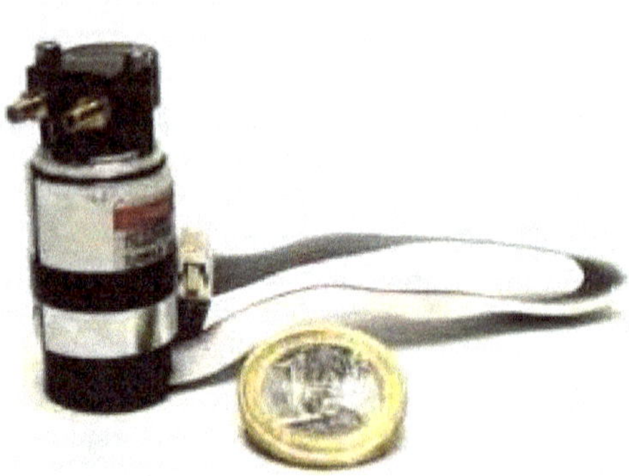

Fig. 21. A custom-made hydraulic pump.

4. References

Bien Z. Zenn; Stefanov Dimitar (Eds.) (2004). *Advances in Rehabilitation Robotics. Human friendly Technologies on Movement Assistance and Restoration for People with Disabilities.* Springer-Verlag Berlin, Heidelberg, New York, Hong Kong, London, Milan, Paris, Tokyo, 2004.

Venkataraman Subramanian T.; Iberall Thea (Eds.) (1990). *Dextrous Robot Hands.* Springer-Verlag New York, Berlin, Heidelberg, London, Paris, Tokyo, Hong Kong, 1990.

Muzumdar Ashok (Ed.) (2004). *Powered Upper Limb Prostheses. Control, Implementation and Clinical Application.* Springer-Verlag Berlin, Heidelberg, New York, 2004.

Shin'ichi Yuta; Hajime Asama; Sebastian Thrun; Erwin Prassler; Takashi Tsubouchi (Eds.) (2006) *Field and Service Robotics. Recent Advances in Research and Applications.* Springer-Verlag Berlin, Heidelberg, New York, 2006.

DeLaurentis KJ, Mavroidis C (2000). Development of a shape memory alloy actuated hand. In: Actuator `2000, S. 281-284, Bremen, Germany, 2000.

Pons JL, Rodriguez H, Ceres R, Van Moorleghem W, Reynaerts D (1998). Study of SMA Actuation to develop a Modular, User-adaptable Hand Prosthesis. 6th Int. Conference on New Actuators, 490-493, Bremen, Germany, 1998.

Pons JL, Rodriguez H, Duarte A, Luyckx, Reynaerts D, Ceres R, Van Brussel H (2000) High torque ultra-sonic motors for hand prosthetics: current status and trends. 7th Int. Conference on New Actuators, 285-288, Bremen, Germany, 2000.

Lee YK, Shimoyama I (2000). A micro rubber artificial muscle driven by a micro compressor for artificial limbs, Actuator 2000, 7th Int. Conf. on New Actuators, Bremen, Germany S. 272-275, 2000.

C.M. Light, P.H. Chappell, (2000). Development of a Lightweight and Adaptable Multiple-axis Hand Prosthesis, Med. Eng. & Phys., 10, 679-84, 2000.

Weir R.F. *ff*, Grahn E.C., Duff S.J., (2001). A New Externally-Powered, Myoelectrically Controlled Prosthesis for Persons with Partial Hand Amputations at the Metacarpals, J. Prosth. & Orth., 12(2), 26-31, 2001.

Kyberd P.J., Pons J.L. (2003). A Comparison of the Oxford and Manus Intelligent Hand Prosthesis. Proceedings of the IEEE (ICRA), Taipei, Taiwan, September 14 - 19, 2003.

Walker Rich (Shadow Robot Company) (2003). Design of a dextrous hand for advanced CLAWAR applications, In: Proceedings of the 6th International Conference on Climbing and Walking Robots (CLAWAR2003), Catania, Italy, 17.-19. Sept. 2003.

Boblan, I. Bannasch R., Schwenk H., Prietzel F., Miertsch L., Schulz A. (2004). A human-like robot hand and arm with fluidic muscles: Biologically inspired construction and functionality Embodied Artificial Intelligence Lecture Notes In Artificial Intelligence 3139: pp. 160-179, 2004.

Lee Y.K., Shimoyama I. (1999). A Skeletal Framework Artificial Hand Actuated by Pneumatic Artificial Muscles, Proceedings of the 1999 IEEE Int. Conf. On Robotics & Automation, Detroit, Michigan, May 1999.

Plettenburg DH (2002). A sizzling hand prosthesis. On the design and development of a pneumatically powered hand prosthesis for children. PhD-thesis, Delft University of Technology, The Netherlands, ISBN 90-370-0196-3, 2002.

Hirzinger G., Sporer N., Schedl M., Butterfaß J., Grebenstein M. (2004). Torque-controlled lightweight arms and articulated hands: do we reach technological limits, The International Journal of Robotics Research, vol. 23, No. 4-5, April-May 2004, pp. 331-340.

Jacobsen S., Iversen E., Knutti D., Johnson R., and Bigger K. (1986). Design of the Utah/MIT Dextrous Hand. In Proceedings of the 1986 IEEE International Conference on Robotics and Automation, pp. 96-102, 1986.

Townsend WT (2000). The BarrettHand grasper - programmably flexible part handling and assembly-Industrial Robot - An International Journal, 27(3), pp. 181-8, 2000.

Kargov A., Pylatiuk C., Schulz S (2006). Study of fluidic actuators in prosthetic hands. Proceedings of the 10th international conference on new actuators "Actuator 2006", Bremen, Germany, 14-16 June 2006. pp. 312-315.

Hollerbach J., Hunter I., Ballantyne J. (1992). A comparative analysis of actuator technologies for robotics, In: O. Khatib, J. Craig, Losano-Perez (Eds.), The robotics review 2, MIT Press, Cambridge, MA, USA, pp. 299-342, 1992.

Schulz S., Pylatiuk C., Bretthauer G. (1999). A New Class of Flexible Fluidic Actuators and their Applications in Medical Engineering. At 47 (8), Seite 390-395, 1999.

Martens C., Ruchel N., Lang O., Ivlev O., Graeser A. (2001). A FRIEND for Assisting Handicapped People, IEEE Robotics & Automation Magazine, Vol. 7, No.1, March 2001, pp. 57-65.

Ivlev O. Martens C., Graeser A. (2005). Rehabilitation Robots FRIEND-I and FRIEND-II with the dexterous lightweight manipulator. Technology and Disability (Special Issue), Vol. 17, 2, 2005, pp. 111-123.

Seraji H. (1989). Configuration Control of Manipulators: Theory and Implementation, IEEE Trans. on Robotics and Automation, Vol. 5, No.4, 1989, S. 472-490.

Ivlev O., Graeser A. (2000). The Optimized Kinematic Configuration Control Algorithm for Redundant Robots. Proc. 16th IMACS World Congress on Scientific Computation, Applied Mathematics and Simulation, Lausanne, Switzerland, August 21-25, 2000.

Dahm P., Joublin F. (1997). Closed form solution for the inverse kinematics of a redundant robot arm. Technical Report 8, Institut für Neuroinformatik, Ruhr-Universität Bochum, 1997.

Asfour T., Berns K., Albiez J., Dillmann R. (1999). Programming of Manipulation Tasks of the Humanoid Robot ARMAR. The 9th International Conference on Advanced Robotics (ICAR'99), Tokyo, Japan, October 25-27, 1999, pp. 107-112.

Ivlev O, Graeser A. (1997). An Analytical Method for the Inverse Kinematics of Redundant Robots. Proc. 3d ECPD International Conference on Advanced Robots, Intelligent Automation and Active Systems, Bremen, 1997, pp. 416-421.

Ivlev O., Graeser A. (1999). Explicit Symbolic Solution of the Inverse Kinematics for Redundant Robotic Systems, at-Automatisierungstechnik, 47, 11, 1999, pp. 523-531 (*in German*).

Ivlev O., Rixen K., Graeser A. (2004). Kinematic Configuration Control of Redundant Robots with 7 Joints, Robotik 2004, VDI-Report Nr. 1841, pp. 543-550 (*in German*).

Feuser J., Ivlev O., Graeser A. (2005). Mapped Virtual Reality for a Safe Manipulation in Rehabilitation Robotics", Assistive Technology: From Virtuality to Reality (AAATE 2005); IOS Press, Amsterdam, 2005, pp. 666-671.

Martens C., Ivlev O., Graeser A. (2001). Interactive Controlled Robotic System FRIEND to Assist Disabled People. 7th International Conference On Rehabilitation Robotics (ICORR 2001); Evry Cedex, France, April 25-27, 2001, pp. 148-54.

Volosyak I., Ivlev O., Graeser A. (2005). Rehabilitation Robot FRIEND II - The General Concept and Current Implementation", Proc. of the IEEE 9th Int. Conf. On Rehabilitation Robotics (ICORR 2005); Chicago, Illinois, pp. 540-544.

Gilbert E. G., Johnson D. W., Keerthi S. S. (1988). A Fast Procedure for Computing the Distance between Complex Objects in Three Dimensional Space. IEEE Journal of Robotics and Automation, Vol. 4, No. 2, April 1988, pp. 192-203.

Atkins DJ, Heard DCY, Donovan WH (1996). Epidemiologic overview of individuals with upper-limb loss and their reported research priorities. J Prosthet Orthot 8(1):2–11, 1996.

Englehart K, Hudgins B (2003). A robust, real-time control scheme for multifunction myoelectric control., IEEE Transactions on Biomedical Engineering, 50(7):848- 854, 2003.

Kargov A, Pylatiuk C, Martin J, et al. (2004). A comparison of the grip force distribution in natural hands and in prosthetic hands. Disabil Rehabil 26(12):705–711, 2004.

Keller A, Tyalor C, Zahm V (1947). Studies to Determine the Functional Requirements for Hand and Arm Prosthesis. Dept. of Engineering, UCLA, July 1947.

Kyberd PJ (2004). Research and the future in myoelectric prosthetics. In: Ashok Muzumdar (ed) Powered upper limb prostheses: control, implementation and clinical application. Springer, Berlin Heidelberg New York, pp 175–190, ISBN 3540404066, 2004.

Asfour, T., Regenstein, K., Azad, P., Schröder, J., Bierbaum, A., Vahrenkamp, N. and Dillmann, R. ARMAR-III (2006). An Integrated Humanoid Platform for Sensory-Motor Control. In IEEE-RAS International Conference on Humanoid Robots (Humanoids 2006), Genoa, Italy, December 2006.

Azad, P., Asfour, T. and Dillmann, R. (2006). Combining Appearance-based and Model-based Methods for Real-Time Object Recognition and 6D Localization. In Proc. International Conference on Intelligent Robots and Systems (IROS 06), Beijing, China, October 2006.

Asfour, T.; Ly, D.N.; Regenstein, K.; Dillmann, R. (2005). Coordinated Task Execution for Humanoid Robots. In Experimental Robotics IX, STAR, Springer Tracts in Advanced Robotics, Vol. 21, pp. 259-267, 2005.

Morales, M., Asfour, T., Azad, P., Knoop, S. and Dillmann, R. (2006). Integrated Grasp Planning and Visual Object Localization for a Humanoid Robot with Five-Fingered Hands. In Proc. International Conference on Intelligent Robots and Systems (IROS 06), Beijing, China, October 2006.

Schulz, S. , Pylatiuk, Ch., Kargov, A., Oberle, R. and Bretthauer, G. (2004). Progress in the development of anthropomorphic fluidic hands for a humanoid robot, In IEEE/RAS International Conference on Humanoid Robots, Los Angeles, Nov 2004.

6

Task-oriented and Purposeful Robot-Assisted Therapy

Michelle J Johnson, PhD[1,2,3], Kimberly J Wisneski, MS[3], John Anderson[1,3], Dominic Nathan[2,3], Elaine Strachota[4], OTR, PhD, Judith Kosasih, MD[1,3], Jayne Johnston, OTR, RN[3], Roger O. Smith, OTR, PhD[5]
Medical College of Wisconsin[1], Marquette University[2], Clement Zablocki VA[3], Concordia University[4], University of Wisconsin, Milwaukee[5]
Milwaukee, Wisconsin, USA

1. Introduction

Robot-assisted therapy devices are available for rehabilitation of persons after stroke, which is the leading cause of disability among adults in the United States (AHA 2006, Volpe et al. 2002). Improving upper extremity function after stroke is critical for performance of one's life-role and the completion of unilateral and bilateral activities of daily living (ADLs). Carryover to real-life activities after rehabilitation training cannot be assumed (Sterr et al. 2000; Maclean et al. 2000; Ma and Trombly 2002; Trombly and Ma 2002; Prange et al. 2006). For example, the existence of learned non-use behavior indicates that motor gains after rehabilitation therapies may not transfer to long-term functioning on ADLs (Taub et al. 1994; Taub et al. 1999; Sterr et al. 2000). This behavior is present when persons with hemiparesis due to strokes demonstrate significant differences between residual movement capabilities and spontaneous use of the impaired arm in real world. There is a need to address barriers to the carryover of motor gains during training to stroke function in real life.

This chapter reviews examples of current upper arm robot-assisted therapy environments and present findings from case study experiments with a new task-oriented, robot therapy system focused on improving carryover of motor improvements to functional activities of daily living. We draw attention to influence of function on arm movements during robot training and explore how future environments can be more functional and engaging.

Robot-assisted therapy devices are now being used more frequently in the rehabilitation of persons with physical disabilities due to neurological trauma caused by stroke and spinal cord injury. These therapy robots provide semi- or fully-autonomous training and permit patients using them to engage in repeated and intense practice of goal-directed tasks (Volpe et al 2002; Prange et al 2006; Burgar et al. 2000; Loureiro et al. 2003; Patton et al. 2006; Krebs et al. 2003; MacClellan et al. 2005, Kahn et al. 2006). Typically, the automation of therapeutic exercises involves generating trajectories that guide reaching movements and the application of forces directly or indirectly to the impaired arm to assist, resist, and/or passively support it during the reaching exercise. For example, the MIT-MANUS (Krebs et al. 2003; MacClellan et al. 2005) therapy robot permits stroke survivors to practice two-dimensional (2-D) point-to-point (PTP) movements while systems like the Gentle/s (Loureiro et al. 2003) and MIME (Burgar et al. 2000) robots are capable of three dimensional (3-D) PTP training. Studies have shown that these early robotic therapy systems improve motor function as quantified by motor performance measures such as movement time and smoothness during reaching (Rohrer et al. 2002) and standard clinical measures of motor impairment such as the Upper Extremity Fugl-Meyer (UE-FM (Fugl-Meyer et al. 1975). Despite this, they have mixed impact on learned non-use and the ability to use the impaired arm in real tasks (Prange et al 2006). Given the promise of robot-assisted therapies, it is important to further investigate the mapping between practice and real-world ADL function and determine what mechanisms influence it.

Recent evidence from neuroscience literature suggests that enriched environments (Will et al 2004; Fisher and Sullivan 2001; Nudo et al. 2003), highly functional and task-oriented practice environment (Carr et al. 1985;Ada et al. 1995; Trombly et al. 1995; Aycock et al. 2004, Bayona et al. 2005; Wu et al. 2000; Woldag et al. 2003; Theilman et al. 2004), and highly motivating fun and game-based environments that increase task engagement (Bach-y-rita et al 2002, Wood et al. 2003) are important for motor re-learning, recovery after stroke and reduced learned non-use behavior. Task-oriented therapies facilitate the practice of a variety of simple and complex functional movements within a real context, with environment feedback to cue task success or failure. Occupational therapists Wu and colleagues have shown that the presence of real objects as the target of reach significantly influences the reaching kinematics of both neurologically normal and stroke impaired persons (Wu et al. 2000, 1998). In fact, reaching towards a real object is more likely to result in smoother movements, lower movement times, and higher peak velocities. These results were also verified by Wisneski and Johnson (Wisneski and Johnson 2006, 2007) for complex ADLs such as drinking and eating. Successful examples of novel task-oriented therapy are forced-use and Constrained-Induced Movement Therapy (CIMT) (Taub et al. 1994; Taub et al. 1999; Sterr et al. 2000; Liepert et al. 2002; Page et al. 2004; Aycock et al. 2004). The training is intense and repetitive, requiring the use of the impaired arm. Data indicate that CIMT therapies reduce learned non-use, increase ADL function, and often increase the size and change the location of the cortical area representative of a muscle function (Liepert et al. 2002). These forced-use therapies often induce changes in the motor areas especially in the motor cortex and the cerebellum.

A natural question is whether combining robot-assisted therapies with a task-oriented approach involving the practice of real ADLs would improve real world functional outcomes and whether current trajectory planning processes support functional retraining on complex ADLs such as drinking and eating. The trend in the field has been towards the development task-oriented, biofeedback mechanical systems with virtual environments that permit the practice of real ADL tasks and some form of biofeedback (Huang et al. 2006). Examples of such environments include Jiping He and colleagues's RUPERT upper arm exoskeleton (He et al. 2005) and Riener and colleagues's ARMIn upper arm exoskeleton (Nef et al. 2006) that embed robot assisted training into patient-centered, engaging, and focused on daily living activities with virtual functional objects.

Currently few clinical trials exist that test whether robot-assisted therapies can be more effective when combined with a highly task-oriented therapy paradigm that focuses on the practice of ADLs in virtual or real environments. One study did examine the effect of adding grasping to the planar manipulation environment of the MIT-MANUS (Fasoli et al 2005). No additive effect for the reach-to-grasp practice was found but this was most likely due to differences in the intensity of training administered to the two groups and the use of motor impairment measures (the UE-FM was used to judge motor gains) to evaluate between group differences. It is still not clear what gains were made in ADL functioning on real-world tasks or how robot-assisted practice may have influenced the CNS cortical changes.

The rehabilitation robotics lab at the Medical College of Wisconsin and Marquette University has developed the Activities of Daily Living Exercise Robot (ADLER) stroke training environment, which was inspired by the Gentle/s system set-up to accommodate reaching and grasping activities in the three-dimensions (Johnson et al. 2006). Here robot-assisted training is focused on improving carryover of motor gains to real life through ADL task practice and the trajectory models used to implement movement plans in 2-D and 3-D space. The chapter presents the design and several case studies to evaluate some of the main design concepts of the robot system. The ADLER was developed to train functional ADL-like tasks with and without physical objects. It capitalizes on the existing benefits of robot-assisted therapies while supporting more natural movements to position the wrist during ADL practice. Three case studies with a few able-bodied and stroke adults were conducted to evaluate the performance of the ADLER system. Case study 1 examined issues in repeatability and stability of kinematic measures such as movement time and smoothness. Case study 2 examined issues in modeling and trajectory planning of wrist movements for a real ADL task, the drink task. Case study 3 examined ADLER system's ability to reduce motor impairment and improve ADL function during the practice of point-to-point (PTP) movements that mimic real ADL tasks. Overall, these case studies show that the system has the potential to be effective in training of the upper arm after stroke with future work focused on the ability to improve both reaching and grasping abilities in the long-term.

2. Activities of Daily Living Exercise Robot (ADLER)

2.1 Hardware

ADLER is a robot therapy environment developed to permit training of real-life functional tasks involving reach, grasp, and object transportation in both 2-D and 3-D space (Fig. 1ab) (Johnson et al. 2006). The system is designed to support seated functional tasks such as grooming, drinking, eating, and desktop vocational tasks such as game playing tasks including tic-tac-toe. ADLER uses a HapticMaster robot (FCS Robotics) to assist an impaired arm along trajectories for real-life tasks and administer customized forces along programmed trajectories. The HapticMaster is an admittance-controlled, 6 degrees of freedom (DOFs) robot. Three active DOFs position the hand in space. The end-effector of the robot can pivot 1 full radian and has a vertical range of 0.40 m. The arm pivots about a post, with end-effector positions ranging between a radius of 0.28 m and 0.64 m. A three-axis force sensor located at the end-effector measures interaction forces (3 DOF) generated during the tasks. The three remaining DOFs orient the wrist passively through rotation of a three-axis gimbal. Fig. 1b illustrates the range of gimbal position in the ADLER environment with an approximation of the actual task space, which is often extended beyond the end-effector, depending on the orthosis used.

Several custom-designed orthoses have been designed for attaching an impaired limb to the gimbal at either the wrist or the forearm (close to the elbow) without impeding grasp. The configuration permits the subject to orient freely their hand as needed to grasp and use an object (Fig. 2ab). Orthoses have also been constructed to support lower-functioning stroke survivors that have no grasp capability, i.e. those that need to begin training in the reaching phase only (Fig. 2c).
A custom-made glove is designed to assist in functional grasping as needed (Nathan and Johnson 2007). The glove uses bend sensors (Flexpoint Sensor Systems) to detect finger joint angle changes between 0 and 90 degrees. Sensors measure the joint angles of the 2nd interphalangeal joint (PIP) of the index finger and the distal interphalangeal joint of the thumb during the tracking movements. At present only the index finger and thumb is incorporated since these are most often involved in ADLs to complete whole arm grasp, pinch and cyinder grips (Ada et al. 1995). The glove can be used with a functional electrical stimulation (FES) unit to assist in voluntary grasp and release or passive grasp and release. The current glove design is minimally evasive and does not interfere during task performance and to allow appropriate hand shaping before and during grasp with open-ended finger tips to allow haptic feedback and better grasping and shaping of the hand.
Patients using the ADLER system are asked to sit on a rail-mounted chair that can be easily pushed into position. The chair can be positioned on either side of the table. The table height is adjustable, and a custom-made harness is available to restrain motion of the trunk. To ensure subject safety during robot therapy, three safety systems are integrated into ADLER. First, power to the robot can be cut (halting any motion of the arm) and all systems shut down with the use of an emergency stop button held by an experimenter. The second safety system, controlled by the subject, is a foot pedal placed under the dominant foot that must be depressed during any operation of the robot. If at any time the subject lifts his or her foot off the pedal, the robot halts all motion. Finally, all orthoses attach to the gimbal magnetically with a pair of solenoids. Current through the two solenoids is automatically stopped if a force overload is detected and the orthoses detaches.

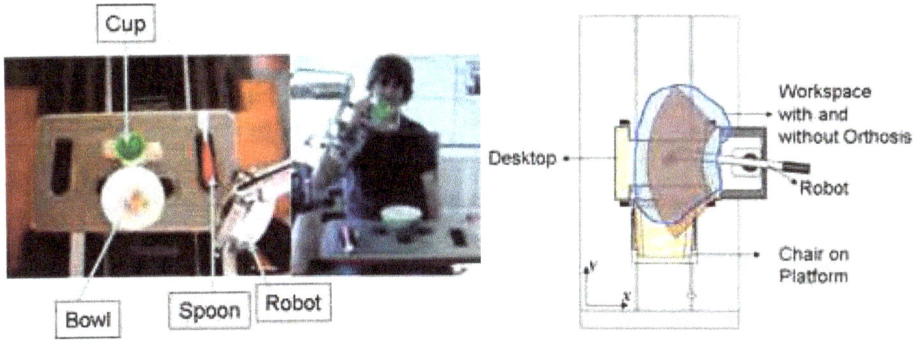

Fig. 1. The set-up for the ADLER stroke therapy system.

The system consists of an activity table and tray for selfcare-like tasks such as eating. The chair is on guide rails that permit it to be adjusted and mounted on either side of the table. The HapticMaster robot is the main system used and is customized wrist orthosis that permits the hands to be free for 3-D spatial functional movements such as drinking.

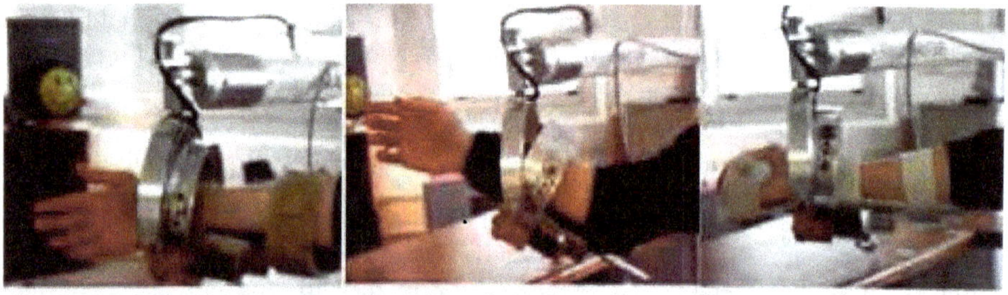

Hands Free: Wrist Orthosis   Hands Free: Elbow Orthosis   Hand-Not Free

Fig. 2a-c. The ADLER Orthoses.

Three orthoses for ADLER; depending on the protocol used and tasks, these orthoses are interchangeable with the system.

2.2 Software

The ADLER system uses a custom-designed software called HERALD to implement various upper arm functional movements. The HERALD software, flow-charted in Fig. 3a, uses HapticAPI (FCS Robotics Manual 2003) to control the HapticMaster robot and Crystal Space v0.98 (Tyberghein et al. 2004), a freeware for creating graphical user interfaces (GUIs), to render the simulated environment. Crystal Space is an open-source engine that is platform and application programming interface (API) independent. In the ADLER system, we use this engine within a PC-based Windows XP environment. The safety signals from the foot pedal and emergency stop are also monitored by HERALD. The glove signals are also monitored so that the glove collection rate can be synchronized with the robot system.

In HERALD, the experimenter can define all the parameters for a task and the training modes. The experimenter is able to program arm movements on-the-fly using start, end, and multiple via points or upload the data from a file storing real or pre-defined trajectories. HERALD can also be used to set boundaries within the robotic workspace, for example, to prevent the gimbal from scraping against the table.

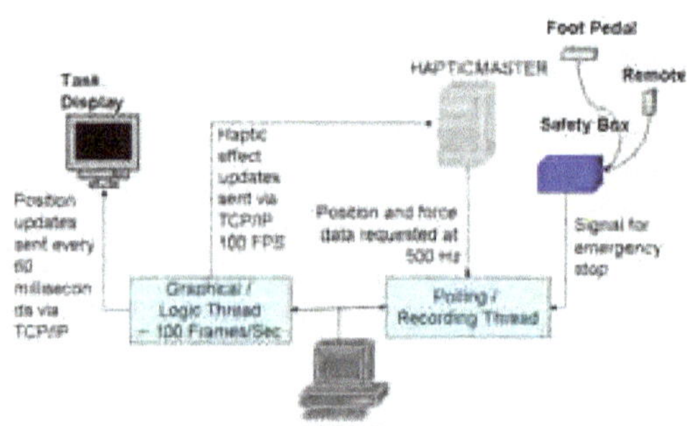

A.

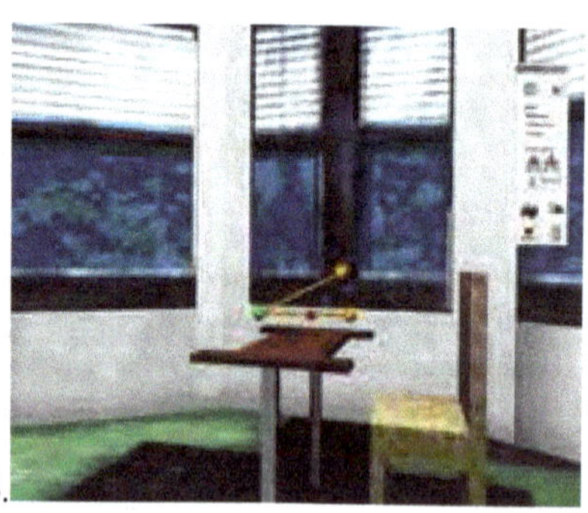

B.

Fig. 3. HERALD Control software.

a. Signal flow to and from HERALD. b. Graphical interface where spheres denote via-points with straight line trajectories. Colored dots indicate the gimbal position and the current target via-point.

HERALD's graphical interface displays a one-to-one mapping of the task environment, which consists of the platform, table, chair, and straight-line or curved connections to the key points in the trajectories (Fig. 3b). Typically, one of the experimenters operates the computer and monitors the therapy on-screen. Audio cues signal acquisition of key events that correspond to pre-programmed points in the real task, providing feedback to the user and experimenters. The system actively acquires the position and the orientation of the gimbal center as well as the forces on the end-effecter at up to 1250 Hz. Training session data are stored automatically.

2.3 Training Paradigms in ADLER

In order to accommodate a range of training protocols, ADLER is able to operate in three modes: normal, form, and function. Normal mode permits unconstrained subject motion anywhere within the robot workspace. In form mode the subject is constrained to move along a defined path between via-points. When a via-point is reached, the robot emits an audible cue and continues along a new path to the next point. The robot pulls the user with a spring force traveling at a minimum velocity set by the experimenters. In function mode the subject is constrained to a cylindrical space around the defined path between via-points, allowing more freedom than form mode. A spring force, again with a minimum velocity, pulls the user towards and along the axial path. When the user moves into a defined spherical volume around each via-point called a pull zone, a spring force pulls the user radially towards the via-point. Form and function modes are illustrated in Fig. 4. Assistance can be provided in form and function modes by increasing the spring constant, or removed entirely by setting the spring constant to zero. The robot can also resist user motion in any mode by setting a velocity-dependent damping coefficient.

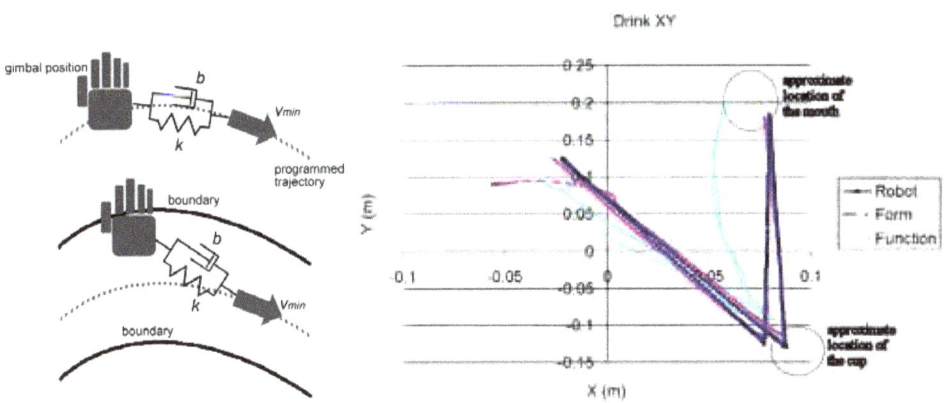

Fig. 4. Movement Modes.

Form (a) versus function (b) concept implemented in the ADLER training modes. The subject performed in function and form modes. The subject starts at location in upper left quadrant. The functional mode allowed for more natural trajectories.

Subjects using ADLER may be classified as high, medium, or low functioning. ADL training protocols have been developed for each. High functioning subjects train with tasks that involve grasping and manipulating objects. Medium and low-functioning subjects may begin by performing PTP tasks that mimic functional ADLs and then progress to performing reaching and grasping tasks with the FES Grasp glove integrated with ADLER. Table 1 displays some of the training tasks currently programmed in ADLER. Subjects are evaluated in the normal mode with the tasks from Table 1 or additional evaluation tasks as shown in Table 2.

2.3.1 Point-to-Point Reaching Robot Training

Two-dimensional reaching movements are guided by a flat-screen computer monitor on the activity table (Fig. 5a). Subjects move from one highlighted point to another, tracing predefined shapes and paths. While the entire monitor is contained within the robotic workspace, certain points can be excluded if the subject is not able to reach them. Three dimensional reaching movements are designed to be similar to those of functional activities. For instance, to mimic the actions of drinking from a cup, the subject may be asked to touch a point on the activity table, reach up to his/her mouth, touch the table again, and return his/her hand to rest. Subjects can practice these tasks repeatedly and at different levels of assistance or resistance.

2.3.2 Task-oriented Robot Training

Task-oriented robot training consists of functional, self-care tasks such as eating, drinking (Fig. 5 and Tables 1 and 2), combing hair, game-playing tasks such as tic-tac-toe (against the experiment or against the computer, and household manipulation tasks such as ringing a bell or opening doors and locks. Typically, game-playing tasks are only performed in normal mode, but robot impedance characteristics can be modified to react faster or slower in response to the forces on the end-effector. Task-oriented robot-assistance can be performed in any of the three modes.

	Task Name	High-ADL	Low-ADL
ADLs	Drink	Subject reaches, grasps and lifts a cup; drinks; returns cup.	Subject reaches, touches red dot; touches mouth; touches red dot.
	Comb	Subject reaches, grasps, and lifts a comb; lifts comb to side of head; combs up and down twice; returns comb.	Subject reaches, touches blue dot; touches side of head; touches blue dot.
PTP	Reaching	Subject reaches straight out, presses a buzzer	Subject reaches straight out to a colored dot
	Point-to-point	Subject traces a 2-D pattern with a pointer.	Subject follows a 2-D pattern without a pointer.
Other tasks	Doors	Subject performs a sequence of tasks that unlocks and opens nine different doors.	Subject reaches and touches nine sets of colored dots in specific sequences.
Fun	Tic-tac-toe	Subject plays tic-tac-toe in normal mode with custom-designed board and pieces	N/A
	Plinko	Subject plays drops a ping pong ball into plinko game in normal mode	N/A

Table 1. Examples of training tasks on ADLER.

ADLER supports several categories of task from selfcare tasks such as feeding and drinking, reaching tasks in 2D and 3D space and fun tasks.

Task Name	Description
Reach	Subject reaches outward to six points
Drink	Subject reaches, grasps and lifts a cup with one hand; drinks; returns cup.
Bilateral Drink	Subject reaches, grasps and lifts a cup with both hands; drinks; returns cup.
Point-to-Point	Subject traces circle and cross patterns
Jebsen-Taylor	Subject performs a Jebsen-Taylor evaluation task

Table 2. Evaluation tasks supported on ADLER.

ADLER supports several evaluation tasks that are performed without forces in the normal mode. From selfcare tasks such as feeding and drinking, reaching tasks in 2D and 3D space and fun tasks.

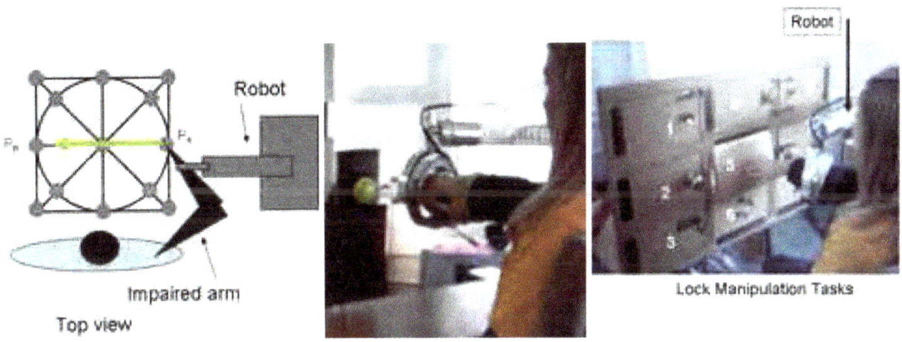

Fig. 5. ADLER Activities.

The ADL activity table set up in the ADLER environment; a. 2-D PTP reaching; b. patient practicing functional reaching; c. patient practicing manipulation.

2.4 Trajectory Planning for Functional and More Natural Wrist Movements

Typically, robot-mediated movements between via-points in reaching tasks are modeled on the minimum jerk theory of movement (Flash & Hogan, 1985; Flash & Hogan, 1987; Amirabdollahian et al. 2003; Loureiro et al. 2003). The minimum jerk algorithm defines straight-line movements and bell shaped velocity curves with zero starting and ending velocities. However, more complex models may be necessary to describe reaching during ADLs. The presence of a real object modifies the orientation of the wrist for the reach-to-grasp movement (Gentilucci et al. 1991, 1996, 2002; Gentilucci, 2005; Wu et al. 1998; Wu et al. 2000). Loureiro and colleagues, in their study of 3-D tracking in the Gentle/s robot-assisted therapy environment, proposed the use of 7th order polynomial curves with varying boundary conditions to better approximate reaching towards real objects (Loureiro et al. 2003; Amirabdollahian et al. 2003).

We had investigated the influence of objects on reaching movements and compared the results to a popular current trajectory model called the minimum-jerk model (Wisneski &

Johnson 2007). Wrist movements were significantly curved away from a predicted straight line and they were curved to accommodate task constraints such as the table, a cup handle, or an obstacle. Supporting real task trajectories means identifying trajectory planning models that better account for curvatures observed in real tasks. We have also developed a 5th order model based on curvature equations reported by Flash and Hogan with modified input conditions (Flash & Hogan, 1985; Flash & Hogan, 1987). The models are described in Fig. 6 and show the contrast in how accurately the models approximate the actual trajectories. Wisneski & Johnson demonstrated that the model with curvature consideration is adequate for functional task planning (providing the input conditions in Table 4 are well defined) however the basic minimum-jerk model without curvature is adequate for PTP movement and planar movements (Wisneski & Johnson 2007). Table 3 shows the relevant equations for these raw data along with the raw subject data. The minimum jerk model with curvature considerations combined with the model inputs for via points was a better fit than the basic model (Model A in Table 3). The model inputs lead to significant reduction of area between data curves; these area reductions were seen for all events as compared to the original minimum jerk paradigm (Model C - 5th order with initial conditions such as those seen in Table 4 for the drink task).

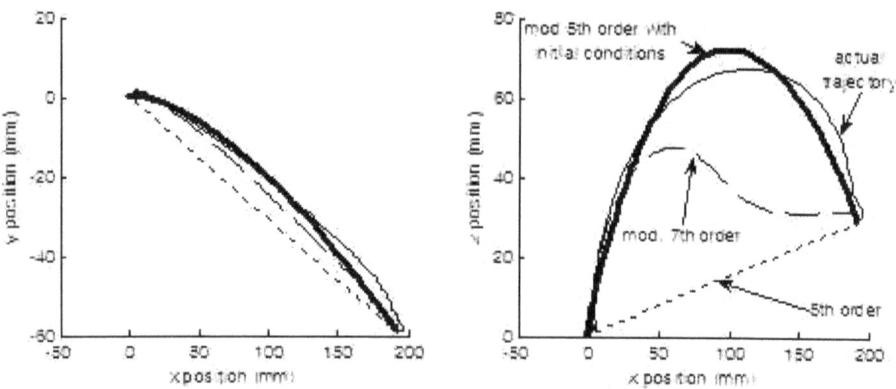

Fig. 6. Trajectory Planning Fits.

Three trajectory models supported by ADLER and an actual trajectory defined from motion analysis studies for a reach to a cup during drinking. Model C based on the 5th order trajectory with curvature and end-point considerations was the best fit for X-Y and X-Z planes.

3. Case Studies

3.1 Methods

Three case studies presented below examine how two healthy, right-handed normal-functioning adults and a low-functioning stroke survivor used and experienced ADLER and its various modes. All subjects gave informed consent for the study, which was approved by the Institutional Review Board of the Clement J. Zablocki VA Medical Center. Table 5 summarizes the able-bodied subjects in this case study.

Case study 1 examines issues in repeatability and stability of kinematic measures such as movement time and smoothness. Able-bodied subjects (age 59 - S1 and age 55-S2) experienced the ADLER robot three times at the beginning and end of one week. The tasks for this study were defined using the 5th order minimum jerk model (Model A, Tables 3). The subjects completed both reaching and grasping phases of a battery of ADLs. Only the drink task is shown and analyzed for kinematic parameters.

Model	Defining equations and boundary conditions	
A. 5th order minimum jerk	$x(t)=x_o+(x_o-x_f)(15\tau^4-6\tau^5-10\tau^3)$ $y(t)=y_o+(y_o-y_f)(15\tau^4-6\tau^5-10\tau^3)$ $z(t)=z_o+(z_o-z_f)(15\tau^4-6\tau^5-10\tau^3)$ Zero velocity, acceleration at initial and final points	The 5th order minimum jerk model for reaching is widely used in robotic therapy (Flash & Hogan, 1985; Flash & Hogan, 1987).
B. Modified 7th order minimum jerk	$p(\tau)=a+b\tau+d\tau^3+f\tau^5+h\tau^7$ where $a=\frac{1}{2}\sum p; b=v_{mid}; d=-3v_{mid}+\frac{35}{16}\Delta p$ $f=3v_{mid}-\frac{21}{8}\Delta p; h=-v_{mid}+\frac{15}{16}\Delta p$ $\sum p=p_f+p_s; \Delta p=p_f-p_s$ Zero velocity, acceleration at initial and final points. Maximum velocity and zero acceleration at 50% reach.	This modified 7th order model was developed by Loureiro and colleagues as a better approximation of actual reach towards an object (Loureiro et al. 2003; Amirabdollahian et al. 2003).
C. 5th order curvature model	$x^-(\tau)=\frac{t_f^5}{720}\left(\pi_1\left(\tau_1^4\left(15\tau^4-30\tau^3\right)+\tau_1^3\left(80\tau^3-30\tau^4\right)\right.\right.$ $\left.-60\tau^3\tau_1^2+30\tau^4\tau_1-6\tau^5\right)+c_1\left(15\tau^4-10\tau^3-6\right.$ $x^+(\tau)=x^-(\tau)+\pi_1\frac{t_f^5(\tau-\tau_1)^5}{120}$ where $c_1=\frac{1}{t_f^5\tau_1^2(1-\tau_1)^5}\left(\left(x_f-x_0\right)\left(300\tau_1^5-1200\tau_1^4+1600\tau_1^3\right)\right.$ $+\tau_1^2\left(-720x_f+120x_1+600x_0\right)+\left(x_0-x_1\right)\left(300\tau_1-2\right.$ $\pi_1=\frac{1}{t_f^5\tau_1^5(1-\tau_1)^5}\left(\left(x_f-x_0\right)\left(120\tau_1^5-300\tau_1^4+200\tau_1^3\right)-20(x_1-\right.$ Zero velocity, acceleration at initial and final points. Via point (x_1,y_1,z_1) defined at time $\tau_1 = 0.4$ (40% of reach).	This modified 5th order model is based on equations developed by Hogan and Flash to describe reaching. We have applied special inputs to the equations based on motion analysis studies to approximate functional reaching.

Table 3. Summary of Trajectory Planning Models Investigated.

Three trajectory models supported by ADLER and an actual trajectory defined from motion analysis studies. The critical time for via points and the Cartesian inputs are as X1, Y1, and Z1.

Model Input#	Purpose	Applicable Events	t1	X1	Y1	Z1
1	Table Constraint (TC)	'Reach' 'Rest'	.40 .40	N/A N/A	N/A N/A	42 mm 28 mm
2	TC+Cup Manipulation	'Reach' 'Rest'	.40 .40	39mm 39mm	N/A N/A	T.C. + 12 mm T.C. + 7mm
3	Movement out-of-the-plane (MOP)	'To Mouth' 'Return Object'	.40 .40	N/A N/A	N/A N/A	59mm 59mm
4	MOP + a cup-type object	'To Mouth' 'Return Object'	.23 .40	16mm 16mm	N/A N/A	10.5mm 10.5mm

Table 4. Settings of Model C for A Drink Task.

Summary of input and output points used to define Model B for a drinking task using a cup with one hand. This setting is also used with Case Study 2.

Case study 2 examines issues in modeling and trajectory planning of wrist movements for a real ADL task, the drink task. An able-bodied subject (age 22 - S3) experienced the ADLER robot with two different trajectory planning models in the same day and compared the results. The tasks for case study 2 were defined using either Model A or the curved model Model C with input as shown in Tables 4. These tasks were drink and feed (with spoon). They were repeated at least three times. First, the subject completed the reaching and grasping phases of the tasks without a trajectory model, i.e., the subject completed the task in normal mode with no assistance from the robot and the ADLER is only recording movement and forces. Next, the subject repeated the tasks with Models A and C and then answered questions about their experiences. Only the drink task is shown and analyzed for kinematic parameters.
Case study 3 examines ADLER system's ability to reduce motor impairment and improve ADL function during the practice of Low ADL movements (Table 1). The stroke survivor was 48 years old and sustained an ischemic stroke four years before with hemiparesis of the left side (Fig. 7).

Subjects	Gender	Trained with	Age	Mode	Robot Mode Assist/Resist	Motor Functional level	Trajectory Model Used
S1	Female	Left hand	59	Function	Assist	Able-Bodied	Model A (Table 3)
S2	Male	Left hand	55	Form	Assist	Able-Bodied	Model A (Table 3)
S3	Male	Left hand	22	Form	Assist	Able-Bodied	Model A Model C (Table 4)
S4	Male	Left Impaired hand	48	Form	Assist	Stroke(RCVA) UE-FT: Level2 UE-FM: 22	Model A (Table 3)

Table 5. Subjects for Case Studies 1-3.

Summary of able-bodied and stroke subjects ran on ADLER. The stroke survivor had a right CVA and motor functional level (UE-FM) of 22 of 66 and an ADL functional (UE-FT) of level 2 of 7.

The stroke subject participated in the reaching aspects of the functional tasks but was not able to participate in the grasping portion (the FES glove was not worn in this instant). The training was conducted in form mode using 2-D and 3-D PTP reaching tasks mimicking ADLs. These tasks were programmed using Model A. As the subject improved, the force assistance (gains on the spring forces) was gradually decreased. Training sessions were administered three times per week for six weeks, with each lasting for approximately one hour. Clinical and robotic evaluations sessions using tasks in Table 2 were completed in the first, third, and last weeks of training. Clinical evaluations included upper-extremity Fugl-Meyer (UE-FM) and functional test (UE-FT) evaluations administered by an occupational therapist (Fugl-Meyer et al. 1975; Wilson et al. 1994). A follow-up evaluation was conducted about one month after the final training period. The ADLER evaluations, completed in normal mode (without force assist), allow for quantification of kinematic improvement without the aid of robotic assistance.

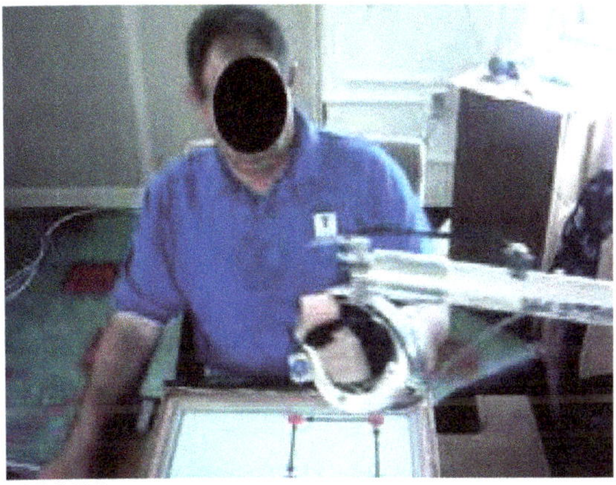

Fig. 7: Stroke Subject in ADLER.

Training takes place using ADLER to complete several low ADL tasks. The low functioning stroke is completing a 2-D PTP.

Force and position data recorded by HERALD were filtered (10 Hz Butterworth low pass) and analyzed using Matlab software (The MathWorks, Inc.). Several kinematic dependent variables were calculated for Case Studies 1 and 2. Total displacement (TD) is the total distance traveled during a given task. The total time required to complete a given task is the movement time (MT). Peak Velocity (PV) is the maximum velocity used in the task. Several measures of smoothness are calculated from the velocity profile, including the ratio of peak velocity (PV) to mean velocity. The movement smoothness (MS) is defined as the peak velocity divided by the average velocity (PV/MeanV) (Rohrer et al. 2002). Trajectories are charted on two position plots, where the initial starting position is normalized to point (0, 0, 0). The x-y plane is parallel to the activity table top, while the z axis points up. The responses to questions about Model A and C for case study 2 were analyzed and compared using t-test.

3.2 Results and Discussion of Cases

3.2.1 Case Study 1: Repeatability and Short-term Learning

Table 6 shows the results of the drink evaluation sessions. We expected that able-bodied subjects may have some short-term learning but that, in general, they would have minimum changes across the key kinematic variables. Subject 1 had consistent kinematics across all kinematic variables with low standard deviations. The fact that S2 had more variance than S1 may indicate that some subjects may require more time during training than others. In addition, we realized that a possible source of error is in the placement of artifacts during it repeatable task trial. It is important the artifacts are placed in the same location during these trials. On the other hand subject 2 only had consistent kinematics across total displacement and peak velocity. Figure 8 shows an example of the results for subject 1.

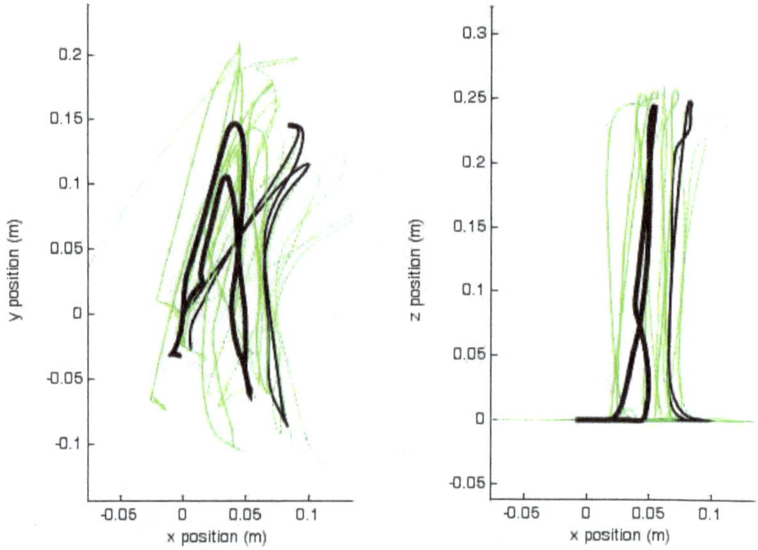

Fig. 8. XY and XZ plane data of the drink task for subject 1 for all trials for 1st and last evaluations.

The graphical data show all three trials and averages for days 1 and 4. Day 1 is solid lines (thick average line) and Day 4 is dash lines (thin line average). XY is the plane of the table and XZ in out of the plane of the table in the plane of the person's torso.

Subject	Initial				Final			
	MT (s)	TD (m)	PV (m/s)	MS	MT (s)	TD (m)	PV (m/s)	MS
S1	7.26	2.36	0.40	3.04	7.38	2.41	0.40	2.95
	±0.39	±0.13	±0.04	±0.23	±0.67	±0.13	±0.01	±0.23
S2	17.51	2.65	0.21	3.06	4.31	2.02	0.33	2.24
	±8.22	±0.65	±0.02	±0.38	±1.09	±0.12	±0.04	±0.18

Table 6. Able-bodied subjects' kinematics are shown. The evolution of Movement Time (MT), Peak Velocity (PV), Total Displacement (TD) and movement smoothness (MS) are shown across two evaluation sessions. S1 was more stable that S2

3.2.2 Case Study 2: Model Evaluation on ADLER

The results from the case study are presented in Figures 9 and 10. The area between curves was significantly reduced for all the drink events. The new model provides a more accurate prediction of the desired functional trajectory than the old paradigm of the minimum jerk model. These results show that this trajectory generation scheme provides more appropriate wrist center paths for implementing functional tasks in the ADLER environment. This improvement was noted by the subject as well.

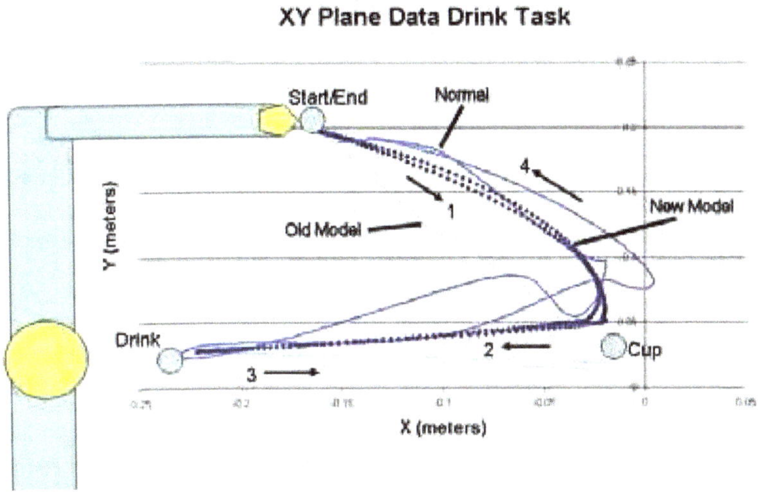

Fig. 9. XY plane data of (from top to bottom) the drink task on ADLER.

The data collected in normal mode is represented by a thick solid line, the data collected when using the old model is represented by a thin solid line (cyan), and the data collected when using the new model is represented by a dotted line. MT = 8.97 ±4.03 seconds, TD =2.23±0.33, PV= 0.29±4.03, and MS 3.70±0.73.

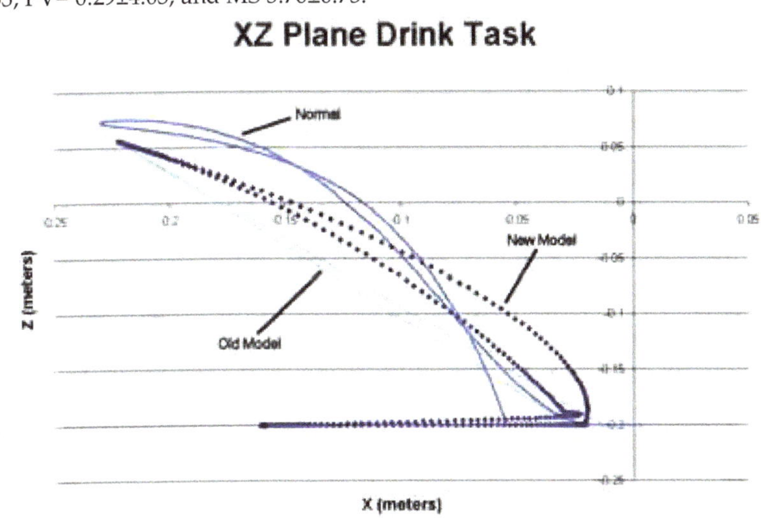

Fig. 10. XZ plane data of (from top to bottom) the drink task on ADLER.

The data collected in normal mode is represented by a thick solid line, the data collected when using the old model is represented by a thin solid line (cyan), and the data collected when using the new model is represented by a dotted line.

Table 7 shows the average responses to the questions presented to the subject after each trial. When using the new model and asked if the robot was moving the way he would have liked to move he answered with an average value of 7. This is a more positive response than for the old model, with which he answered 3. When using the new model and asked if he felt as though he had to work against the robot to complete the task he answered with an average value of 2. This is a more positive response than for the old model, with which he answered 5. His comments reveal that the old model did produce movements that did not feel natural.

Question	Response Range (1-10)	Average Response
Do you feel as though the robot is moving the way you would like to move?	10 = Yes, completely; 5 = About half the time; 1 = No, not at all	Model A: 3 +/-1 **Model C: 7 +/- 1 ***
Do you feel as though you need to fight against the robot to complete the task?	10 = Yes, all the time; 5 = About half the time; 1 = No, not at all	Model: 5 +/- 1 **Model: 2 +/- .5 ***

Table 7. Subject survey at the end of each trial.

The questions, possible responses, and average responses are listed. Representative comments were chosen for each model. If a result was statistically more successful by means of a t-Test it is marked with an asterisk and in bold.

The results from the questionnaire show that the differences seen between the new and old model can be felt by the subject and that using the new model provides for a more comfortable experience and more natural feeling movements. The obvious next step is to complete this analysis with stroke survivors to determine their response to the changes. Since stroke survivors are more likely to have decreased proprioception that affects their ability to sense their arm in space, we anticipate less sensitivity to changes in arm position in space. The question of whether training using these more accurate and natural movement paths will translate into the ability to dynamically position and orientate the impaired arm for various ADL artifacts (e.g., spoon, comb etc.) and the ability to use any performance improvements seen in less supervised environments.

3.2.3 Case Study 3: Training Evaluation on ADLER

Training improved the subject's ability to perform more functional reaching. The result of the 4 main evaluation sessions using the drink 3-D PTP patterns are illustrated in Fig. 11 and the biomechanical measures for kinematics and the clinical measures of ADL and motor function are shown in Table 8. The subject's UE-FT improved by two levels, while UE-FM scores did not change during training. However, this subject was low functioning and did not practice grasping objects, so improvement in UE-FM testing was not expected. A clinical evaluation 1 month (at about 6 weeks) after the end of training showed that the subject maintained a UE-FT score of level 4 and a UE-FM score of 24/66.

Table 8 summarizes the evolution of the key kinematic variables derived for S4. We expected that the kinematic variables of movement time and smoothness (Peak V/mean V) would consistently decrease as evaluation proceeded from pre to post to follow-up and approach normal values (Rohrer et al 2002; Krebs et al. 2002; Wu et al 2000). In general this expectation was met and can be seen from the data for S1 and S2 in Tables 7and S4 in Table 8.

We expected that the peak velocity and total displacement would consistently increase as evaluation proceeded from pre to post to follow-up and approach normal values. Table 8 clearly shows the gain in peak velocity over time. Overall total displacement was not consistent from pre- to post-training and follow-up because this measure as calculated evaluated the entire movement included those that were not useful to accomplish the task.

From Figure 11, it is clear that the subject's height off the table increased and the range of motion on the table also increased. This implies that although overall TD did not behave consistently, therefore, in the future, a better and more sensitive kinematic measure could be derived in terms of increases in height (z) and table top range of motion (x-y area). We anticipate that when we include the FES grasp glove, especially for low-functioning stroke survivors, we will add the inclusion of a curvature and orientation measure to detect changes in dynamic orientation of the hand during functional reaching to an ADL artifact such as the cup in the drink task.

The subject used the normal mode to complete the evaluation tasks and the training modes to complete the training tasks. The drink task is shown.

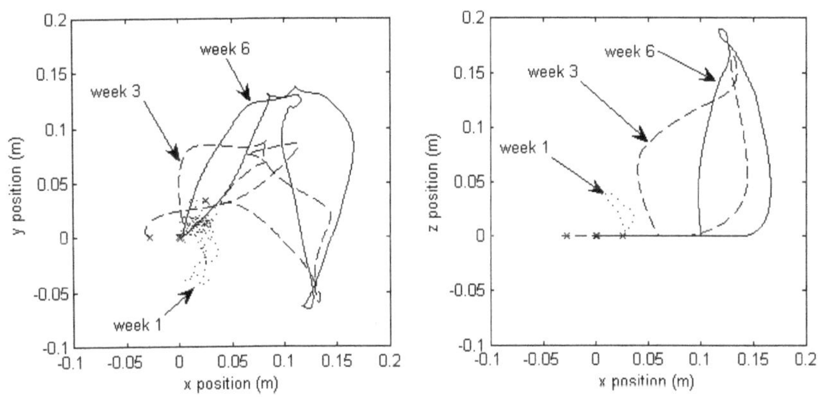

Fig. 11. Drinking Task Changes in XY and XZ planes.

The evolution of movement for the drink task are shown for the evaluation sessions from pre-training (Week 1) to follow-up (Week 6) for the drink task. The subject had increasingly more height in the Z direction as time passed and covered more table area in the X-Z area.

The key changes seen translated mainly into increased shoulder and elbow movement, which lead to change from level 2 to 4 on ADL function. This result is typical of systems that training only reaching performance (Loureiro et al. 2003; Krebs et al. 2002; Prange et al. 2006). Since grasp function did not improve and is required for ADL function on levels 5 through 7, we anticipate that training to assist opening and closing of the hand for grasping as well as reaching via the full integration of the FES game glove into the ADLER system will improve these results. In addition to gaining data from lower functioning stroke subjects, we are also evaluating the performance of higher-functioning stroke survivors with low to medium grasping capability on the ADLER system (with and without FES glove). We hope to see improvement in the UE-FM and UE-FT scores of these subjects due to more functional training. We also anticipate greater improvement following the full implementation of curved trajectory models (Model C especially). The first stroke subject was trained using PTP trajectories defined by the straight-line, 5th order minimum jerk model. We expect that the curved trajectories, which approximate better actual movements, will result in improved recovery.

Evaluation Session	Biomechanical and Clinical Measures					
	MT (s)	TD (m)	PV (m/s)	MS	UE-FM	UE-FT
Initial	15.78 ±5.65	2.51 ±0.46	0.26 ±0.01	3.90 ±0.68	23	Level 2
Week 1	12.75 ±4.01	2.05 ±0.23	0.23 ±0.10	4.32 ±1.32	27	Level 2
Week 3	8.14 ±1.42	1.88 ±0.37	0.28 ±0.031	2.93 ±0.20	23	Level 2
Week 6	6.38 ±0.13	2.08 ±0.13	0.27 ±0.03	2.97 ±0.54	23	Level 4
Follow-up	12.59 ±1.01	2.89 ±0.59	0.36 ±0.05	3.27 ±0.94	24	Level 4

Table 8. Evolution of the Kinematics of S3 (Stroke) on PTP drink task.

The table shows the changes in movement time (MT), total displacement (TD), smoothness (PV/MeanV), and clinical values for motor impairment (UE-FM with 66 as maximum) and ADL function (UE-FT: Level 7 maximum).

4. Conclusion

This chapter discussed the development of a task-oriented therapy robot focused on real ADL training and performance. The development of the software, HERALD, and the hardware platform and FES grasp glove has been discussed. We also presented training and trajectory planning models that have been implemented with the system along with defining the pros and cons of three possible models that can be used to accurately reflect natural movement of the wrist during ADL task. We presented three case studies that briefly examined how the system has repeatable performance and has the ability to train stroke survivors. A low functioning stroke survivor was successfully trained on the system using PTP ADL-like movement. The subject's kinematics, especially movement time and movement smoothness decreased reflecting motor impairment reduction and increased motor control. The ADL functioning was improved on tasks involving more shoulder and elbow function but not on task involving grasp. In the future, the FES glove will be fully integrated in the ADLER system to allow stroke clients on all levels of motor function and ADL ability to be trained in both reaching and grasping ADLs. As such we anticipate that a major impact will then be seen on both motor impairment and functional scales.
We also presented via case study 2 different trajectory models for planning and assisting movement of the wrist using ADLER. We demonstrated that models that included curvature and had customized inputs can improve a subject's movement kinematics for an ADL tasks such as drinking and can affect their perception of the ease or difficulty of the movement. In the case study performed on the ADLER system, the subject reported a "more natural" feel when operating with the new model rather than the old model. This shows that the model appears to meet the goal of providing a more natural prediction of functional

wrist paths. Although these results are promising it is understood that much more work to be done and there is a need to examine movements from the perspective of the stroke survivor.

In the near future, we will be improving our models for trajectory planning of ADL movements as well as examining whether the ADLER system including the FES glove can improve both motor and ADL function.

5. References

(AHA) American Heart Association. Heart Disease and Stroke Statistics - 2005 Update. Dallas, TX: American Heart Association; 2005

Ada L., Canning C.G., Carr J.H., Kilbreath S.L., Shepherd R.B. "Task-specific training of reaching and manipulation." In Insights into Reach to Grasp movement. K.M.B. Bennett and U. Castiello (Editors). Elsevier Science B.V. 1994

Abend W, Bizzi E, Morasso P: Human arm trajectory formation. *Brain* 1982, Vol 105, pp. 331-348.

Amirabdollahian, F, (2003). An investigation of roboti-mediated therapies and therapy effects on the recovery of upper limb post stroke. *University of Reading, Department of Cybernetics, Dissertation Thesis.* September.

Amirabdollahian, F.; Loureiro, R. & Harwin, W., (2002). Minimum jerk trajectory control for rehabilitation and haptic applications. *Proceedings of IEEE Int Conf on Robotics Automation*, Washington DC, May, pp. 3380-3385.

Atkeson CG, Hollerbach JM: **Kinematic features of unrestrained vertical arm movements.** *Journal of Neuroscience* 1985, 5(9): 2318-2330.

Aycock DM. Blanton S. Clark PC. Wolf SL. What is constraint-induced therapy? *Rehabilitation Nursing*. 29(4):114-5, 121, 2004

Bach y Rita P, Wood S, Leder R, Paredes O, Bahr D, Bach-y-Rita EW, Murillo N. "Computer assisted motivating rehabilitation for institutional, home, and educational late stroke programs." *Top Stroke Rehabil*, Vol. 8, Issue 4, pp. 1-10, 2002

Barton, L. A. & Wolf, S. L., (1993). Learned nonuse in the hemiplegic upper extremity. In Gordon WA, Editor. *Advances in Stroke Rehabilitation.* Boston: Butterworth-Heinemann; pp. 79-87, 1993

Bayona, NA.;Bitensky, J.; Salter, K. & Teasell, R. (2005a). The role of task-specific training in rehabilitation therapies. *Topics in Stroke Rehabilitation,* Vol. 12, Issue 3, pp. 58-65, 2005a

Burgar, C.G.; Lum, P.S.; Shor, P.C. & Van der Loos, H.F.M., (2000) Development of robots for rehabilitation therapy:the Palo Alto VA/Stanford experience, *Journal of Rehabilitation R&D*, Vol. 36, Issue 6, November/December.

Carr J, Shepherd R. *A Motor Relearning Programme For Stroke.* 2nd edn. Heinemann Medical, Oxford; 1987

Calautti, C. & Baron, J., (2003). Functional neuroimaging studies of motor recovery after stroke in adults. A review. *Stroke*, Vol. 34, pp. 1553-66.

Fasoli, S.; Krebs, H.I.; Stein, J.; Frontera, W.R. & Hogan, N., (2003). Effects of robotic therapy on motor impairment and recovery in chronic stroke. *Archives of Phys Med Rehabil,* vol. 84, pp. 477-84.

Fasoli, S.;Krebs, H. I.; Hughes, R., Stein J. & Hogan N., (2005). Functionally-based rehabilitation: Benefits or Buzzwrod? *Proceedings of International Conference on Rehabilitation Robotics ICORR),* Chicago, IL, June 28-July 1, pp. 223-226, 2005.

FCS Control Systems HapticAPI Programming Manual, Version 1.2, Schipol, The Netherlands: FCS Control Systems, 2003.

Fisher, B. E. and Sullivan, K. J., "Activity-Dependent factors affecting poststroke functional outcomes." *Top Stroke Rehabil*, Vol. 8, Issue 3, pp. 31-44, 2001

Flash, T. & Hogan, N., (1985). The coordination of arm movements: An experimentally confirmed mathematical model. *The Journal of Neuroscience*, Vol. 5, pp. 1688-1703.

Fugl-Meyer, A.R.; Jaasko L. & Leyman I:, (1975). The post-stroke hemiplegic patient. A method for evaluation of physical performance. *Scandinavian Journal of Rehabilitation Medicine*, Vol. 7, pp. 13-31.

Gentilucci, M.; Castiello, U.; Corradini ML., Scarpa M., Umilta C., & Rizzolatti G., (1991). Influence of different types of grasping on the transport component of prehension movements. *Neuropsychologia.* Vol. 29, Issue 5, 361-78.

Gentilucci, M., (2002). Object motor representation and reaching-grasping control." *Neuropsychologia.* Vol. 40, Issue 8, pp. 1139-53.

Gentilucci, M.; Daprati, E.; Gangitano, M.;Saetti, M.C. & Toni, I., (1996). On orientating the hand to reach and grasp an object. *Neuroreport.* Vol. 7, pp. 589-592.

Hogan, N. & Flash, T (1987). Moving gracefully: quantitative theories of motor coordination. *TINS.* Vol. 10, Issue 4, pp. 170-174.

Hogan, N. (1984) An organizing principle for a class of voluntary movements," *Journal of Neuroscience*, Vol. 4, pp. 2745-2754.

He Huang, H., Wolf, S.L. & He J. (2006) Recent developments in biofeedback for neuromotor rehabilitation. *Journal of NeuroEngineering and Rehabilitation.* Vol. **3**, Issue 11. doi:10.1186/1743-0003-3-11

He, J.; Koeneman, E.J.; Schultz, R.S.; Huang, H.; Wanberg, J.; Herring, D.E.; Sugar, T.; Herman, R.; & Koeneman, J.B., **(2005).** Design of a robotic upper extremity repetitive therapy device. *9th International Conference on Rehabilitation Robotics, 2005. (ICORR 2005)* Volume, Issue , 28 June-1 July 2005, pp. 95 - 98

Hunter, P.; Peckham, P. & Knutson, J.S., (2005). Functional electrical stimulation for neuromuscular applications. *Annu. Rev. Biomed. Eng.* Vol 7: pp. 327–60,

Johnson, M.J.; Wisneski, K.J.; Anderson. J.; Nathan, D., & Smith. R., (2006) Development of ADLER: The Activities of Daily Living Exercise Robot. *IEEE-EMBS Biomedical Robotics (BioRob 2006)*, February 2006, Pisa, Italy, pp. 881-886.

Kahn, L. E., Zygman, M. L., Rymer, W. Z. & Reinkensmeyer, D.J., (2006). Robot-assisted reaching exercise promotes arm movement recovery in chronic hemiparetic stroke: a randomized controlled pilot study. *Journal of NeuroEngineering and Rehabilitation* 2006, Vol. 3, Issue 12, doi:10.1186/1743-0003-3-12

Krebs, H.I.; Palazzolo, J.J.; Dipietro, L.; Ferraro, M.; Krol, J.; Rannekleiv, K.; Volpe, B.T. & Hogan, N., (2003). Rehabilitation robotics: Performance-based progressive robot-assisted therapy. *Autonomous Robots*, Vol. 15, pp. 7-20.

H.I. Krebs, B.T. Volpe, et al., "Robot-aided neurorehabilitation: from evidence-based to science-based rehabilitation," *Top Stroke Rehabil*, vol. 8, no. 4, pp. 54-70, 2002.

Latash, M. L. & Nicholas, J.J. (1996). Motor control research in rehabilitation medicine. *Disability & Rehabilitation.* Vol. 18, Issue 6, pp. 293-9.

Liepert, H.; Bauder, W., Miltner, H.R. ; Taub, E. & Weiller, C., (2002). Treatment-induced cortical reorganization after stroke in humans. *Stroke*, Vol. 31, pp. 1210-1216.

Loureiro, R.; Amirabdollahian, F.; Topping, M.; Driessen, B. & Harwin, W., (2003). Upper limb robot mediated stroke therapy-GENTLE/s approach. *Autonomous Robots* Vol. 15, Issue 1, pp. 35-51.

Ma, H. & Trombly, C. A. (2002). A synthesis of the effects of occupational therapy for persons with stroke, Part II: Restoration of roles, tasks, and activities. *Am J Occup Ther*, Vol. 56, No. 3, pp. 260-74

Maclean N, Pound P, Wolfe C, Rudd A: Qualitative analysis of stroke patients motivation for rehabilitation. British Medical Journal 2000, 321(7268):1051-1054.

MacClellan, L.R.; Bradham, D.D.; Whitall, J.; Volpe, B.; Wilson, P.; Ohlhoff, J.; Meister, C.; Hogan,N.; Krebs, H.I. & Bever Jr, C., (2006) Robotic upper-limb neurorehabilitation in chronic stroke patients. *Journal of Rehabilitation R&D*, Vol. 42, No. 6, November/December, pp. 717-722

Merians, A.S.; Jack, D.; Boian, R.; Tremaine, M.; Burdea,G.C.; Adamovich,S.V.; Recce, M. & Poizner H., (2002).Virtual Reality-Augmented Rehabilitation for Patients Following Stroke. *Physical Therapy*. Vol. 82, No. 9 . September 2002, pp. 898-915

Michaelsen, S.M.; Jacobs, S.; Roby-Brami, A. & Levin, M.F. (2004) Compensation for distal impairments of grasping in adults with hemiparesis." *Experimental Brain Research*, Vol. 157, Issue 2, pp. 162-73.

Nathan and Johnson - ICORR 2007

Nelles, G., W. Jentzen, et al. (2001) Arm training induced brain plasticity in stroke studied with serial positron emission tomography. *Neuroimage*, Vol. **13**, Issue 6 Pt 1, pp. 1146-54

Nef T, Mihelj M, Colombo G, Riener R. "ARMin - Robot for Rehabilitation of the Upper Extremities." *IEEE International Conference on Robotics and Automation*, pp. 3152—3157, Orlando, Florida, May 15-19, 2006

Page, S.J.; Sisto, S.; Levine, P.; & McGrath, R.E., (2004). Efficacy of modified constraint-induced movement therapy in chronic stroke: a single-blinded randomized controlled trial. *Arch Phys Med Rehabil* , Vol. 85, pp. 14-8.

Patton, J.L.; Kovic, M. & Mussa-Ivaldi, F.A. (2006). Custom-designed haptic training for restoring reaching ability to individuals with stroke. *Journal of Rehabilitation Research and Development*, In press, 2006.

Patton, J.L.; Stoykov, M.E.; Kovic, M. & Mussa-Ivaldi, F.A., (2006). Evaluation of robotic tr aining forces that either enhance or reduce er r or in chronic hemipar etic stroke survivor s. *Exp Brain Res*, Vol. 168, pp. 368-383.

Patton, J.L. & Mussa-Ivaldi, F.A. (2004) Robot-assisted adaptive training: custom force fields for teaching movement patterns. *IEEE Transactions on Biomedical Engineering*. Vol. 51, Issue 4, pp. 636-46.

Prange, G. B.; Jannink M. J. A; Groothuis-Oudshoorn, C. G. M.; Hermens, H. J. & IJzerman, M. J., (2006). Systematic review of the effect of robot-aided therapy on recovery of the hemiparetic arm after stroke. *Journal of Rehabilitation R&D*, Vol. 43, No. 2, March/April, pp. 171-184

Reinkensmeyer, D.J.; Takahashi, C.D.; Timoszyk, W.K.; Reinkensmeyer, A. N. & Kahn, L.E., (2001). Design of robot assistance for arm movement therapy following stroke. *Advanced Robotics*, Vol. 14, No. 7, pp. 625-637.

Roby-Brami, A.; Jacobs, S.; Bennis, N. & Levin, M.F., (2003) Hand orientation for grasping and arm joint rotation patterns in healthy subjects and hemiparetic stroke patients." *Brain Research*, Vol. 969, issues 1-2, pp. 217-29.

Rohrer, B.; Fasoli, S.; Krebs, H.I.; Hughes, R.; Volpe, B.; Frontera, W.R.; Stein, J. & Hogan, N., (2002). Movement smoothness changes during stroke recovery. *Journal of Neuroscience*, Vol. 22, Issue 18, pp. 8297-304.

Schaechter, J.D., (2004) .Motor rehabilitation and brain plasticity after hemiparetic stroke. *Progress in Neurobiology*. Vol. 73, Issue 1, pp. 61-72.

Simone, L.K. & Kamper, D.G., (2005) . Design considerations for a wearable monitor to measure finger posture. *Journal of NeuroEngineering and Rehabilitation*, Vol 2, Issue 5, doi:10.1186/1743-0003-2-5

Sterr, A.; Freivogel, S. & Schmalohr, D. (2000). Neurobehavioral aspects of recovery: Assessment of the learned nonuse phenomenon in hemiparetic adolescents. *Arch Phys Med Rehabil*. Vol. 83, No. 4, pp. 1726-31

Thielman G.T., Dean C.M., Gentile A.M. "Rehabilitation of reaching after stroke: task related training versus progressive resistive exercise.," *Arch Phys Med Rehabil*, Vol. 85, pp. 1613-1618. 2004.

Trombly, C. A. & Ma, H. (2002). A synthesis of the effects of occupational therapy for persons with stroke, Part I: Restoration of roles, tasks, and activities. *Am J Occup Ther*, Vol. 56, No. 3, pp. 250-59.

Trombly C. Occupational Therapy of Physical Dysfunction. Trombly C, editor. Baltimore (MD): Williams & Wilkins; 1995

Taub E, Uswatte G, Pidikiti R. Constraint-induced movement therapy: a new family of techniques with broad application to physical rehabilitation -- a clinical review. J Rehabil Res Dev. 36(3): 1-18, 1999

Taub, E.; Crago, J.E.; Burgio LD, et al., (1994). An operant approach to rehabilitation rehabilitation medicine: overcoming learned nonuse by shaping. Journal of Experiment Analysis of Behavior. Vol. 61, pp. 281-93.

Taub, E.; Lum, P. S.; Hardin, P.; Mark V. & Uswatte. G., (2005). AutoCITE, Automated delivery of CI therapy with reduced effort by therapists. *Stroke*, Vol. 36, pp. 1301.

Tyberghein J., E. Sunshine, (2004, Aug 13). "Crystal Space 0.98 manual," available: http://www.crystalspace3d.org/docs/online/manual-0.98/.

Wilson DJ, Baker LL, Craddock JA: Functional test for the hemipar etic upper extremity. *Am J Occup Ther* 1984, 38(3):159-164.

Wisneski, K.J. & Johnson, M.J. (2006) Insights into Modeling Functional Trajectories for Robot-Mediated Daily Living Exercise Environments." *IEEE-RAS Biomedical Robotics* (BioRob 2006), February 2006.

Wisneski K. Development of a Model for Functional Upper Extremity Trajectory Generation and Implementation on the Activities of Daily Living Exercise Robot (ADLER). Masters Thesis, *Marquette University, Department of Biomedical Engineering*, August 2006.

Wisneski, K.J. & Johnson, M.J. (2007). Quantifying kinematics of purposeful movements to real, imagined, or absent functional objects: Implications for modelling trajectories for robot-assisted ADL tasks. *Journal of NeuroEngineering and Rehabilitation*, Vol 4, Issue 7, doi:10.1186/1743-0003-4-7

Woldag, H.; Waldmann, G.; Heuschkel, G. & Hummelsheim, H., (2003). Is the repetitive training of complex hand and arm movements beneficial for motor recovery in stroke patients?. *Clinical Rehabilitation*. Vol. 17, Issue 7, pp. 723-30.

Wood, S. R., N. Murillo, et al., (2003). Motivating, game-based stroke rehabilitation: a brief report. *Top Stroke Rehabil*, Vol. 10, Issue 2, pp. 134-40.

Wu C., Trombly C.A,. Lin K, & Ticke-Degnen L. (1998). Effects of object affordances on reaching performance in persons with and without cerebrovascular accident. *Am J Occup Ther* 1998

Wu C., Trombly C.A., Lin K, et al., (2000). A kinematic study of contextual effects on reaching performance in persons with and without stroke: Influences of object availability. *Arch Phys Med Rehabil*, Vol. 81, Issue 1, pp. 95-101.

Volpe BT, Ferraro M, Lynch D, Christos P, Krol J, Trudell C, Krebs HI, Hogan N., (2002). Robotics and other devices in the treatment of patients recovering from stroke. *Current Neurology & Neuroscience Reports*, Vol. 5, Issue 6, pp. 465-70.

7

Robotic Solutions in Pediatric Rehabilitation

Michael Bailey-Van Kuren
Miami University
USA

1. Introduction

The rehabilitation of pediatric patients involves unique constraints in comparison to adult rehabilitation. Therefore, the utilization of robotic technology in the rehabilitation of pediatric patients provides unique challenges. Research focusing on the application of robotic technology to pediatric cerebral palsy patients with spasticity is searching for flexible solutions that can address a wide range of patient capabilities. A variety of solutions are being investigated that place robotics in different roles in relation to the patient.

Cerebral palsy describes a group of neuro-muscular disorders that are caused by injury to the brain during the brain's developmental period. Cerebral palsy hinders motor skills and control of movement. According to the United Cerebral Palsy Research and Educational Facility, there are at least 550,000 persons in the United States with the disorder. Furthermore, there are approximately 9,750 new cases per year. Substance abuse and other factors also help increase the chances of the affliction (Matthews and Wilson, 1999; Styer-Acevedo, 1999).

Cerebral palsy affects the Basal Ganglia which is responsible for coordinating motion in the muscles. This affects all muscles of the body. The most noticeable muscles affected in children with cerebral palsy are the arm and leg muscles resulting in reduced motor skills, and the tongue which affecting speech and swallowing (Matthews and Wilson, 1999; Styer-Acevedo, 1999).

Cerebral palsy is usually diagnosed within the first two years after birth. Therefore, rehabilitative therapy for cerebral palsy patients may initiate shortly after birth. Although there are three main types of cerebral palsy: spastic, athetoid, and ataxic, the most common form of cerebral palsy is spastic cerebral palsy where high muscle tone constrains motion. Rehabilitation for pediatric cerebral palsy patients includes physical therapy, occupational therapy, and interventional medicine such as the injection of Botulinum-A Toxin paired with serial casting. Physical therapy early in the child's development prevents contractures and help to keep the muscles from becoming weakened or from deteriorating due to lack of use. Pediatric physical therapy differs from adult therapy in that patients often can not (or may not be willing to) follow direct instructions of a therapy routine thus therapy is incorporated in play. Furthermore, therapists must consider the natural progression of fine and gross motor skills in conjunction with developmental delays caused by cerebral palsy as a patient grows from infancy to adolescence.

2. Previous Work Related to Robotic Pediatric Rehabilitation

Robotics provide a reprogrammable flexible platform for manipulation and interaction with the robot's environment. The role of robotics in adult rehabilitation is well established. Robotic applications in adult rehabilitation have centered on the neuro-muscular difficulties experienced by stroke patients. Robotic devices to assist patients with their gait have been used to re-establish neuro-muscular pathways (Sawicki et al., 2006). Furthermore, robots have been developed that increase the bilateral range of motion of patients performing reach tasks (Burgar et al., 2000). In other related work, there is a variety of research investigating the use of gaming (Merians et al., 2002) or virtual reality to motivate adult patients in performing rehabilitative tasks. This research points to three capabilities that robotics can provide to pediatric patients with cerebral palsy: aiding the establishment of neuro-muscular pathways, extending range of motion, and providing patient motivation.

Previous pediatric devices have focused on the motivational capability of robots with children. Robots have been designed to target children with speech, learning, and physical disabilities (Plaisant et al., 2003). These robots mimic the actions of pediatric patients based on signals from armbands or leg bands. In addition, the robots used games and activities to encourage the children to continue their exercises.

The use of autonomous robots has been studied with autistic children (Michaud et al., 2003). It was hypothesized that "mobile robots can serve as an appropriate pedagogical tool to help children with PDD[autism] develop social skills because they are more predictable and less intimidating" than an adult or therapist. The project consisted of six different robots, each with a unique look and set of abilities. Three of the prototype robots are shown in Fig. 1. It was found that positive reinforcement was an affective tool for the children to improve their skills. They explain; "having the robots behave in particular ways (like dancing, playing music, etc.) when the child responds correctly to requests made by the robot becomes an incentive for the child to continue playing with the robots". The research found that the best and most effective robots appealed to the children's visual sense, auditory sense, sense of touch, spatial perception and use of language. The use of lights, music, and short vocal messages excited the children and encouraged continued play. Unique problems were found in dealing with the pediatric population including possible damage to the robots and the danger of small parts as choking hazards with younger children.

In further research, a robot named "Roball", shown in Fig. 2, was designed to develop the language, affective, motor, intellectual and social skills for children ages 12 to 24 months (Michaud et al., 2004). The robot has the ability to perform autonomous movement, sense, illuminate, and generate sound. A study of eight children investigated the development of each child's motor skills, stimulation of intellectual skills, social interaction and language skills. This study focuses on the development of healthy children; however, the similar research could be compared and applied to children with disorders such as autism and various physical disabilities.

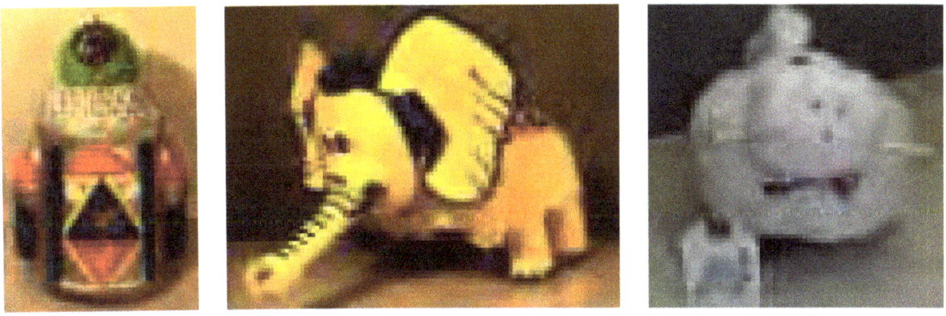

Fig. 1. Three Robots Used in Therapy for Autistic Children (Michaud et al., 2003).

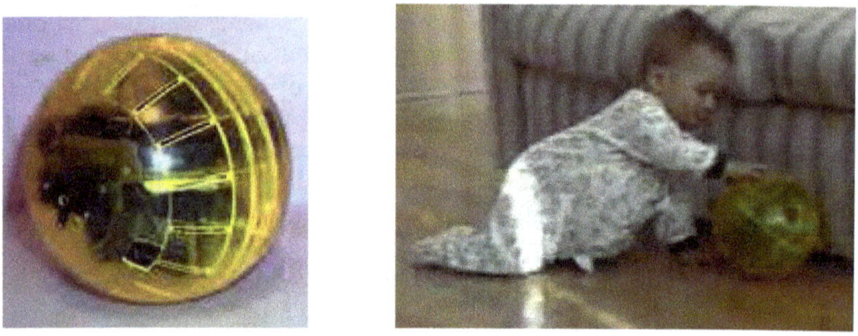

Fig. 2. Prototype Roball and infant interacting with Roball (Michaud et al., 2004).

Pediatric related robotic systems that extend beyond motivational capability include the blocks assembly robot that provides the ability for blocks play children without the physical capability to manipulate blocks with their hands (Plaisant et. al., 2003). This system utilizes customized interfaces to provide children with a command structure that can be used to control a prismatic actuator. Some children with cerebral palsy may be a candidate for this type of robotic interaction. However, this is not directly a therapy related activity.

Although robotics has been successfully applied to rehabilitation and interaction with children, these systems have not been designed to meet the specific needs of children with cerebral palsy. Therefore, three different pediatric robotic therapy approaches are being investigated to take of advantage of reprogrammable platforms including an active rehabilitative boot, motivation robots, and an assistive robotic trainer.

3. An Active Rehabilitative Boot

An active rehabilitative boot is the application of a programmable platform to the stretching of the lower leg to maximize range of movement for children with spastic cerebral palsy. The most commonly occurring form of CP is spastic CP. Spastic refers to high muscle tone (tightness) which constrains motion. When both legs are affected by this condition it is classified as spastic diplegia. Children with spastic diplegia often will walk on their toes. This is caused by the contraction of the gastronemus muscle in the leg.

The most common rehabilitative method for spastic diplegia is interaction with a physical therapist to stretch the muscle in order to increase the range of motion for the patient's gait. Physical therapy early in the child's development prevents contractures and helps to keep the muscles from becoming weakened or from deteriorating due to lack of use.

A second rehabilitation method is an ankle foot orthosis. An ankle foot orthosis forces the ankle into a preferred position while the patient wears the device. This is often achieved through the use of fastening straps. It has been found that ankle-foot orthosis are beneficial to children with spastic diplegia during sit to stand transitions (Park et. al., 2004).

Another method of therapy is the use of Botulinum-A Toxin, also called Botox, paired with serial casting. The Botox safely and effectively reduce spasticity in specific muscle groups. Botox is administered by direct injection into a shortened muscle (for example a spastic calf muscle causing a tight heel cord) to temporarily weaken that muscle and allow it to stretch. The effects of Botox are not permanent; weakness typically lasts for a few months. In some cases, patients may require repeated injections to treat a shortened muscle. The Botox helps relax the muscles so the therapist can stretch the muscle group by securing the foot into position with a standard plaster or fiberglass cast. After approximately one week, the cast is removed, the ankle is stretched to the new limits, and a new cast is applied. This process is repeated throughout a period of four to six weeks. The serial casting procedure can be uncomfortable and modify the patient's behavior. A set of casts restricts the child's gait, which may lead young patients to revert to crawling. A set of serial casts for a 3 year old child was weighed and the average weight of a cast was 377g per foot. Cast materials can also lead to skin irritations causing the cast to be removed and the effective therapy window for the Botox injection may be wasted.

A new active orthotic boot is being constructed to assist in the rehabilitation of children with cerebral palsy that have spastic diplegia typically manifested by toe-walking. A new dynamic or active orthotic boot can assist in walking and gradual rehabilitation of the associated muscle group. The programmability of a microcontroller based device provides the boot with the flexibility to address the needs of different patients as well as different therapeutic applications.

In previous work, an active ankle foot orthoses to treat drop-foot has been devised (Blaya and Herr, 2004). The actuator modulates the stiffness of the low muscle tone ankle joint. Although this work proved the feasibility of an active orthotic boot, the actuator mounting on the back side of the calf would be problematic for pediatric patients. Furthermore, this previous boot required fast actuator response times in order to facilitate active ambulation of the patient. Our proposed boot for pediatric rehabilitation requires a much slower system response which enables the investigation of different actuation solutions. By incorporating new materials and technology, the boot can be more compact and lightweight resulting in increased patient comfort. Some important functional requirements of this new boot are the ability to adapt to changing rehabilitation requirements, the ability to store a history patient/boot interaction data for the therapist, and safety for daily use.

Thus, the rehabilitation of patients with spastic diplegia can benefit from the development of a new active orthotic boot that can provide a more flexible alternative to serial casts and also provide in home stretching therapy.

3.1 Rehabilitative Boot Design Concept

The active boot design targeted a thin wall boot similar to current orthoses with integrated actuators and feedback sensors to provide the proper stretch or set to a fixed "cast" position. Feedback on the patient is collected in terms of the foot angle and the pressure that the foot exerts against the boot and is monitored by a microcontroller. The microcontroller analyzes input signals and provides output voltage to the system actuators. The magnitude and duration of the system output can be tuned and customized for each patient. Based on the input of a pediatric physical therapists, an approximation of three times the patient's body weight provides an upper bound for the magnitude of force needed to be exerted on the patient's foot. The relationship of system components is depicted in Figure 3.

The boot design is based on existing DAFO configurations. Current manufacturing methods can be utilized to custom fit durable, lightweight plastic to the geometry of the foot and ankle. Figure 4 shows the final design and the original prototype. A thin film pressure sensor is located at the ball of the foot to detect the pressure resulting from the patient's tendency to walk on their toes. The sensor pads depicted in Figure 4 provide a stiffened package to improve the repeatability of the signal from thin film sensors. The objective of the pressure sensor is to determine whether the foot is bearing weight so that the brace flexibility can be increased to facilitate ambulation. An angle sensor is located at the hinge point of the boot. This can be used for dynamic feedback or verification that the boot is in a set "cast" position. Pediatric physical therapists have stated that +/- 10 degree range is typical for the target population.

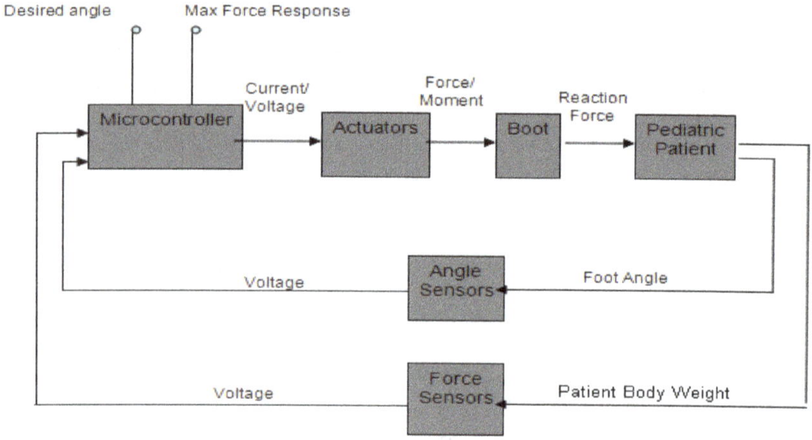

Fig. 3. System Block Diagram for a Pediatric Rehabilitative Boot.

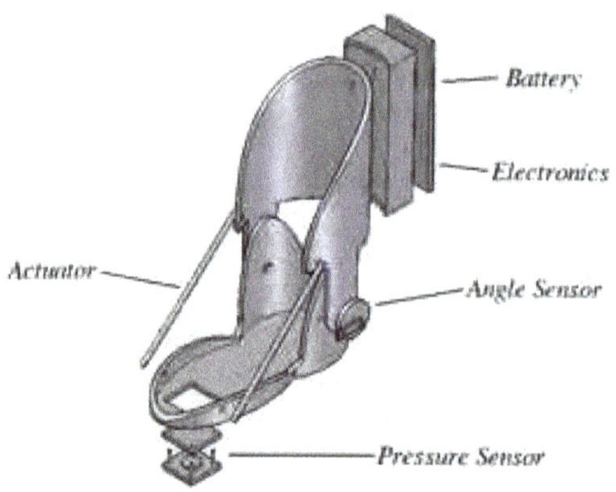

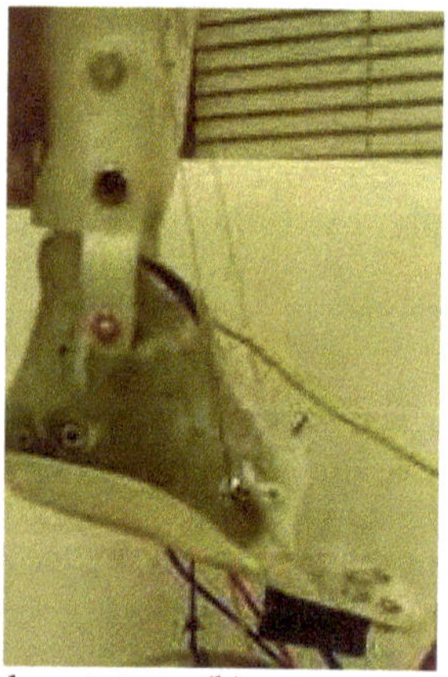

Fig. 4. A comparison of the rehabilitative boot design (a) and prototype (b).

Further development of a lightweight compact design integrates the actuators into the boot materials. Actuation can be achieved through contraction or bending. The microcontroller, interface circuitry, and battery are located on the back side of the boot to create an autonomous wearable device.

3.2 Prototype Rehabilitative Boot Design

System actuators must be able to move and stretch the leg muscles as part of a daily physical therapy routine. The concept of smart materials for use in orthotic and prosthetic devices has been investigated (Herr and Kornbluh, 2004) but not implemented. The use of electroactive polymer artificial muscles for assisting ambulation is discussed. Whereas the ambulatory system requires a high speed system response, the rehabilitation system benefits from a slow actuator response.

A smart material that meets the design requirements well is Shape Memory Alloys. Their unique pseudo-elastic and shape memory effects would provide the structure and motion needed in the therapy, along with the flexibility desired for safety. The heat being supplied to the wire is essentially the power that drives the molecular arrangement. This particular effect would be useful in the orthotic device as a way to change and set the desired distortion (length and angle). However, the pseudo-elastic properties are only exhibited when the alloy is composed of austenite phase and a load is applied. As the load is increased, the alloy transforms from austenite to martensite. The load strain is absorbed by the softer martensite, then as the load is reduced, the martensite transform back into austenite and returns to its original shape. In conjunction with the shape memory effect, the pseudo-elastic effect would be useful in the orthotic device as a general comfort and safety level assurance since the material would ideally give flexibility in its movement while still maintaining the needed shape. Some advantages the shape memory alloys have over other actuators include high power density (>1000 W/kg), large stress (>200 MPa), and large strain (~5%).

System sensors monitor the interaction between the patient and the boot. Force sensors are required to monitor that actuation forces are stretching the leg muscles while ensuring that the muscle is not torn. This is performed indirectly by measuring the force applied by the brace on the patient's foot. The sensor will be placed at the ball of the foot because the spasticity is often exhibited by the extension of the child's foot, as when the child is walking on his/her toes.

Since the boot is controllable it is possible to facilitate walking when the patient is ambulating by reducing the boot stiffness. In order to perform this function, the sensor must be able to differentiate when the patient is standing versus when the patient is sitting.

By placing sensors at the ball of the foot, the type of sensors that can be used are limited by the comfort of the user. Therefore a thin flexible sensor is required. Second, it should give consistent readings over a range of temperatures. As an approximation, the lowest temperature the sensor will experience would be during the winter months (0°C) and the highest temperature the sensor will experience would be during the summer months (45 °C). Finally, the sensor must give accurate measurements over the required range of forces, 0-108kg. Negative force measurements are not required since we are only concerned when pressure is being applied. The highest force will occur either when the patient is standing or when the brace is applying forces to the patient to stretch the leg muscles. The highest force will vary from patient to patient however an estimate of the force needed to stretch the leg muscles is no more than three times the body weight of the child. This gives a maximum force of 108 kg.

A thin film force sensitive resistor can meet the design requirements. This sensor was chosen because it has a thickness of 0.2 mm, high durability, and low cost. The ability of the sensor to detect small forces, indicating the patient is sitting, versus large forces, indicating the child is standing, will require the sensor to give a measurement within approximately 0 to 5 kg of the actual force. This can be achieved because the sensor has a repeatability of 2.5%, a hysteresis of 4.5%, a linearity of 5%, and a temperature error of 0.36% / °C.

The angle of the foot relative to the leg is an important measurement in the therapy. The objective is to stretch the leg so that the range in foot angle of the patient will match the range of a person who does not have spastic diplegia. Currently the angle of the foot is measured during visits to the therapist using a goniometer. The active boot will track the angle for active control of the boot. Furthermore, the availability of this data over time greatly enhances the physical therapist's insight into the ankle behavior. This information will give a more accurate picture of the patient's progress and can be used in future diagnosis.

An angle measurement sensor needs to be constrained to planar motions. Since the ankle joint can move with three degrees of freedom, the boot needs to measure a planar movement containing the calf and foot. In addition to this, the brace itself should be designed to limit rotation of the foot to only one axis. For this application, the range of angles is between -10° to +10°.

Finally, in order to meet the design objective for comfort, the sensor should be as small as possible and easily attached to the boot. Potentiometers provide a simple solution that meets the design objectives. This results in resistive elements for both the pressure sensor and the angle measurement sensor. The use of resistive elements provides for easy interface with a system microcontroller.

In order to provide a boot that can adapt to different patient requirements and support a wearable device, an embedded programmable controller is required. The system microcontroller has two modes: serial casting and therapeutic stretching. In the serial casting mode, a desired angle is maintained until the force sensor detects that the foot is supporting a load, such as walking. The boot then allows flexure of the angle by the patient to facilitate walking. Once, the boot comes to rest, the desired angle for stretching the calf muscles is restored. In home therapy mode, a therapy sequence can be initiated when the patient is at rest. The boot is slowly cycled through a stretching exercise that has been set by the physical therapist. The safety functions of the boot system require a fast monitoring rate, so there will be no muscle damage. However, a high speed microcontroller is not required. The Parallax BS2-IC microcontroller was selected for development of a prototype rehabilitation boot based on familiarity with the device, no need for numerous I/O pins, cost and ease of programming.

3.3 Rehabilitative Boot Conclusions

Bench testing of the boot proved that the proposed actuator is sufficient for the stretching task. However, the prototype achieved a range of motion of 8-10 degrees short of the device goal of +/- 10 degrees. This discrepancy can be accounted for by changes to the actuator and boot geometry. Furthermore, heat generated by the actuator presents safety concerns which are being addressed.

Overall, it can be concluded that the concept of a wearable active rehabilitative boot is feasible. Continuation of the project will model and test candidate materials with and without embedded sensors.

4. Physical Therapy Robot Study

As stated earlier, there have been instances of motivational robots in physical therapy. However, it does not appear that the design of robot activities has been designed as a tool for the pediatric physical therapist. Therfore, motivational robot sessions were investigated by reprogramming commercially available robots to perform some standard therapy routines and instructing children to mimic the robots actions. These robots were designed for children who suffer from Cerebral Palsy. It should be noted that these children tend to have more physical difficulties. Everyday activities such as walking, crawling, or stretching are a struggle for these children. A child's physical impairments can lead to a low perception of self-efficacy and self-competence due to having difficulties engaging in play activities (Miller and Reid, 2003). To address these issues, proposed therapy routines for CP patients will focus on walking, stretching, and positive reinforcement for motivation.

After preliminary interviews with pediatric physical therapists, it was revealed that therapists often have difficulty keeping a child's attention during physical therapy sessions. Furthermore, they often have difficulty persuading the child to perform his or her required exercises. The goal of this project is to fully create, program, and implement therapy routines using the Sony AIBO robotic dog (model ERS-220) focused on the needs of Cerebral Palsy and Autism patients in the age range of 3 to 12. More specifically, the robotic dog will be used to improve children's motor skills and social interactions during physical therapy sessions.

The group has thoroughly investigated several pediatric disorders and found that both Autism and Cerebral Palsy (CP) will benefit most from AIBO's capabilities. Therapists and professionals were consulted to aid in developing several proposal routines that can be programmed into AIBO and implemented during therapy sessions. These proposals consist of motivational games, stretches, exercises, and social activities designed to enhance the current sessions. The Sony AIBO, a robotic dog, was chosen as prototype due to its vast capabilities, intricate programmability, and its highly sophisticated components. The autonomous robot is fully programmable and responds to its surroundings. Its performance is enhanced with colorful LEDs and the ability to play music and sound clips.

A user friendly interface will ensure ease of use for the therapist and parents. Overall, the project hopes to aid children suffering from these diseases by improving their physical, cognitive, and social skills, all while enhancing their overall well-being.

4.1 Physical Therapy Robot Activity Design Concept

The physical therapist centered design methodology was implemented using seven design criteria. These criteria required the final designs to: 1) be within AIBO's physical capabilities, 2)correspond with the desired age group, 3) address a pertinent or common physical, cognitive, or emotional problem, 4) have a high predicted effectiveness, 5) be relatively simple to program, 6) pose no risk of harm to the child, and 7) be easy to evaluate the effectiveness. These criteria wereapplied to activities targeting two distinct populations of children: children with autism and children with cerebral palsy. The proposed therapy routines for autistic children focus on speech, interaction, and play. The proposed therapy routines for cerebral palsy patients will focus on walking, stretching, and positive reinforcement for motivation.

Under the guidance of professional therapists, several Autism routines have been developed and each evaluated based on the seven feasibility criteria described above. One proposed activity is a voice activation game in which the child can command the dog to perform a certain action such as "sit," "stand," "move forward," "walk right," etc. Children with Autism typically have trouble asking questions or with speech in general. This will encourage the child to not only speak, but also ask a question or make a command. The child will be further motivated to play with AIBO when he or she sees AIBO successfully perform the desired action.

Another proposed activity is a game that involves throwing and kicking AIBO's pink ball (a special ball that comes with the robot). The child will gently throw or kick the ball to AIBO and the robot will locate the ball and kick it back to the child. This activity could involve more than one child to further encourage social interaction for the Autistic child.

The last activity is a sensory exercise that utilizes AIBO's pressure sensors. Autistic children often cannot distinguish between touching something hard and touching it lightly. This activity begins with the therapist (or adult) telling the child to touch one of AIBO's buttons "hard." If the child touches lightly and lifts his or her finger, AIBO will shake his head "no" and the child can try again. If the child succeeds, AIBO performs a celebration dance.

Several routines for cerebral palsy patients were developed. The first routine is a game that will be used to motivate children to walk. Most cerebral palsy patients have trouble walking and many patients do not have any motivation or desire to try to walk. To address this, AIBO can be programmed to walk in front of the child a set distance (approximately 1 meter). AIBO will then turn around and face the child. The robot will use its distance sensor to determine whether the child has walked closer (within ¾ of a meter from AIBO). Next, AIBO will complete a celebration dance if the child succeeds or sit and wait until the child does. This process can be repeated the desired number of times as specified by the therapist or parent.

To aid the cerebral palsy patient in his or her stretches, a "Follow the Leader" set of activities is proposed. This set of activities will involve AIBO performing a stretch and the child mimicking the robot for the desired number of repetitions as specified by the therapist. One example stretch is referred to as the "Airplane," which requires the child to lie on his or her stomach. The child will then lift all four limbs into the air. This stretches and works the abdominal muscles and is often recommended for cerebral palsy patients (see Figures 5 and 6). Other proposed mimicking activities include arm extensions, balancing, hamstring curls, leg extensions, sitting up tall, pushups, rolling over, and stair climbing.

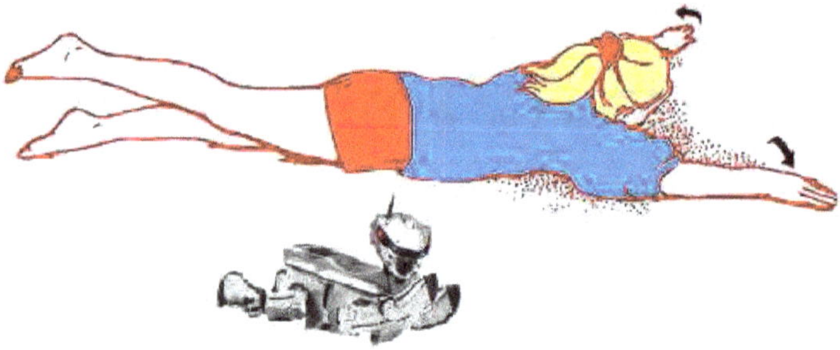

Fig. 5. A physical therapy document showing the airplane stretch along with the robot implementation.

An important aspect of the robotic therapy tool is ease of use for the therapist. A colorful user interface with detailed directions and an instructional computer program ensure that the therapist can perform the desired routine without delaying a therapy session (see Figure 7). Each routine can be accessed by pressing a combination of colored buttons on AIBO's back side. For instance, to instruct AIBO to perform the leg extension activity, the user must simply push the blue button and then the red button.

Evaluations of the project will be based on each child's level of motivation to participate in the activity, overall emotional effect that the activity has on the child, and the child's performance and overall improvement when completing a routine.

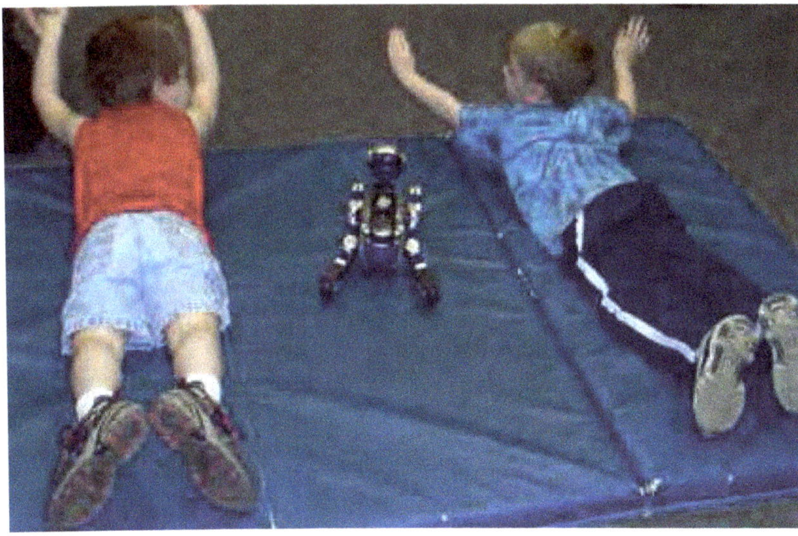

Fig. 6. Children Performing Airplane Stretch with AIBO.

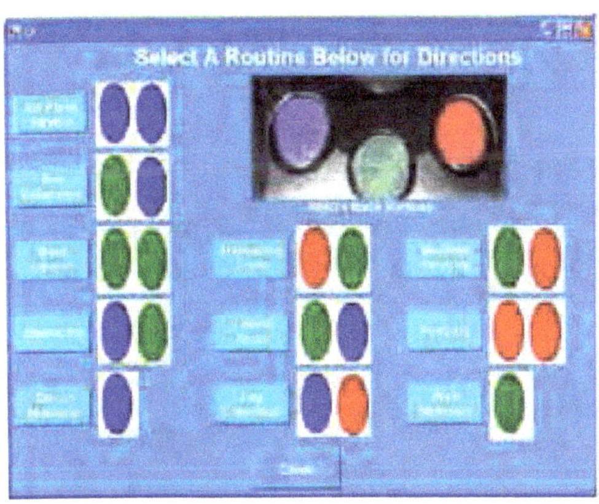

Fig. 7. Color code routine selection designed for therapist use.

4.2 Physical Therapy Robot Testing

After selecting various routines to be implemented, several programming designs were created for each routine. Smooth, human-like movements were desirable for each routine. When determining the best program design, robot positioning and stability were considered. This initial testing ensured that AIBO would remain stable throughout the routines and would look life-like to the users.

Pilot testing was conducted for the cerebral palsy routines during therapy sessions at a preschool, which is designed for children ages three to five with various developmental delays. Half of the test population at the preschool were typically developed. Testing was conducted by a physical therapist familiar with the project who also evaluating the robotic tool. Five groups were tested for 10-15 minute sessions. The sessions were video taped. A second set of sessions was performed a month after the first.

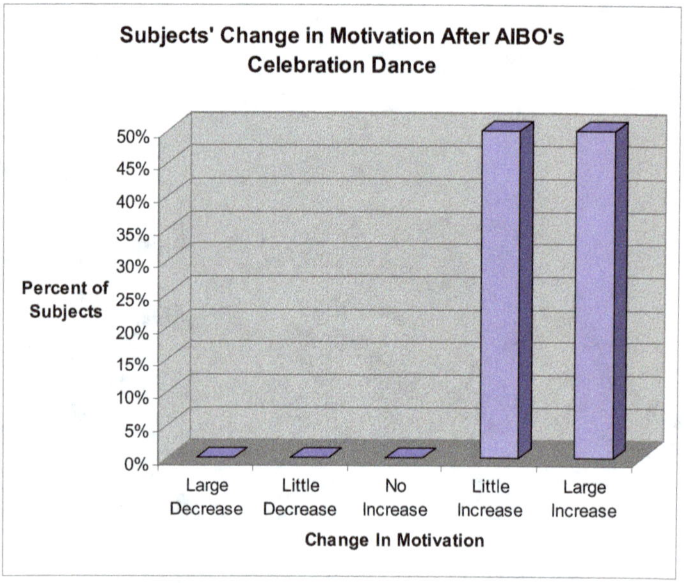

Fig. 8. Pilot study results regarding motivation.

Therapist evaluation of the tool was collected with a survey. Furthermore, video tape of the sessions were reviewed for visual cues. Results presented in Figure 8 and Figure 9 include a increased willingness to imitate body positions and a high level of enthusiasm for all participants. Most participants correctly mimicked the robot movements. In exercises that separately moved limbs on the right and left, some participants moved the wrong limb. Participants that were exposed to the robot therapy a second time did not lose motivation or enthusiasm with the second exposure.

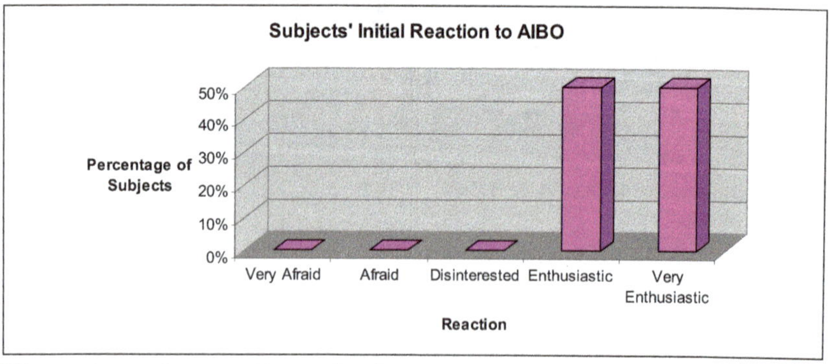

Fig. 9. Pilot study results regarding enthusiasm.

3.3 Physical Therapy Robot Conclusions

Programming a robot to aid pediatric physical therapists provides an effective tool for the therapist. The programmable platform can be used to provide an alternate method of performing existing therapy tasks. A robotic solution provides a tool that can be applied to a wide range of patients with little set up time. Further studies need to be conducted in order to test the long term effects in therapy.

4. Final Conclusions

The results of the two studies provide evidence that there are wide ranging opportunities in the area of pediatric rehabilitation for the application of robotic platforms. Two very different platforms were presented addressing two distint therapy outcomes. In both cases, the inclusion of rehabilitation professionals was essential in the deign of the device or activity. System design considerations need to be based on direct therapy goals and robotic systems need to be evaluated on medical outcomes.

5. References

Matthews, D.J. and Wilson, P., Cerebral Palsy. *Pediatric Rehabilitation,* 3rd ed., G. E. Molnar and M. A. Alexander, Ed. Philadelphia: Hanley & Belfus, 1999, pp. 193-217.

Styer-Acevedo, J., Physical Therapy for the Child with Cerebral Palsy. *Pediatric Physical Therapy,* 3rd ed., J. S. Tecklin, Ed. Philadelphia: Lippincott Williams & Wilkins, 1999, pp. 107-162.

Sawicki, G. S., Domingo, A., and Ferris, D. (2006) The effects of powered ankle-foot orthoses on joint kinematics and muscle activation during walking in individuals with incomplete spinal cord injury. *Journal of Neuroengineering and Rehabilitation,* Vol. 3, 1743-0003 (Electronic)

Burgar, C.G., Lum, P. S., Shor, P.C., and Van der Loos, H.F.M. (2000) Development of robots for rehabilitation therapy: The Palo Alto VA/Stanford experience. *Journal of Rehabilitation Research and Development,* Vol . 37 No . 6 (November/December 2000), 663-673, 03425282.

Merians, A.S., Jack, D., Boian, R., Tremaine, M., Burdea, G.C., Adamovich, S.V., Recce, M., and Poizner, H. (2002) Virtual Reality-Augmented Rehabilitation for Patients Following Stroke. *Physical Therapy,* Vol. 82 No. 9 (September 2002), 898-915, 00319023

Plaisant , C., Druin, A., Lathan, C., Dakhane, K., Edwards, K., Maxwell Vice, J., and Montemayor, J. (2000) A Storytelling Robot for Pediatric Rehabilitation. Proceedings *of ASSETS'00: The Fourth International ACM SIGCAPH Conference on Assistive Technologies,* pp. 50-55, 1-58113-314-8, Arlington, Virginia, November, 2000, ACM, New York.

Michaud, F., Duquett, A. and Nadeau, I. (2003) Characteristics of Mobile Toys for Children with Pervasive Developmental Disorders. *Proceedings of IEEE International Conference on Systems, Man and Cybernetics, Vol.3,* pp. 2938-2943, 0-7803-7952-7, Washington, D.C., Ocotober, 2003, IEEE, Piscataway, NY

Michaud, F., Laplante, J-F., Larouche, H., Duquette, A., Caron, S., Letourneau, C. and Masson, P. (2004) Autonomous Spherical Mobile Robot for Child Development Studies. 34(4) (2004) 1-10. , *IEEE Transactions on Systems, Man and Cybernetics, Part A,* Vol. 35, No. 4 (July 2005), 471- 480, 1083-4427

Park, E. S., Park, C. I., Chang, H. J., Choi, J. E. and Lee, D.S. (2004) The effect of hinged ankle-foot orthoses on sit-to-stand transfer in children with spastic cerebral palsy. *Archives of physical medicine and rehabilitation,* Vol. 85, No. 12 (December 2004), 2053-2057, 0003-9993

Blaya, J. A. and Herr, H., (2004) Adaptive Control of a Variable-Impedance Ankle-Foot Orthosis to Assist Drop-Foot Gait. *IEEE Trans. Neural Systems and Rehabilitation Engineering,* Vol. 12, No. 1 (March 2004), 24-31, 1534-4320

Herr, H. M. and Kornbluh, R. D. (2004) New horizons for orthotic and prosthetic technology: artificial muscle for ambulation. *Proceedings of SPIE -- Volume 5385 Smart Structures and Materials 2004: Electroactive Polymer Actuators and Devices,* pp. 1-9, 2004, pp. 1-9 , 07393717, San Diego, CA, March 2004,

Miller, S. and Reid, D. (2003) Doing Play: Competency, Control, and Expression. *Cyber Physiology and Behavior, Vol.* 6, No. 6 (December 2003): 623-630, 10649506

8

Cyberthosis™: Rehabilitation Robotics With Controlled Electrical Muscle Stimulation

Patrick Métrailler, Roland Brodard, Yves Stauffer, Reymond Clavel & Rolf Frischknecht
Fondation Suisse pour les Cyberthèses, Monthey, Switzerland
Laboratoire de Systèmes Robotiques, EPFL, Lausanne, Switzerland
Unité de Neuroréhabilitation, CHUV, Lausanne, Switzerland

1. Introduction

Each year, following an accident or illness, over 200 new cases of paraplegia occur in Switzerland, and 1000 in France. This makes 7'000, respectively 40'000 para-tetraplegic patients in these countries. Since the Second World War, methods available for the treatment of medullar trauma at the moment of lesion, and for re-education, have evolved considerably. Nowadays, these methods allow in around 80% of medullar injuries, limitation of the damage to a partial lesion of the spinal cord. Unfortunately, only 10% of these patients ever recover autonomous walking [Zäch G.A., 2000].

Today paraplegics often benefit from walking re-education programmes on treadmills. Two, occasionally three physiotherapists are required to mobilise the patient's legs and pelvis. Unfortunately this work is extremely hard on the staff, and the movements are difficult to reproduce and obviously non-quantifiable. These manual treatments are slowly being replaced by robotic rehabilitation [Reinkensmeyer et al., 2004], much more capable of providing the repetitive and precise exercises demanded by modern methods. However, in cases where residual voluntary capacity is absent, or where there is muscular atrophy, the movements made are purely passive. The Cyberthosis Project presented below, allows active re-education, and preliminary testing has confirmed its great efficacy.

2. Cyberthosis Project

An orthosis is a device intended to correct or improve a deficient function or compensate for incapacity of a part of the body - trunk, member or segment of a member. A hybrid orthosis has the addition of one or several motors and sensors. The latter serves as a mechanical interface with the patient and allow the measurement of a limb's position, as well as the force generated by the subject. Its motors assist or resist the movement according to the therapy being applied. A new dimension has appeared with cyberthosis, this being a hybrid orthosis assisted by controlled neuromuscular electrostimulation.

Initiated by the Fondation Suisse pour les Cyberthèses (FSC), the Cyberthosis Project aims to combine closed-loop electrical muscle stimulation with motorised orthoses. This innovative concept not only allows automation of the treatment, but also an active participation of the patient's muscles. From this concept new devices have been developed in a general re-

education process where recovery of walking did not feature as the only aim. It also integrated the benefits of electro-stimulated physical activity within an improvement to the quality of life for sufferers from medullar trauma and hemiplegics [Takahashi & Reinkensmeyer, 2003] through the reduction of complications due to immobilisation of the lower limbs.
The benefits of such treatment are obvious for the patient, but also for physiotherapists by releasing them from difficult and repetitive mobilisations.
The philosophy of Cyberthosis is founded on treatment in three stages. A dedicated re-education device corresponds to each phase; they are described in part 3, 4 and 5 of this chapter.

2.1 Medullar lesion

Medullar lesion is the result of an injury to the spinal cord. Its origin is usually traumatic, but it can also originate from an illness or an anomaly in the development such as discal hernia, tumour and spina bifida for example. The term paraplegic covers patients with paralysis of the lower limbs (dorsal, lumber or sacral lesions) as well as quadriplegics with paralysis of the four limbs (cervical lesions). Most patients with para- or quadriplegia have to get about in wheelchairs, but this is only the most visible consequence [Maury, 1981], [Grundy et al., 2002]. Several deficiencies, often hidden, result from the paralysis. At motor system level, these complications can be cardiovascular (adaptation to effort), muscular (atrophy), articular (limited movements), osseous (osteoporosis) and sensory. The resulting physical condition in these patients is insufficient for the recuperation of walking. The active muscular participation of the patient [Fitzwater, 2002] as well as their verticalisation [Postans et al., 2003], (basic principles of the Cyberthosis concept), permits the reduction of these secondary effects and in certain cases of incomplete lesions, to regain voluntary mobility.

2.2 CLEMS™[1]

CLEMS™ (Closed Loop Electrical Muscle Stimulation) is one of the basic principles of the Cyberthosis concept.
The benefits of the addition of functional electrical stimulation (FES) to mobilisation have been shown for the last 10 years [Frischknecht & Chantraine, 1989], [Belanger et al., 2000], [Rushton, 2003]. FES is used to stimulate the recuperation of a certain voluntary activity, especially in cases of incomplete paraplegia, as well as to reduce muscular atrophy and spasticity. To maximise the chances of recuperation, controlled electro-induced contractions are essential. They allow the respect of coherence between movement and the proprioceptive impulses generated by the muscular-tendinous system (Golgi apparatus and neuromuscular spindles). Information about amplitude and position supplied to the nervous system during a movement resembles as closely as possible to that produced by muscular contractions observed during a voluntary movement.
Classical FES, as it is open loop, is capable of following the activation sequences of muscles concerned in a movement. However, it is unable to adapt its intensity during the execution of the movement. A closed-loop control of the FES is therefore necessary to accomplish complex and repetitive movements such as the leg-press, pedalling, or walking in a similar manner to that produced naturally. Thus, CLEMS technology allows the closest possible reproduction of the kinematics and dynamics of natural movements. This can have considerable impact on the plasticity of the nervous system at both spinal and cerebral levels.

---

1 Cyberthosis™, CLEMS™, StimMaker™, MotionMaker™, WalkTrainer™ and WalkMaker™ are commercial trade marks belonging to the Swiss Foundation for Cyberthosis

2.3 The Cyberthosis devices

The aim of research conducted for the Cyberthosis project is the re-education of paraplegic and hemiplegic patients; ideally as soon as possible after stabilisation of the acute phase so as to avoid muscular atrophy, but also during the chronic phase. For this, a process in three stages has been evolved.

MotionMaker™ is the first element in the process of rehabilitation [Schmitt et al., 2004a]; it is described in part 3 of this chapter. The patient's limbs can be mobilised passively or work actively in an electro-stimulated manner and/or voluntarily against resistance loads created by the motors. The aim of MotionMaker is to treat patients as quickly as possible, so as to limit the effects of an absence of movement. This means maintaining, or increasing muscular volume and capacity for patients in the chronic phase, to reinstate mobility of the joints, to train cardiac capacity and prevent neurological osteoporosis.

Once the subject has successfully completed training on MotionMaker, and attained sufficient physical condition, re-education of the motor patterns for over-ground walking can begin using the mobile device WalkTrainer™. This device is presented in part 4 of this chapter. Equipped with orthoses for the legs and pelvis, body weight support, and with CLEMS, this system allows near perfect mimicking of walking movements with the aim of stimulating nervous system plasticity.

WalkMaker™ is the third cyberthosis. This is a walking assistance device using CLEMS type electrostimulation. It offers people who have not regained sufficient walking autonomy with WalkTrainer, a functional orthotic gait [Goldfarb et al., 2003].

3. MotionMaker™

It consists of a couch and two orthoses enabling a controlled movement of the hip, knee, and ankle joints. The feet move in arcs parallel to the sagittal plane.

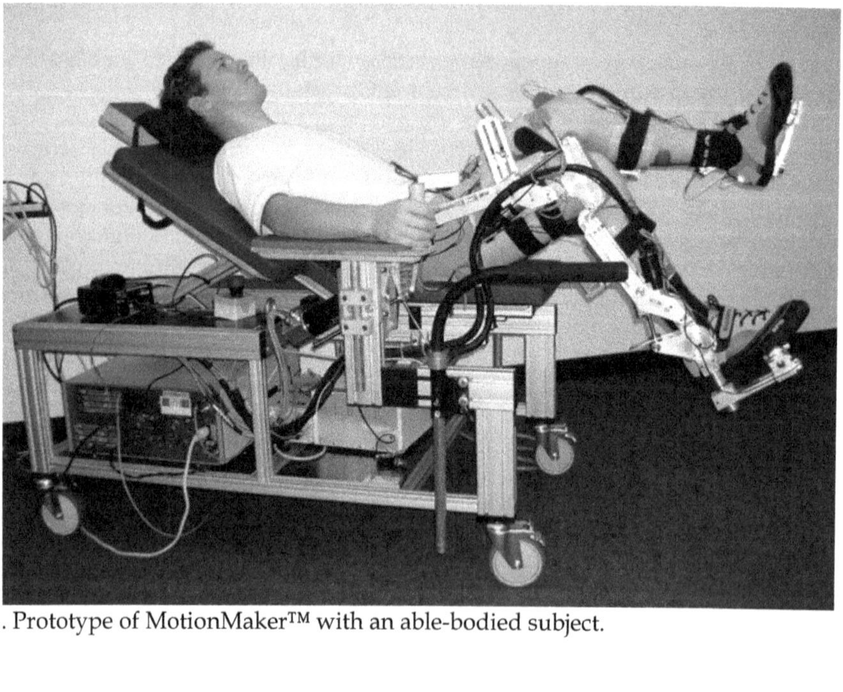

Fig. 1. Prototype of MotionMaker™ with an able-bodied subject.

MotionMaker is marketed by SWORTEC SA, a company dedicated to production and commercialization of the methods developed by the FSC.

3.1. An innovative concept

What is new about MotionMaker is essentially the coupling between the motorised orthoses, and the electrostimulation with closed-loop control. Each joint is motorised and equipped with sensors of position and articular moment. The sensors provide the control unit with the necessary information for the real-time adjustment of the electrical stimulation (CLEMS), during the execution of the movement. This adjustment takes into account the forces developed by the effect of electrostimulation, as well as the voluntary efforts made by the patients themselves. The aim of this control is to attain the level of force prescribed by the practitioner at the beginning of the exercise. According to the patient's muscular participation, the motors either assist or resist the movement. This allows active training throughout the articular range even in cases of great physical deficiency.

3.2. Technical description

The articulations of the orthosis are based on the principle of the variable length connecting rod and crank as shown in Fig. 2.
This type of orthotic joint allows the non-linear physiological curve of moment to be followed, according to the articular angle, and thus optimisation of the actuators' size. Calculation of the articular moments is made through the force sensors measuring axial amplitude in the actuator screw.

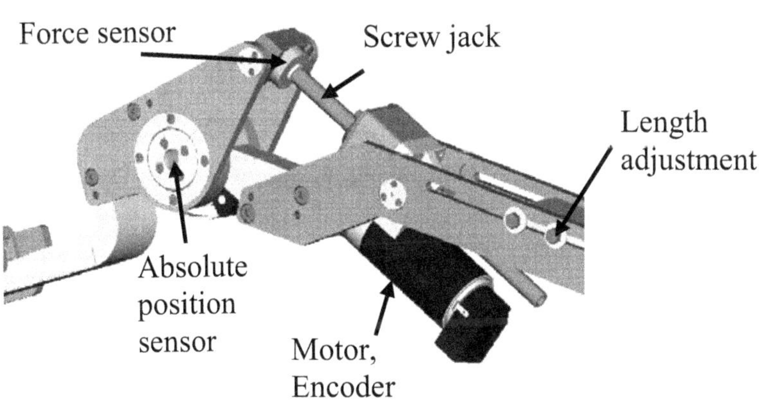

Fig. 2. Details of a MotionMaker joint.

Geometrical alignment between the robot and the patient's legs is ensured by adjustment to the length of the orthosis segments.
A dedicated electrostimulator has been developed to attain the performance required by the CLEMS control. The StimMaker™ has 20 channels of stimulation and allows modification of the electrostimulation parameters on 20 muscles with a reaction time of 0.5ms per channel.
Two systems are monitored on MotionMaker: the orthosis and the leg. Both being rigidly linked, their respective control loops must be uncoupled so that each system has its own physical

quantity to adjust. The choice is based on verification of the robot's position, and on the force of the legs. The CLEMS algorithm calculates the articular moments corresponding to the force prescribed at the level of the foot, or gets them from the initial instruction for a purely articular movement. The CLEMS algorithm uses these moments to define which muscles are to be stimulated, and then adjusts the amplitude of stimulation current supplied to these muscles throughout the movement. The stimulation technique is carried out by surface electrodes.
The comparison between the prescribed moments and those measured on the orthosis allows the adjustment of the electrostimulation but also the detection of disruptive elements such as spasms and clonus. In fact, electrostimulation and mobilisation can encourage involuntary reflex contractions that in certain patients can be considerable. To ensure the safety of the patient during an exercise, the system behaves in a carefully programmed manner following detection of a spasm. MotionMaker reacts to interrupt this spasm by reducing stimulation current, and lessening the osteo-tendinous constraints engendered by a compliant adjustment of the orthosis.

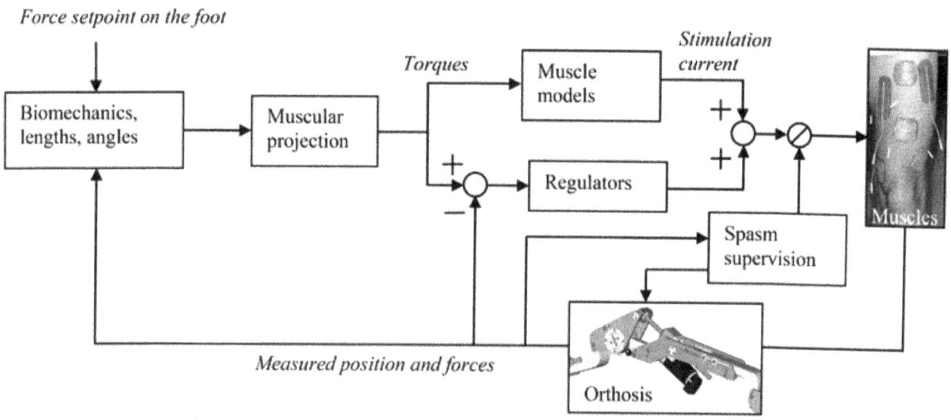

Fig. 3. Diagram of the CLEMS electrostimulation control unit.

3.3 Pilot clinical study

After having evaluated CLEMS with paraplegic patients using a simple knee orthosis [Schmitt et al., 2004b], the algorithm was tested using MotionMaker on able-bodied subjects [Metrailler et al., 2006a] with a leg-press type movement of extension-flexion. The results being satisfactory, a pilot clinical study was carried out [Metrailler et al., 2006b].
5 paraplegic patients (with lesions over 4 years old) - 4 with incomplete lesions and 1 with a complete lesion - conducted training sessions of 60 minutes on MotionMaker, 2 to 3 times a week over 2 months. The movements were leg-press type with alternate stimulation of the extensor muscles (Gluteus Maximus, Quadriceps and Gastrocnemius) and the flexors (Hamstrings and Tibialis Anterior). The principal aims of these tests were:

1. To confirm the inoffensiveness of the device.
2. To evaluate the possibility of carrying out controlled movements with paraplegic patients,
3. To confirm the possibility of increasing voluntary force and electro-induced force of subjects with incomplete medullar lesions,
4. To study the effect of movements with CLEMS on spasticity.

3.4 Results

All subjects were able to complete the whole training, there was no drop out. None of the participants felt unsafe at any time during the training sessions and they all appreciated the safety features of the MotionMaker™.

Fig. 4 shows the position of the patient during leg-press exercises. The patient is lying in dorsal decubitus position and pushes or pulls on his feet on a horizontal movement. Torque is measured on each joint and the resulting forces on the feet are obtained through biomechanical calculus.

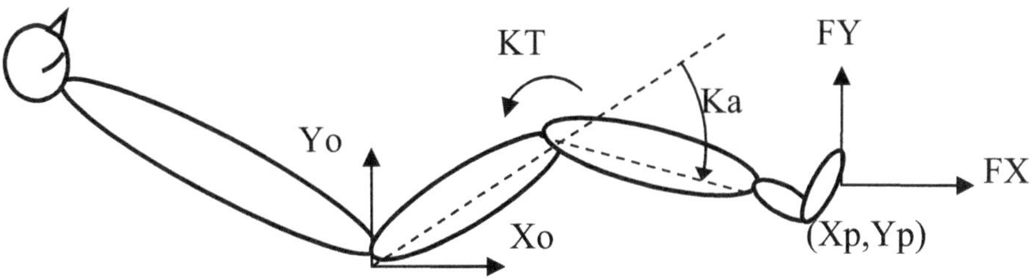

Fig. 4. Position of the foot (Xp, Yp), angle of the knee (Ka) and torque at the knee (KT).

The result of controlling the electro-induced force during extension and flexion of a leg-press exercise with a completely paraplegic patient is presented in the following diagrams. Fig. 5 (a) shows the X position of the foot (Xp), the horizontal force setpoint (FXs) and measured (FXm), the vertical force measures (FYm). The vertical setpoint force stays constant at 0N, the vertical (Yp) position remaining constant. Fig. 5 (b) shows the effects of theses forces on the foot at knee level. There one finds the torques setpoint (KTs) and measured (KTm), the angle (Ka) and the stimulation current of the quadriceps (KSc). It should be noted that the great differences between setpoint and measured values are due to saturation of the stimulation current at 70mA for safety reasons.

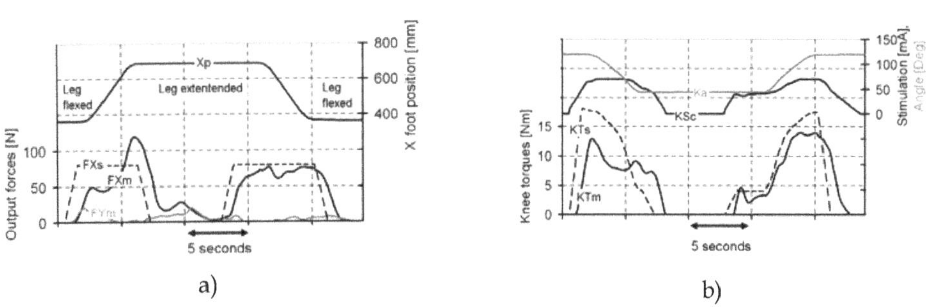

Fig. 5. a) Extension and flexion, with the position of the foot (Xp), the command force (FXs) the measured forces (FXm) horizontal and (FYm) vertical. b) Torques setpoint (KTs) and corresponding measurements at the knee (KTm), angle of the knee (Ka) and stimulation current of the quadriceps (KSc).

Through these measurements, it has been demonstrated that the force resulting from several muscular contractions can be controlled in amplitude and in direction and that the CLEMS algorithm is judicious.

During mobilisation exercises with CLEMS stimulation and voluntary force, the subjects with incomplete lesions experienced greater awareness in their limbs than when doing purely voluntary exercises. This increase in sensation seems to be due to better stimulation of the proprioceptive receptors with CLEMS stimulation. Thus, they could develop greater voluntary force with electric stimulation. The improvement in perception of their limbs enabled them also to increase their purely voluntary force in the course of the exercises.

After the two months of training, all the subjects with incomplete lesions (P1, P2, P4 and P5) had more than doubled their voluntary force, without electrostimulation, on at least one leg. Fig. 6 shows the evolution of their average voluntary force by series of exercise, in % between the first and last sessions. This increase in performance can be explained by an improvement of muscular function, by improved function of the spinal motor system linked to the neuronal plasticity, to a central motor control improved by the reactivation of dormant motor patterns or by a combination of these three elements.

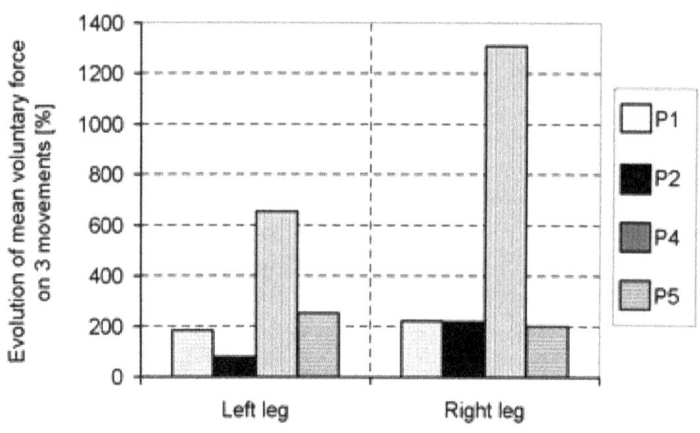

Fig. 6. Evolution, in % between the first and the last session, of the mean force developed voluntarily by the 4 incomplete paraplegic subjects, for the left and right legs, without electrical stimulation.

Fig. 7 shows the evolution of their average electro-induced force, in % between the first and last session. This increase in performance can be explained by an improvement of muscular function and by the increased stimulation current allowed by the patient's accommodation to electrical stimulation and the diminution of occurrence of spasms along the training program.

The activation of muscles in exercises of neurological re-education brings patients not only the recovery/conservation of good physical condition, but also the proprioceptive information essential for recovering the ability to activate of their own muscles. The example of patient P4 in our pilot study is particularly revealing. Fig. 8 shows the mean output power developed according to the type of exercise and the number of training sessions. The grey curve corresponds to the results of exercises with electrostimulation but without voluntary contribution, and the black curve shows the results of exercises with voluntary contribution but without electrostimulation.

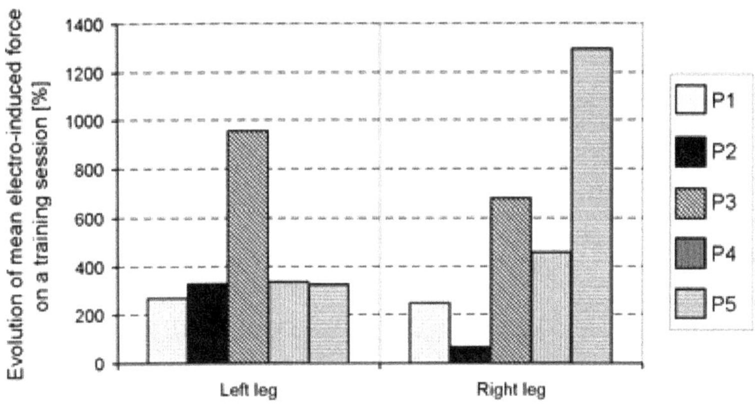

Fig. 7. Evolution, in % between the first and the last session, of the mean electro-induced force developed without voluntary participation, for the left and right legs.

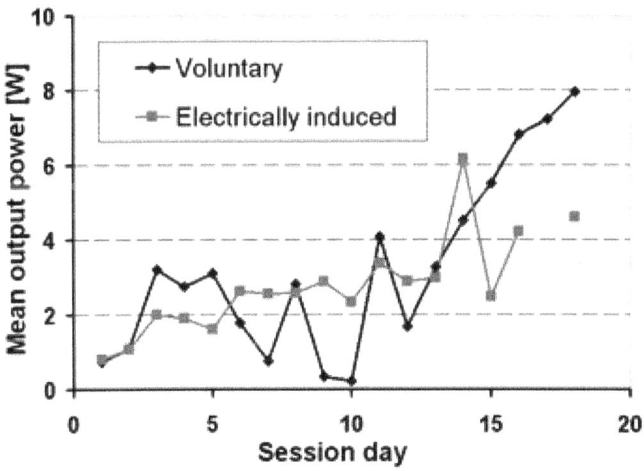

Fig. 8. Evolution of voluntary and electro-induced power for subject P4 in the clinical trial.

The evolution of voluntary force from session 10 shows a sudden and significant improvement in P4's voluntary power. This progress, being not related to the electrically induced evolution, tends to demonstrate the recovery of P4's motor pattern. This hypothesis was consolidated by the comments made by P4 concerning his capacity to use the muscles affected by his injury.

The mobilisation of the legs with electrostimulation has also had beneficial effects on the reduction of rigidity in the limbs due to hypertonia. Three of the five subjects were known to have considerable spasticity. Fig. 9 shows the evolution of mean spasticity measurements before and after each exercise session. The physiotherapists carried out manual mobilisations and graduated the resistance to movement according to the modified Ashworth Scale [Bohannon & Smith, 1987]. The reduction of spasticity lasted 2 to 3 hours after the session. This reduction was significant, hypertonia returning to levels close to those of able-bodied subjects, and it was felt to be most pleasant by the subjects concerned.

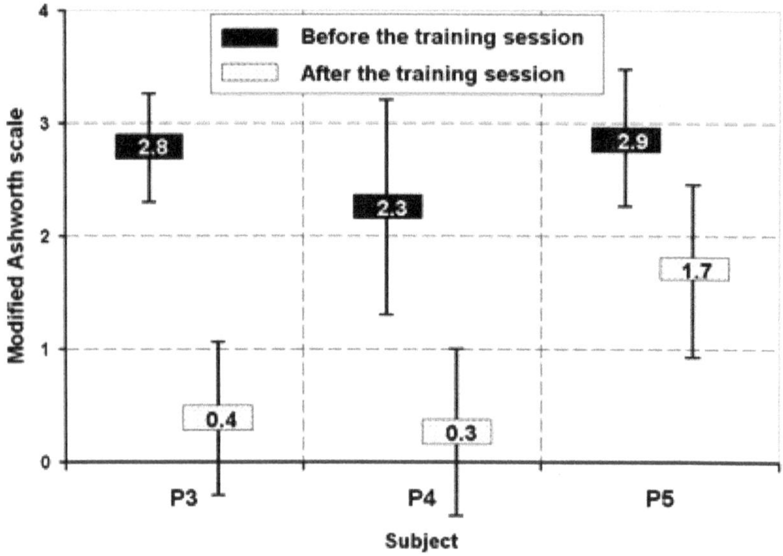

Fig. 9. Mean and standard deviation measures of spasticity before and after an exercise session.

4. WalkTrainer™

4.1. Concept

The technological developments and the promising results obtained from the clinical tests of MotionMaker, have led to the development of the second phase of the Cyberthosis project: WalkTrainer™.

The basic principle, namely closed-loop electrical muscle stimulation in conjunction with robotic assistance, is common to both these projects. The re-education of the walking motor patterns demands perfect emulation of the natural gait, which is why WalkTrainer offers training for over-ground walking. In fact, the kinematics and dynamics of the walking movement being different on a treadmill (modification of stride length [Dingwell et al., 2001] and of Electromyogram EMG [Arsenault et al., 2001]), the proprioceptive information differs. Motor patterns trained like this find themselves disrupted for over-ground walking. Locomotion with the subject moving in his environment, will not only stimulate the re-learning of over-ground walking functional motor patterns in the best possible way, but also its motivation, which constitutes an indispensable factor to the efficacy of re-education. Pelvic movement is essential to guarantee natural gait, which is why a pelvic orthosis was designed.

4.2. Components

WalkTrainer is composed of five mechatronic sub-assemblies that interact with the subject in two ways:

- Mechanically: the walking frame, the leg orthosis, the pelvic orthosis and the active suspension.
- Electrically: the CLEMS.

The main function of the walking frame is to follow the patient while moving. It serves as a mobile support for all the other components. Equipped with two differentially mounted wheels, it can operate in the plane and thus perfectly accomplish its task of following. Future versions will also have batteries on board to allow more freedom during training.

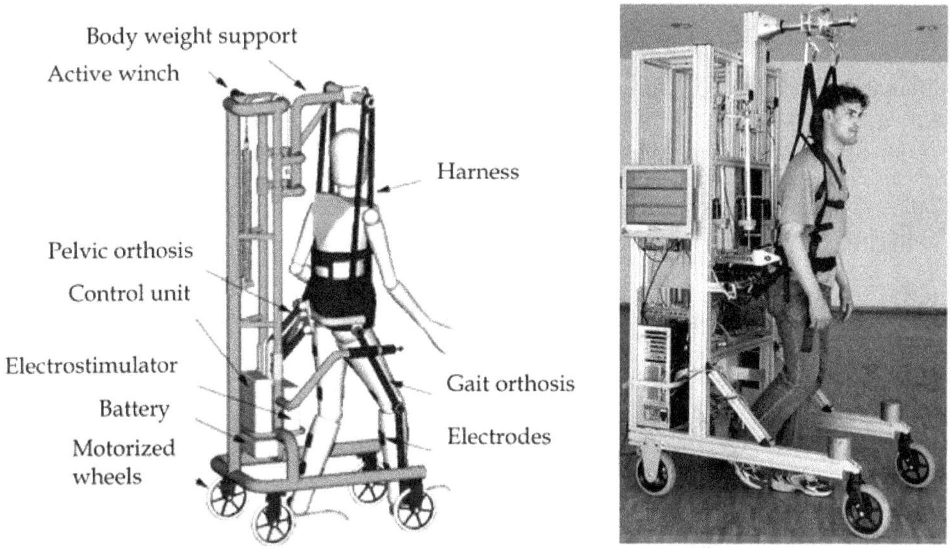

Fig. 10. a) Diagram of the principle of WalkTrainer™, b) partial execution with an able-bodied subject, without the leg orthosis.

The muscular condition of paraplegics, sometimes severe atrophy of the leg muscles, together with poor control of the postural muscles, must be taken into account. A harness allows controlled unloading of the legs, while supporting the patient's trunk. This suspension is termed 'active' as a motor combined with force and position sensors enable compensation of irregularities and force oscillations, due mainly to the preloaded spring and the different inertias at play.

The chosen kinematics for the pelvic orthosis is that of a parallel robot with six degrees of freedom. It is therefore possible for us to accompany the subject according to the three rotations and the three translations of space. The aim is to initiate the movements through the patient's pelvis and to guide it in a similar way to the work of a physiotherapist. The force sensors allow precise monitoring of the forces exerted on the subject. The work done by the pelvic orthosis is thus perfectly quantifiable, and can equally well be used in a diagnostic context.

The leg orthosis fulfils two functions of major importance. Firstly, positional measurement of the limbs of the subject is supplied in real time by the latter through the attached position sensors. The force the subject exerts on the orthosis is also measured by the force sensors. These two types of information are indispensable for the adjustment of the closed-loop muscular stimulation. Secondly, equipped with motors, the leg orthosis allows the patient's movements to be assisted.

The real-time muscular stimulator StimMaker, as described in 3.2 is also used with WalkTrainer. In this application the main muscles responsible for walking are targeted, i.e.:

Gluteus Maximus, Vastus Medialis, Vastus Lateralis, Rectus Femoris, Hamstrings, Tibialis Anterior and Gastrocnemius.

4.3. Global coordination

All the components described under section 4.2 must be coordinated to allow an interactive gait with the active participation of the subject, but without the latter being rushed by the machine.

Different strategies of co-ordination are envisaged. That currently employed consists of a master/slave relationship between the different components. The master component serves as a guiding element to the others. A logical choice for this function is the leg orthosis. In fact this latter is the keystone of CLEMS, thus of active re-education. Moreover, it includes all the necessary sensors for the measurement of the subject's activity (force and position). The master/slave relationship could therefore resemble that shown in Fig. 11.

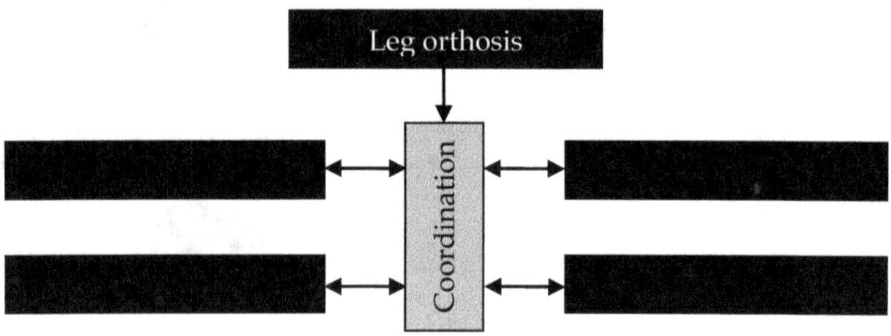

Fig. 11. Strategy of coordination between WalkTrainer's different components.

At the time of writing the leg orthosis was not available. However, an initial installation of the coordination strategy was set up. Instead of the leg orthosis, a footswitch placed under the subject's right leg served as the proprioceptive sensor to establish the position of the leg. Knowing the latter, it was possible to coordinate the movement of the pelvic orthosis with the subject's gait. The contact on the right heel was used to obtain two fundamental pieces of information: the frequency of steps and the phase difference between the legs and the pelvic orthosis. Knowledge of these two values then allows a trajectory of the pelvic orthosis guaranteeing synchronisation to be generated, under the condition that it does not rush the subject. This means that the synchronisation operates on a whole cycle and not instantaneously, which would induce acceleration that would be extremely unpleasant for the user.

The pelvic orthosis, Fig. 13, is able to guide the subject according to the six spatial degrees of freedom. These movements can be obtained with millimetric precision. However, to impose such movements in an inflexible way could generate great force on the subject, so to be considered negative, even counterproductive. It could thus be interesting to make the structure compliant in a controlled manner. One must however control these deviations exactly, and for this reason an algorithm allowing each degree of freedom in the orthosis to be made compliant independently and in a controlled manner, was installed.

This unit can be used to control interaction between the orthosis and the subjects so as not to rush them. Moreover, such an algorithm can be made progressive. It also allows the subject's progress to be evaluated. In fact, it is possible to adapt the compliance to the subject's evolution. If subjects follow good trajectories with a compliant controller, this means that they are capable of generating these trajectories themselves.

The basic principle of this algorithm is the calculation of return forces in the operational space (OP), then their projection into the articular space (ART). In this paragraph, we assume this process takes place around a fixed point, but the same reasoning remains valid for any trajectory.

The OP error of the pelvic orthosis is calculated, then converted into OP force (in the case of a spring : Force = k•error). This force is projected into the ART space by means of the Jacobian matrix of kinematical structure [Sciavicco & Siciliano, 2001]. Finally the ART forces are applied to the pelvic orthosis, as illustrated in Fig. 12. It then remains to measure the ART so as to calculate a new OP error and so on.

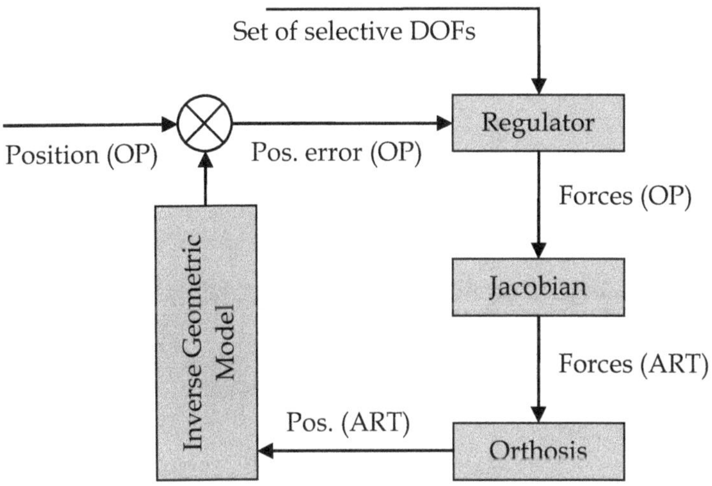

Fig. 12. Principle of selective compliance.

Initially static tests were carried out. A transverse force, Fig. 13, was applied to the orthosis and displacement in the operational space was measured.

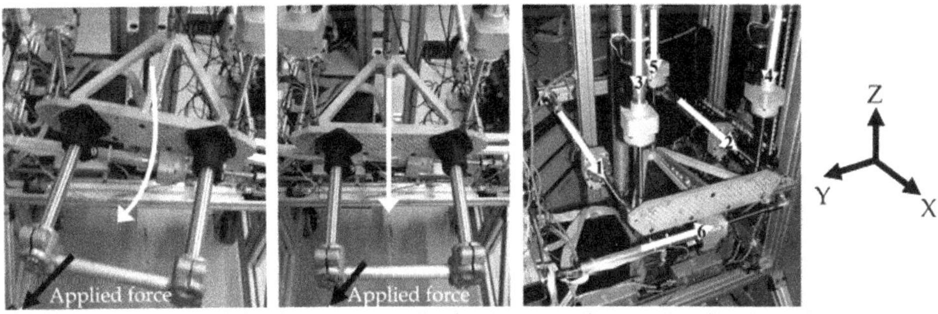

Fig. 13. Illustration of the functioning of selective compliance. Application of a transverse force with algorithm a) non-selective, b) selective, c) actuators responsible for advance (X) and rotation (Y).

In one case, Fig. 13(a), the advance axis (X) was made compliant in a non-selective manner by reducing the rigidity of the motors responsible for this translation. In the other case, Fig. 13(b), the advance axis (X) was made compliant in a selective manner. It can be clearly seen that with non-selective compliance, the translation (X) is added to by rotation around the vertical axis (Y). This originates from coupling of the translation (X) and the rotation (Y). The selective regulator however, guarantees a pure translation.

4.4. WalkTrainer and analysis of pelvic movement

WalkTrainer can also be used as a device for measuring pelvic movement for research or therapeutic purpose. To do this the addition of three sensors is necessary:

- An easyTrack200 6 axes sensor, which allows the real-time acquisition of the six degrees of freedom of the pelvis.
- A footswitch, which is placed under the subject's right heel. This signal is used to identify heel strike and lift and to compute the temporal measures in a repetitive gait cycle.
- Two potentiometric sensors, which link the subject to WalkTrainer, and actuate its servomechanism according to the subject's speed/position.

The easyTrack200 sensor is marketed by Atracsys SA. It enables, through an active tracer and linear cameras, the measurement of the 6 degrees of freedom of an object in space. A flexible pelvic belt, specially developed by an orthopaedist, is worn by the subject to carry the active tracer and also the mounting for the potentiometers, Fig. 14.

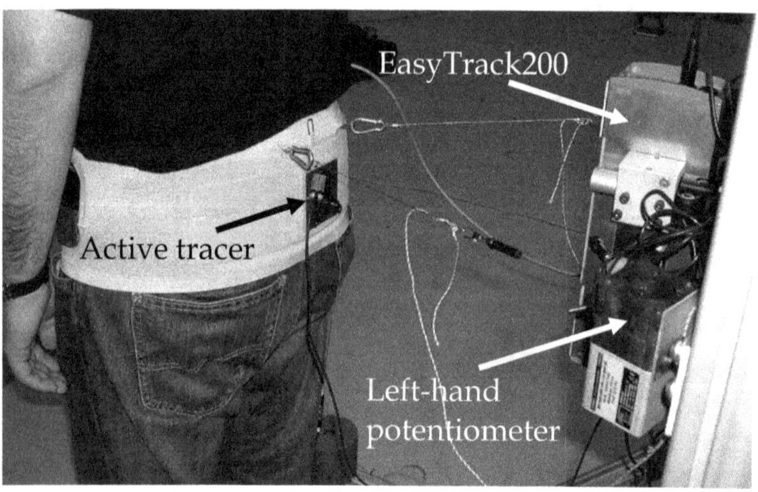

Fig. 14. Subject equipped for the measurement of pelvic movements.

Subjects then make two or three attempts at walking to familiarise themselves with the system. Then they repeat three series of measurements (1.4, 0.8 and 0.4m/s). A physiotherapist walking beside the patient governs the rate of travel, and WalkTrainer measures the effective speed. Several attempts may prove necessary before obtaining the desired walking speed. Each series takes place over a distance of around 20 metres and allows the acquisition of 15 walking cycles. The tracer's position relative to the pelvis is obtained through a calibration process.

The six degrees of freedom of the pelvis are thus measured, then processed with Matlab© using a graphic interface. Twenty people participated in the measuring campaign. These results will be used to generate trajectories for the pelvic orthosis based on a mathematical model including the walking speed and the patient's morphology, age, gender, etc. A typical vertical movement is shown in Fig. 15. The vertical line represents lifting of the right heel (~60% of the gait cycle). All the degrees of freedom are thus rapidly available in graphic form and in Excel© type files to facilitate analysis and exchange.

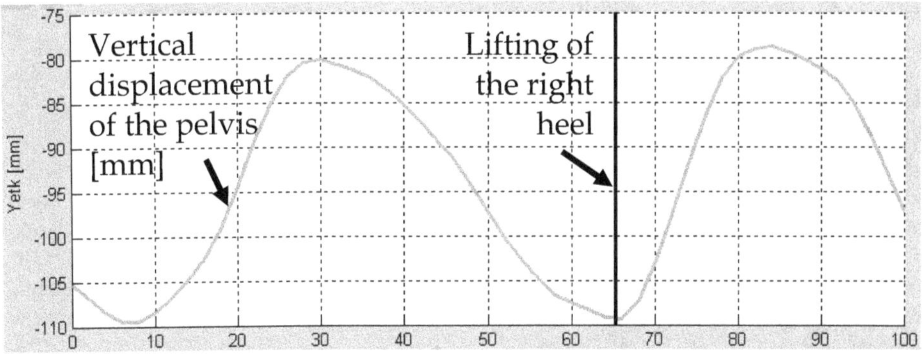

Fig. 15. Results of pelvic measurements, vertical displacement.

To enable the measurement of such movement it is essential to link WalkTrainer's position/speed to that of the subject by servo control. A special algorithm was developed for this task. It allows greater reactivity when necessary, while preventing the whole structure from following the slight oscillations of the pelvis according to the axis of advance.

5. WalkMaker™

5.1. Concept

WalkMaker™ will be a walk assisting cyberthosis using CLEMS type electrostimulation. The orthosis will serve as a mounting for the sensors required to control the electrostimulation, but will also have the function of helping and guiding the movements by active or passive actuators. It is intended for subjects who have not regained sufficient walking autonomy after exercising on WalkTrainer. These patients could benefit from WalkMaker to acquire a functional orthotic autonomous gait.

5.2 Challenges

The challenges in developing such a device are primarily mechanical. It has to provide sufficient rigidity to guide the limbs and pelvis, while also ensuring good compliance of certain degrees of freedom enabling smooth locomotion. The amount of guidance will be dependant on the neurological level of the lesion as well as the degree of paralysis.

The second challenge concerns the CLEMS electrostimulation which has to supply the basic energy of propulsion. The quality of control being directly linked to the quality of the muscular response obtained by training on MotionMaker and WalkTrainer, actuators mounted on the orthosis will probably have to filter the articular moments supplied by the muscles. Propulsion by the muscles and the use of a dynamic gait will permit reduced

energy consumption, be it electrical, pneumatic or other. Systems for recuperating energy during braking are also envisaged.
The final specification can only be established in terms of the results obtained with WalkTrainer. The main difficulty for this system is to propose an alternative at least as good as the wheelchair in functional terms, but also in terms of ease of use and implementation.

6. Conclusion

Cyberthosis brings a new approach to physical and neurological re-education. The patient regains his role as a protagonist in the movement, even if his voluntary mobility is reduced to nothing. This principle allows better emulation of the natural voluntary movements and so doing, places the patient in an ideal situation for relearning his motor patterns.
The first stage with MotionMaker has clearly shown the advantages of combining robotics and controlled electrostimulation to improve voluntary control. The activation of muscles in exercises of neurological re-education brings patients not only the recovery of muscle strength and joint mobility, but also the proprioceptive information essential for recovering the ability to activate by themselves their paralysed muscles. Training with WalkTrainer should allow one to go even further in the relearning of gait patterns by offering over-ground walking with controlled pelvic motion and muscle activity.

7. Acknowledgements

The Fondation Suisse pour les Cyberthèses would like to acknowledge the "Laboratoire de Système Robotique de l'Ecole Polytechnique Fédérale de Lausanne" as well as its associates for their scientific and technical support.
The FSC would also like to thank the "Loterie Romande" for its important financial help. The WalkTrainer™ project benefits from a grant made by the Swiss Innovation Promotion Agency, CTI Project N° 7485.2 LSPP-LS.

8. References

Arsenault, A.B., Winter, D.A. & Marteniuk, R.G. (1986). Treadmill Versus Walkway Locomotion in Humans: an EMG study. *Ergonomics*, Vol. 29, No. 5, 665-676

Belanger, M., Stein, R.B., Wheeler, G.D., Gordon, T. & Leduc, B. (2000). Electrical stimulation: Can it increase muscle strength and reverse osteopenia in spinal cord injured individuals? *Archives of Physical Medicine and Rehabilitation*, Vol. 81, No. 8, 1090-8.

Bohannon, R.W. & Smith, M.B. (1987). Interrater reliability of a modified Ashworth scale of muscle spasticity. *Physical Therapy*, Vol. 67, No. 2, 206-7

Dingwell, J.B., Cusumano, J.P., Cavanagh, P.R. & Sternad, D. (2001). Local Dynamic Stability Versus Kinematic Variability of Continuous Overground and Treadmill Walking. *Journal of Biomechanical Engineering*, Vol. 123, 27-32

Frischknecht, R. & Chantraine, A. (1989). Traitement de la spasticité par les agents physiques. *Annales de Réadaptation et de Médecine physique*, Vol. 32, 475-93

Fitzwater, R. (2002). A Personal View of FES Cycling. *Artificial Organs*, Vol. 26, No 3, 284-286

Goldfarb, M., Korkowsky, K., Harrold, B. & Durfee, W. (2003). Preliminary Evaluation of a Controlled-Brake Orthosis for FES-Aided Gait. *IEEE Transactions on Neural Systems and Rehabilitation Eengineering*, Vol. 11, No. 3, 241-8

Grundy, D., Tromans, A., Carvell, J. & Jamil, F. (2002). Medical management in the spinal injuries unit, In: *ABC of spinal cord injury*, Grundy, D. & Swain, A., 25-32, BMJ Books, London

Maury, M. (1981). *La paraplégie chez l'adulte et chez l'enfant*. Paris, Flammarion Médecine Sciences

Métrailler, P., Brodard, R., Frischknecht, R., Clavel, R. (2006a). Improvement of rehabilitation possibilities with the MotionMaker™. *Proceedings of Biobob2006, the first IEEE/RAS-EMBS international conference on biomedical robotics and biomechatronics*, Pisa, Italy

Métrailler, P., Brodard, R., Clavel, R., Frischknecht, R. (2006b). Closed loop electrical muscle stimulation in spinal cord injured rehabilitation. *Europa Medicophysica, Mediterranean Journal of Physical and Rehabilitation Medicine*, Vol. 42, 72-3

Postans, N.J., Malcolm, H.G., Hasler, J.P. & Douglas, J.M. (2003). FES augmented partial weight-gearing support treadmill training in acute incomplete SCI patients. *Proceedings of the 8th Conference of the International Functional Electrical Stimulation Society*, 135-37, Brisbane, Australia

Reikensmeyer, D.J., Emken, J.L., & Cramer, S.C. (2004). Robotics, Motor Learning, and Neurologic Recovery. *Annual Review of Biomedical Engineering*, Vol. 6, 497-525

Rushton, D.N. (2003). Functional Electrical Stimulation and rehabilitation - an hypothesis. *Medical Engineering & Physics*, Vol. 25, 75-78

Schmitt, C., Métrailler, P., Al-Khodairy, A., Brodard, R., Fournier, J., Bouri, M., Clavel, R. (2004a) The MotionMaker: a rehabilitation system combining an orthosis with closed-loop electrical muscle stimulation. *Proceedings of the 8th Vienna International Workshop in Functional Electrical Stimulation*, 117-20, Vienna, Austria

Schmitt, C., Métrailler, P., Al-Khodairy, A., Brodard, R., Fournier, J., Bouri, M., Clavel, R. (2004b). A study of a knee extension controlled by a closed loop functional electrical stimulation, *Proceedings of the 9th Conference of the International Functional Electrical Stimulation Society*, 135-37, Bournemouth, United Kingdom.

Sciavicco, L. & Siciliano, B. (2001) *Modelling and control of robot manipulators*, Springer-Verlag, New-York

Takahashi, C.D. & Reinkensmeyer, D.J. (2003) Hemiparetic stroke impairs anticipatory control of arm movement. *Experimental Brain Research*, Vol. 149, No 2, 131-40

Zäch, G.A. (2000) Espoir ou illusion. *Paraplégie N0 87*, Bulletin officiel de la Fondation Suisse pour la Paraplégie, Nottwil, 2-3

9

Biomechanical Constraints in the Design of Robotic Systems for Tremor Suppression

Juan-Manuel Belda-Lois, Álvaro Page, José-María Baydal-Bertomeu, Rakel Poveda, Ricard Barberà
Instituto de Biomecánica de Valencia
(Spain)

1. Introduction

The *Movement Disorder Society* defines tremor as an involuntary rythmical oscillation of a body part (Deuschl et al. 1998). This definition excludes other movement disorders with a less cyclic character such as chorea or ataxia. Tremor is the most frequent movement disorder in clinical practice with an estimated prevalence between 3-4% of the population over 50 (Manto et al. 2004).

Everybody has some tremor component, usually invisible for the naked eye, called *physiological tremor*. However, there are other forms of pathological tremor that can be very disabling, and often a cause of social exclusion (Rocon et al. 2004). There are many pathologies that can cause pathological tremor, among others Essential Tremor, Parkinson Disease, brain trauma or multiple sclerosis.

Common treatments of tremor are pharmacological and surgical. Pharmacological treatments depend on the specific pathology that causes tremor. For instance *Parkinson disease tremor* is treated with L-dopa, and common treatments for *Essential Tremo*r are β-blockers (Deuschl et al. 1998). Surgical classical treatment for tremor is thalamic thermocoagulation (Deuschl et al. 2000). However from mid 90's Deep Brain Stimulation (DBS) is preferred to thermocoagulation (Deuschl et al. 2000).

Despite these therapies, there are still an important number of people with pathological tremor resistant to the common treatments (Deuschl et al. 1998). Thus, other alternatives are of interest to help people suffering from different kinds of pathological tremor. Many of these alternatives focus on removing the consequences of tremor rather than its origins. Among others the following approaches can be mentioned:

(a) Removing the tremor from a tremorous signal (Riviere & Thakor, 1996; Gonzalez et al. 2000) (b) Design of assistive devices based in dampers (such as the NeaterEater® or the MouseTrap® (c) Design of robotics systems to suppress tremor.

This chapter focuses the attention on the design of robotics systems to suppress tremor. First of all, we will introduce different strategies to suppress tremor using robotic approaches, then we will show the biomechanical and ergonomics issues to take into consideration in the design of these robotic systems, finally we will introduce a set of guidelines to take into account in the design of robotics systems for tremor suppression.

2. Robotic systems to suppress tremor

Robotic systems allow mechanical tremor suppression while preserving the component of voluntary movement. This approach has been attempted previously by several authors considering different strategies, and using different robotic configurations.

2.1 Methodological introduction

In this chapter we will consider the mechanical system of a body segment with a robotic system attached to it from the perspective of dynamic systems theory. Given a simple mechanical system such as the one in figure 1, we can express the relationship between force and displacement in the form of a differential equation that includes the components of inertia (*M*), stiffness (*K*) and viscosity (*c*) (1)

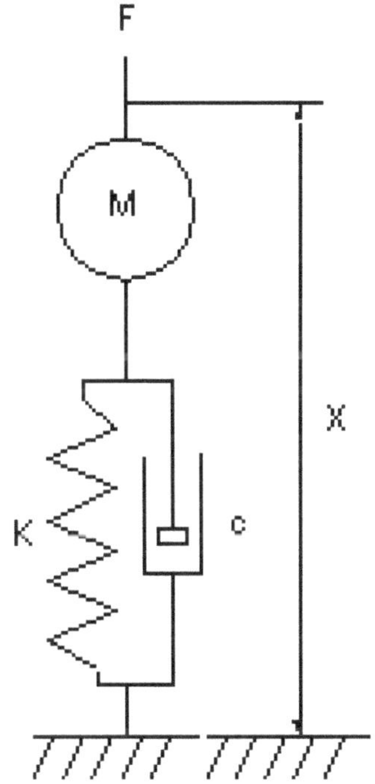

Fig. 1. Simple mechanical system to exemplify the relationship between force (*F*) and displacement (ΔX) depending on the mechanical characteristics of the system.

$$F(t) = M \cdot \frac{\partial^2(\Delta x)}{\partial t^2} + c \cdot \frac{\partial(\Delta x)}{\partial t} + K \cdot \Delta x \qquad (1)$$

Using the Laplace transform (2) we can change a differential equation such as (1) into an expression dependent on the operator s (3), and this kind of transformation allows to obtain expressions in which we can separate the physical charateristics of the system from the inputs and outputs (4). We can refer to these physical characteristics as *dynamic stiffness* (5) in the sense that is an expression of the complex relationship between the force applied and the position of the system.

$$L[f(t)] = F(s) = \int f(t) e^{-st} dt \tag{2}$$

$$F = M \cdot s^2 x + c \cdot sx + Kx \tag{3}$$

$$F = \left(M \cdot s^2 + c \cdot s + k\right)x \tag{4}$$

$$F = B(s) \cdot x \tag{5}$$

Besides, the use of the Laplace transformation has two extra benefits: a) it allows a relationship between an input signal (i.e. force) and an output signal (i.e. displacement) in a mathematical expression known as *transfer function*. b) it allows the identification of the mechanical system from its frequency response.

2.2 Strategies for tremor suppression

One obvious way to supress tremor consists in damping the tremor component: adding viscosity to a joint makes the joint speed dependent. Thus, since a tremor movement is faster than common voluntary movements, the addition of damping should attenuate tremor. This approach has been tested through the use of dampers (Kotovsky & Rosen, 1998) or through the use of actuators based on magneto-rheological fluids (MRFs) (Loureiro et al. 2006).

From a wider perspective, adding viscosity to a joint changes the dynamic stiffness of the joint. But we can change dynamic stiffness by not only adding viscosity but also adding stiffness and inertia.

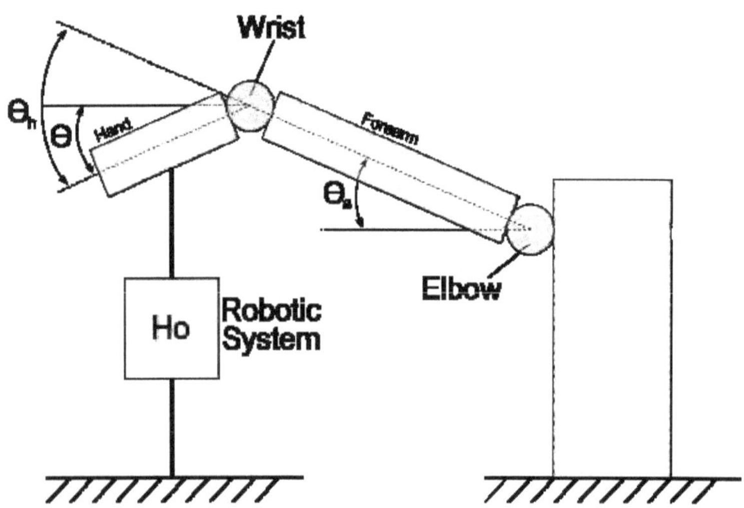

Fig. 2. Simplified diagram of grounded robotic system for tremor suppression.

Pledgie et al. (2000), suggested the use of changes in the dynamic stiffness in order to attenuate tremor. Adding dynamic stiffness the overall bandwith of the system can be changed, if the band of tremor is let out of the band of the overall system (human joint and robotic system) then the tremor should attenuate. This is the approach shown in (6), where B_a is the dynamic stiffness of the body system and B_o is the dynamic stiffness of the robotic system.

$$\theta(s) = \frac{1}{B_a + B_o} \cdot T(s) \tag{6}$$

Another feasible strategy consists in the implementation of a filter in a mechanical system. This has been one of the approaches of Rocon et al. (2005). The main idea of these authors was to track the frequency of tremor using the Weighted Linear Fourier Transform suggested by Riviere & Thakor (1996) and designing a zero-lag notch filter tuned to remove the tremor frequency component.

2.3 Grounded robotic systems

Grounded systems are those which create a mechanical linkage from a body segment to the ground or a fixed external system such as a desktop or a wheelchair. Figure 2 shows a simplified diagram of a grounded robot attached to the hand. For the sake of simplicity we have assumed a 2D model of the arm with only two joints the wrist and the elbow.
A system of these characteristics can efficiently suppress the tremor at the level of the hand. We can simplify the behaviour of the overall system to the diagram blocks of figure 3. We are considering that an input torque at the wrist joint of T_W , H_o is the dynamic response of the robotic system (i.e. the transfer function), and B_e and B_W are respectively the dynamic stiffness of elbow and wrist joints.

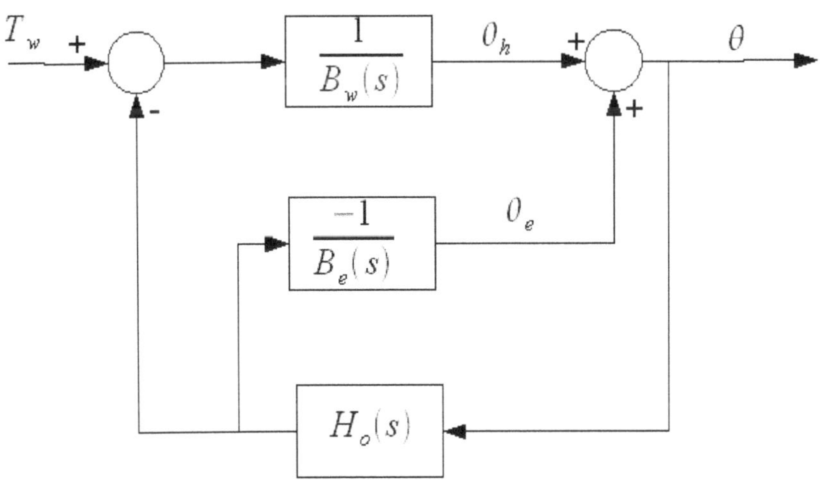

Fig. 3. Linearised model of the grounded robotic system shown in figure 2.

(7) is the be the expression of the overall movement of the hand according to figure 3. As it can be observed in (7) the response of the robotic system can modify the response of the hand.

$$\theta(s) = \frac{B_e}{B_W \cdot B_e + B_W \cdot H_o + B_e \cdot H_o} \cdot T_W(s) \tag{7}$$

However, due to the mechanical coupling introduced by the robotic system, a component of tremor will appear at elbow level such as shown in (8).

$$\theta_e(s) = \frac{-H_o}{B_W \cdot B_e + B_W \cdot H_o + B_e \cdot H_o} \cdot T_W(s) \tag{8}$$

In other words, keeping the tip of the hand steady with a grounded system will introduce a tremor component in the proximal joints. This component of tremor can be potentially dangerous when users perform movements oriented to his/her body such as eating or dressing.

If we considered an strategy based on the addition of dynamic stiffness instead of a generic suppressing strategy represented by a transfer function, we can compare (7) with the approximation of tremor suppression through impedance control suggested by Pledgie et al. (2000) which is shown in (6). At first sight both expressions are very different, but we can rearrange the terms of (7) as shown in (9), and substitute the response of the system, a generic transfer function ,represented by H_o , for a dynamic stiffness represented by B_o .

$$\theta(s) = \frac{1}{B_W + \left(1 + \frac{B_W}{B_e}\right) B_o} \cdot T_W(s) \tag{9}$$

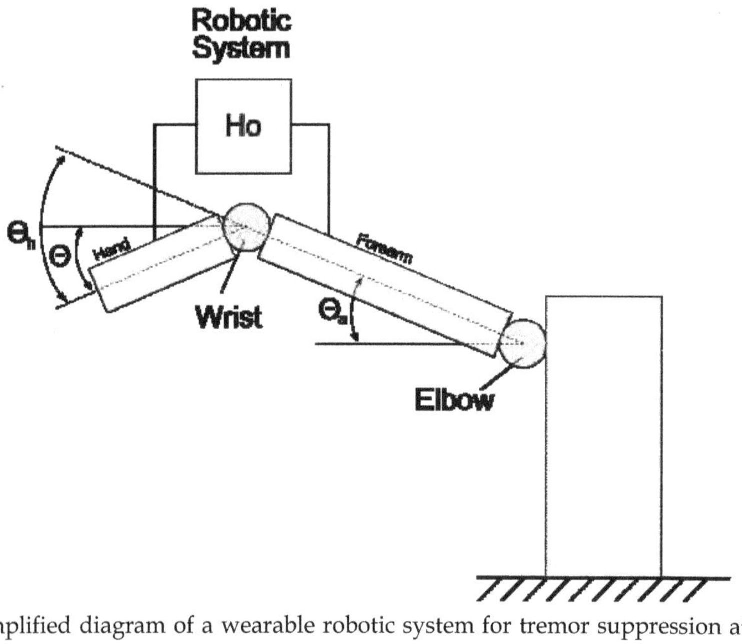

Fig. 4. Simplified diagram of a wearable robotic system for tremor suppression attached to the wrist joint.

But, according to Acosta et al. (2000) the dynamic stiffness of the arm should be considered as a whole due to the coupling of body structures and in particular to the existence of biarticular muscles. This hypothesis provides consistency to the approach of Pledgie et al. (2000) who identify the overall response of the arm as a generic linear second order system. Therefore, if frequency response of the arm is unitary, the dynamic stiffness of different joints can only differ, approximately, in the gain. Consequently, we can simplify further (9) to (10), where K is a positive real number representing the relationship of stiffness of wrist and elbow joints.

$$\theta(s) = \frac{1}{B_w + K \cdot B_o} \cdot T_w(s) \tag{10}$$

As it can be seen, (10) is very similar to (6), and therefore the approximation of Pledgie et al. (2000) can be considered as a special case of the approach shown.

2.4 Exoskeletons and wearable systems

The principles of exoskeletons are very different from grounded robotic systems. figure 4, shows a simplified diagram of exoskeleton to suppress tremor at the wrist joint. As it can be inferred from the figure, in this case there are not mechanical couplings (other than inertial coupling characteristics) able to transmit tremor from distal to proximal joints.
However, this approximation has two main drawbacks: firstly the system doesn't have control over the global position of the hand, just in the movement performed by the joint under control, (in the case of figure 4 the wrist angle), and secondly the system is unable to compensate tremor coming from other joints.
The block diagram for this approximation is much simpler (figure 5).

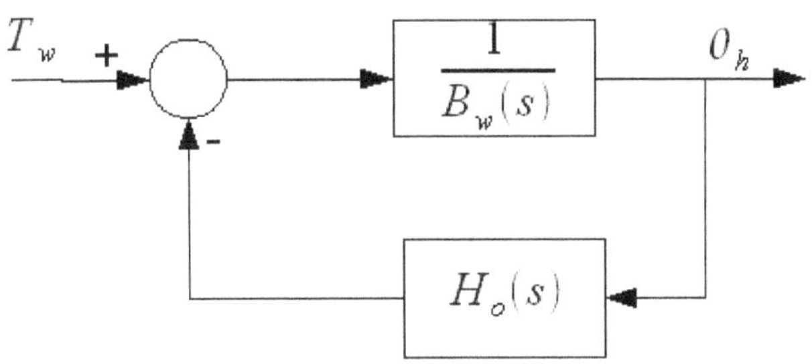

Fig. 5. Linearised model of the exoskeleton system.

Consequently the expression of the position of the hand with respect to the forearm is also simpler (11).

$$\theta_h = \frac{1}{B_w + H_o} \cdot T_w \tag{11}$$

Comparing (11) with (6) we can see that both expressions are identical, therefore the same type of tremor supressing strategy is possible in this configuration.

3. Biomechanical requirements

In the last point we have considered how different strategies and approximations can be effective for tremor suppression. However, in all the development, we have considered ideal conditions in relation to the compatibility between the robotic system and the body segments. Human body segments impose their own constraints to the system and these constraints must be kept into account in order to construct useful devices able to suppress tremor.
One of the key factors when designing these systems is the management of the contact between the body and the system. The systems attached to the body require the

transmission of the loads to the skeletal system, but this transmission is only possible through the layers of soft tissues between the device and the skeleton.
Common orthotic practice has developed procedures for load transmission based mainly on safety and comfort issues. However, many common orthotic procedures are not applicable in the design of systems to suppress tremor because they are successful only in static or quasiestatic conditions, but tremor is a pure dynamic effect and therefore requires other approaches.

3.1 Contact pressures

The transmission of loads from the systems to the skeleton produces contract pressure that can compromise safety and comfort.
Regarding safety, the usual guideline is avoiding pressures above the ischaemia level (the level at which the capillary vessels are not able to conduct blood compromising the tissue). This level has been estimated in 30 mmHg (Landis, 1930).
The relation between pressures and comfort is much more complicated. Touch receptors are sensitive to the deformation of the layers of tissue where they are located (Dandekar et al. 2003), therefore the perception of pressure is indirect: pressure deforms tissues and this deformation is sensed by skin receptors. Besides, the type, density and distribution of skin receptors varies significantly depending on the part of the body implied. Finally, the skin receptors have a dynamic response to the excitation (receptor adaptation). This dynamic response makes the pressure perception dependent on the dynamics of the process of applying pressure.
In orthotic practice the main guideline is reducing the contact pressure as much as possible increasing the contact surface between the system and the body, and reducing the risk of injury for maintained high pressures.
However, this guideline couldn't be appropriate from the point of view of comfort. According to Goonetilleke (1998) there exists an optimal surface to distribute a load and this value is a balance between pressure and number of touch receptors excited, also known as spatial summation theory (Goonetilleke, 1998). Furthermore, in the case of system for tremor suppression, as we will see later, the use of big supports to distribute the load worsen the performance of the system, consequently some kind of increase of contact pressure is needed in comparison with conventional orthoses.
To assess the tolerance of pressure of different parts of the body some authors made indentations to the point where the user feels pain or discomfort (Byström et al. 1995). However, the results of these experiments should be considered as a general indication of discomfort threshold since they depend on dynamics, shape and area of application.

3.1 Shear forces

Shear forces are together with pressure, the most important cause of skin injuries. Besides, compliance of skin in the shear plane is higher than in normal plane and this can cause loss of alignment in actuators which have an action line parallel to the body segment.

3.2 Kinematic compatibility

Body joints never act as pure hinge or ball joints, the geometry of body joints is usually very complex and can differ substantially depending on the person. On the other hand, robotics are commonly composed of inferior pair joints. Therefore, when we place a robotic system acting parallel to a body segment there are loss of alignments between the robotic system joint and body joint Instant Helical Axis (IHA). This loss of alignment is partially

compensated for the flexibility of body soft tissues and partially is transmitted as loads to the structures of the joint, and this can ultimately lead to an injury.
These injuries are relevant in powerful joints which manage an important amount of load such as the knee. In these cases the design of a mechanism able to follow-up as close as possible the body joint IHA is very important.

3.3 Protection of body structures

When applying loads to a body segment it is important to be careful with some structures in order to avoid discomfort, pain or the risk of injuries: Superficial vessels and nerves and bone prominences. Besides, we should keep free the area close to the joints.

3.4 Dynamic stiffness in the contact

In point 2, we have considered ideal contact conditions between the robotic system and the body segment. However, these conditions determine the overall performance of the system.

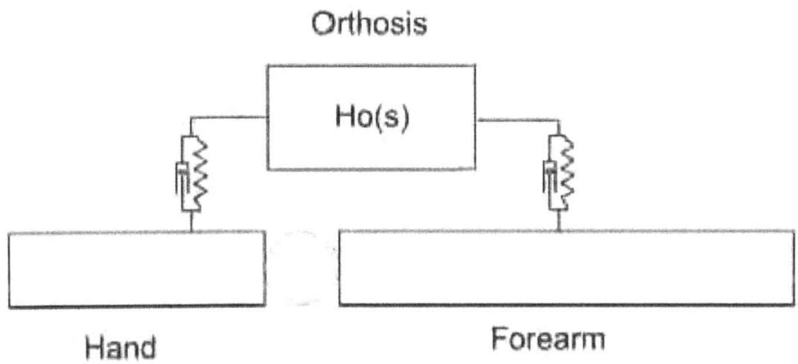

Fig. 6. Simplified view of a robotic system considering the dynamic stiffness in the contact.

If we consider the dynamic stiffness between the system and the body when we model the response of the system (figure 6), and we assume that the effect of the system is to apply a certain amount of dynamic stiffness (B_o), then the overall equivalent stiffness of the system is (12). The dynamical stiffness of the contact points between the robotic system and the body segments, as well as the dynamical stiffness of the actuator are all in serial mode and consequently the overall dynamical stiffness has been reduced.

$$B_t = \frac{B_{s1} \cdot B_{s2} \cdot B_o}{B_{s1} \cdot B_{s2} + B_{s1} \cdot B_o + B_{s2} \cdot B_o} \tag{12}$$

If we consider that dynamic stiffness in both body segments is the same and we neglect the viscous component, then we can simplify (12) into (13) where K is the stiffness of the soft tissues under the contact of the system.

$$B_t = \frac{\frac{K}{2} \cdot B_o}{\frac{K}{2} + B_o} \tag{13}$$

To understand how the contact conditions can affect the performance of a robotic system for tremor suppression the response of an effective system and a sitffness in the contact of

$0.47N/m$ can be considered. As it can be seen in figure 7, the dynamic response of the system has changed considerably. If we consider the contact conditions, even for a well designed system we can lose all the attenuation in the frequency of pathological tremor (4 Hz) due to the stiffness of soft tissue. Thus the system is no longer capable of suppressing tremor due to the conditions of the contact.

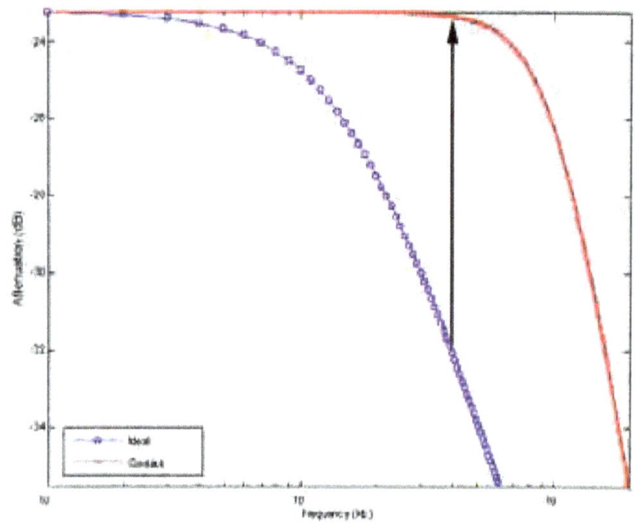

Fig. 7. Effect of the contact. The curve with circles is the response of the system considering an ideal contact between the system and the body segment. The curve with crosses is the response of the system considering the stiffness of the soft tissues. The arrow shows the loss of attenuation at 4 Hz (typical frequency of many pathological tremors) when stiffness of the contact is considered.

If we are able to increase the stiffness of the contact by a factor of 10 (overall stiffness $4.7N/m$), the response of the system (figure 8) will come closer to the ideal behaviour. The system is able to suppress tremor.

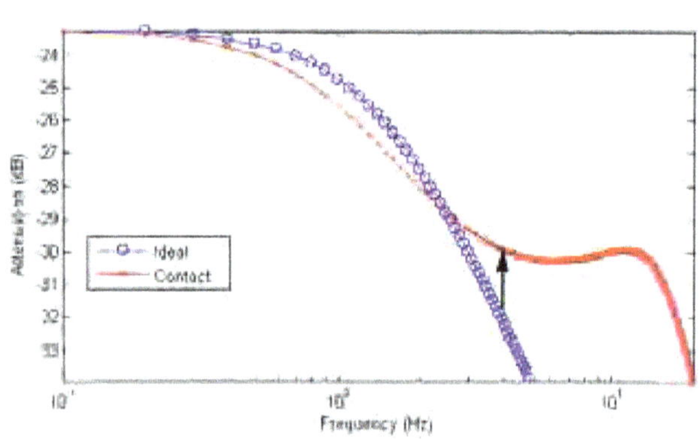

Fig. 8. The effect of increasing the stiffness in the contact. The arrow represents the loss of attenuation at 4 Hz when we consider the stiffness of the contact.

Moreover, the stiffness in the shear plane is considerably lower than in the normal plane. Thus, the response of the system will be worse in the shear plane.
In addition, the loss of alignment between the body segment and the orthosis can also produce a reduction of effectiveness. The stiffness of the soft tissues can produce this loss of alignment (figure 9). In the figure 9(a), the gap between the support system and the body segment is a representation of the contact of stiffness. When the segment corresponding to the hand moves, the orthosis does not act due to the loss of alignment between the fixation and the hand –Fig. 9(b)–

4. Design principles

All the above considerations imply restrictions in the design of robotic systems for tremor suppression. We have summarised these constraints in three design principles:

a) Length restriction
b) Increase of contact pressure
c) Alignments with body segments

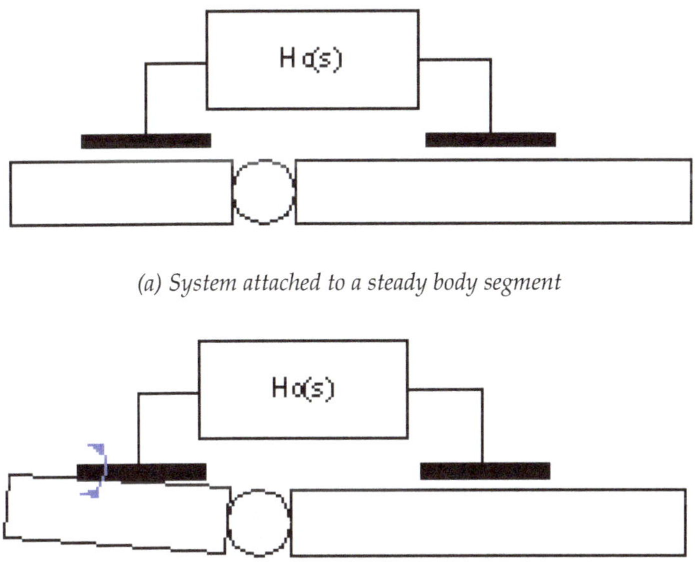

(a) System attached to a steady body segment

(b) Loss of alignment when the body segment moves

Fig. 9. The effect of loss of alignment due to a low impedance.

4.1 Length restriction

This principle is intended to deal with the low stiffness associated with the shear component of stiffness. A constraint in length between the fixation devices (figure 10) increases the overall stiffness of the contact in a factor of 4.
Without this restriction the supports corresponding to each segment can move separately. Therefore, their dynamical stiffness is in serial mode. However, if we restrict the distance between the supports (figure 10), now both supports can only move coordinately.

Consequently, both contacts are now in parallel and the overall dynamical stiffness is higher (14). Therefore, the length restriction affects the overall dynamic stiffness of the system.

$$B_t = \frac{B_o \cdot (B_{s1} + B_{s2})}{B_o + B_{s1} + B_{s2}} \tag{14}$$

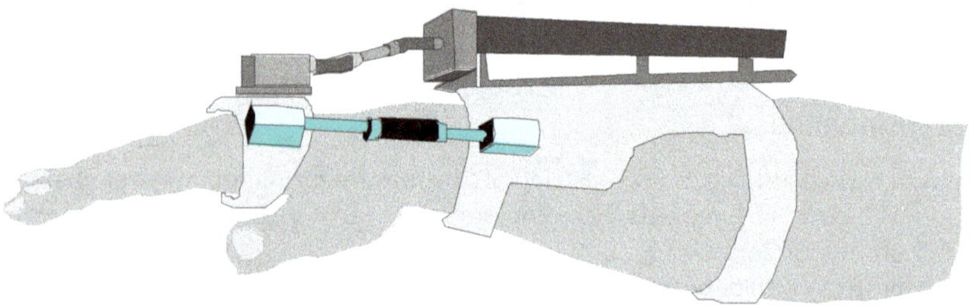

Fig. 10. Length restriction in a device to suppress tremor in the wrist flexion-extension based in a linear actuator.

Using the same simplifications as in (13) (equal impedance in both fixations and neglecting the viscous component), (14) converts to (15).

$$B_t = \frac{2K \cdot B_o}{2K + B_o} \tag{15}$$

Comparing (15) with (13) we can seen that now the equivalent stiffness of the contact is four times higher.

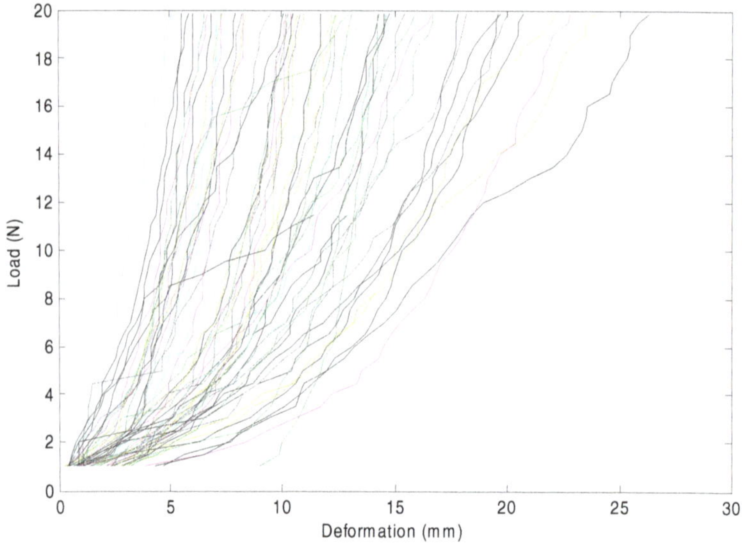

Fig 11. Force deformation characteristics of soft tissues in the forearm.

4.2 Increase of contact pressure

The tenso-deformational characteristics of the soft tissues under the arm are highly non-linear. The stiffness of the tissues increases as contact pressure increases. Figure 11 shows the force-displacement curve measured in the forearm of 10 different young people (5 males and 5 females) measured in 6 points of the forearm (3 in the palmar side and 3 in the volar side).
As we can infer from figure 11, one way to increase contact impedance is increasing contact pressure and moving upwards in the tenso-deformational curve. This strategy has two constraints of safety and comfort that have been dealt with in point 3.1.

4.3 Alignment with body segments

As it has been said before, the loss of alignment between the body segment and the robotic system can reduce the overall performance of the system. One way to ensure the alignment is increasing the number of contact points of each support. Each support part of the system should have at least three contact points to ensure the alignment (figure 12).

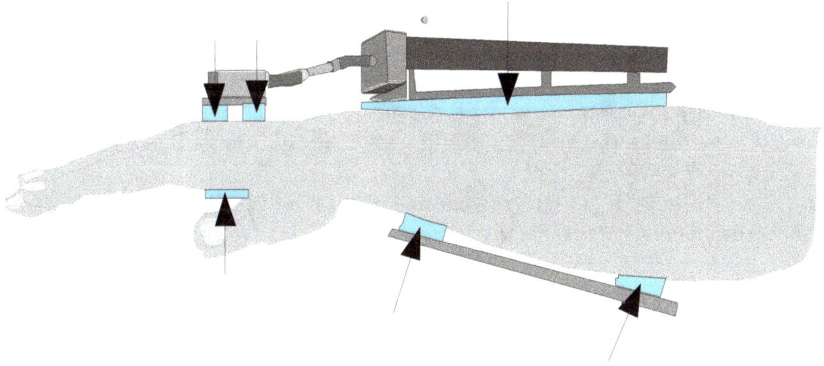

Fig 12. Alignment of the support devices with the body segments once the number of contact points have been increased.

5. Conclusions

Tremor suppression with robotic devices can be an alternative for people with pathological tremor resistant to conventional treatments.
Common orthotic principles don't fit well for tremor suppression due to the inherent dynamic characteristics of tremor.
In the design of robotic systems for tremor suppression the correct design of load transmission to the bones through the soft tissues is one of the key aspects for successful performance.
We have summarised the design specifications into three guidelines:

a) Length restriction to avoid the low stiffness associated in the shear plane.
b) Increase of contact pressure to increase contact stiffness.
c) Increase of the number of contact points to keep the alignments between the orthosis and the body segment.

6. References

Acosta, A M; Kirsch, R F & Perreault, E F (2000) A robotic manipulator for the characterization of two-dimensional dynamic stiffness using stochastic displacement perturbations. *Journal of Neuroscience Methods*, Vol. 102, (177–186), ISSN 0165-0270

Byström, S; Hall, C; Welander, T & Kilbom, A (1995) Clinical disorders and pressure-pain threshold of the forearm and hand among automobile assembly line workers. *Journal of Hand Surgery*, Vol. 20, No. 6, (782–790). ISSN 1753-1934.

Dandekar, K; Raju B I & Srinivasan M A (2003). 3-D Finite-Element Models of Human and Monkey Fingertips to Investigate the Mechanics of Tactile Sense. *Journal of Biomechanical Engineering*, Vol. 125, (682-691), ISSN 0148-0731

Deuschl, G; Bain, P & Brin, M (1998) Consensus Statement of the Movement Disorder Society on Tremor. *Movement Disorders*, Vol. 13, Supplement 3, (2–23), ISSN 0885-3185

Deuschl, G; Wenzelburger, R & Raethjen, J (2000) Tremor. *Current Opinion in Neurology*, Vol. 13, (437–443), ISSN 13507540

Gonzalez, J C; Heredia, E A; Rahman, T; Barner, K E & Arce, G R (2000) Optimal Digital Filtering for Tremor Suppression. *IEEE Transactions on Biomedical Engineering*, Vol. 47, No. 5, (664–673), ISSN 0018-9294

Goonetilleke, R S (1998). The Comfort "Slip". *Proceedings of the First World Congress on Ergonomics for Global Quality and Productivity*, July 8-11, 1998, R Bishu; W Karkowski y R Goonetilleke (Eds.), Hong Kong University of Science and Technology, Hong Kong, pp. 290–293

Kotovsky, J & Rosen, M (1998) A wearable tremor suppression orthosis. *Journal of Rehabilitation Research and Development*, Vol. 35, No. 4, (373–384), ISSN 0748-7711

Landis, E (1930) Micro-injection studies of capillary blood pressure in human skin. *Heart*, Vol. 15, (209–228).

Loureiro, R C V; Belda-Lois, J M; Rocon, E; Pons, JL; Normie, L & Harwin, WS (2006) Upper Limb Tremor Suppression Through Viscous Loading - Design, Implementation and Clinical Validation. *International Journal of Assistive Robotics and Mechatronics*, Vol. 7 No. 2, (11-19), ISSN 1975-0153

Manto, M; Rocon, E; Pons, J; Davies, A; Williams, J; Belda-Lois, J M & Normie, L (2004). An Active Orthosis To Control Upper Limb Tremor: The Drifts Project (Dynamicly Responsive Intervention For Tremor Suppression). *EURO-ATAXIA Newsletter*, No. 26, (2–6)

Pledgie, S; Barner, K E; Agrawal, S K & Rahman, T (2000) Tremor suppression through impedance control. IEEE Transactions on Rehabilitation Engineering, Vol. 8, No 1, (53–59), ISSN 1063-6528

Riviere, C N & Thakor, N (1996) Modelling and cancelling tremor in human-computer interfaces. *IEEE Engineering in Medicine and Biology Magazine*, Vol. 15, No 3, (29–36), ISSN 0739-5175

Rocon, E; Belda-Lois, J M; Sanchez-Lacuesta, J J & Pons, J L (2004) Pathological tremor management: Modelling, compensatory technology and evaluation. *Technology and Disability*, Vol. 16, No. 1, (3–18), ISSN 1055-4181

Rocon, E; Ruiz, A F; Pons, J L; Belda-Lois, J M & Sanchez-Lacuesta, J J (2005) Rehabilitation Robotics: a Wearable Exo-Skeleton for Tremor Assessment and Suppression. *ICRA 2005. Proceedings of the 2005 IEEE International Conference on Robotics and Automation,* pp. 2271 - 2276, ISBN 0-7803-8915-8, Barcelona (Spain), April 2005.

10

Rehabilitation of the Paralyzed Lower Limbs Using Functional Electrical Stimulation: Robust Closed Loop Control

Samer Mohammed, Philippe Poignet, Philippe Fraisse & David Guiraud
LIRMM – CNRS/INRIA – Université de Montpellier II
France

1. Introduction

The reliability, the ease of donning and doffing and the robustness of controllers constitute the primary criteria to evaluate any control strategy based on Functional Electrical Stimulation (FES). This technique is used to excite muscles that are under lesions and no more controlled by paraplegic patients. Consequently, the patient could recover partially some of its lower limb functions, improving the cardiovascular system and bettering the whole quality of life. Many FES based studies; both open loop and closed loop control showed satisfactory results in movement restoration. Although open loop control strategy induces excessive stimulation of the main muscles and consequently fast muscular fatigue, it is still adopted in most clinics till now. This could be explained mainly by their relative simple implantation (Bajd et al., 1981). Actually closed loop control strategies still have several drawbacks, such as overwhelming the patient by sensors' feedback, tuning the parameters of the controllers and identification for every patient, the lack of understanding the muscle contraction phenomena, etc. Closed loop controllers in FES context have been reported in many studies (Riener & Fuhr, 1998); (Mulder et al., 1992); (Donaldson & Yu, 1996). Some authors use a simple PID controller (Wood et al., 1998), Knee Extension Controller KEC (Poboroniuc et al., 2003), a combination of feedback and feed-forward control or an adaptive approach (Ferrarin et al., 2001). Others use a first or a second order switching curve in the state space to control patient movements: The On/Off controller (Mulder et al., 1992) and the ONZOFF controller (Poboroniuc et al., 2002), in the so-called "controller-centered" strategies. The main advantage of these strategies is their low number of parameters to be tuned during stimulation. The so-called "subject centered" strategies, (PDMR: Patient-Driven Motion Reinforcement (Riener & Fuhr, 1998), CHRELMS: Control by Handle REactions of Leg Muscle Stimulation (Donaldson & Yu, 1996)), introduce the voluntary contribution of the upper body of the patient as an essential part of the control diagram. This latter is not yet adopted in clinical use because of the relative high number of parameters to be identified. In order to overcome these drawbacks, we have applied two robust control strategies that are, the High Order Sliding Mode (HOSM) controller (Fridman & Levant, 2002) and the Model Predictive Controller (MPC) also known as receding horizon controller (Allgöwer et al., 1999). These controllers have been evaluated in simulation to highlight i) their performance in terms of capability of tracking a pre-defined reference trajectory and ii) the robustness against force perturbation and model mismatch. Furthermore the MPC technique constitutes an adequate controller for nonlinear multivariable systems and enables us to incorporate explicitly constraints on inputs, outputs and system states. The performances of these controllers have also been compared with a classical pole placement controller. The originality of the presented study comes also from the fact that these control strategies rely on the use of a physio-mathematical based muscle model. In fact, few studies have treated the human muscle as an entire physiological element in a control scheme. Some authors used linear muscle models; others represent the muscle as a non-linear function of recruitment with dynamics activation, angle and angular velocity dependence (Riener & Fuhr, 1998); (Veltink et al., 1992). The muscle model used in this study has been recently published (El-Makssoud et al., 2004-a) and it is based on a complex physio-mathematical formulation of the macroscopic Hill and microscopic Huxley concepts reflecting the dynamic phenomenon that occurred during muscle contraction and relaxation. In this model, the number of recruited motor units increases as a function of both the intensity and the pulse width of the stimulus. This phenomenon is modeled by an activation model (representing the ratio of recruited fibers). The contraction dynamics is expressed by a set of nonlinear differential equations representing the mechanical model. The goal of the present study is to represent the interaction between a closed loop controller and a closely physiological muscle model matching.

In next section, the system modeling is presented; it includes the knee-muscle biomechanical model, its state space formulation and parameter identification based on experimental setup. In the third and fourth sections, simulation results for controllers based on HOSM and MPC are presented. A comparison study of the controller performance is presented in the fifth section.

2. System modeling

Since closed loop control of different muscles actuating the knee joint of a paraplegic patient constitutes a prerequisite step before any upward mobility such as: standing up, standing, walking, climbing stairs, etc., we limited, in this stage, the study to a small scale biomechanical system. It consists of two segments representing respectively the shank and the thigh connected to each other by a revolute joint of one degree of freedom. The thigh is supposed to be fixed with respect to the patient while the shank is free to move around the knee joint (Fig.1). Two agonist/antagonist muscles act on the knee, the quadriceps acts as an extensor muscle while the hamstrings are the flexor muscle group. As a result two forces F_q and F_h cause respectively the extension and the flexion of the knee.

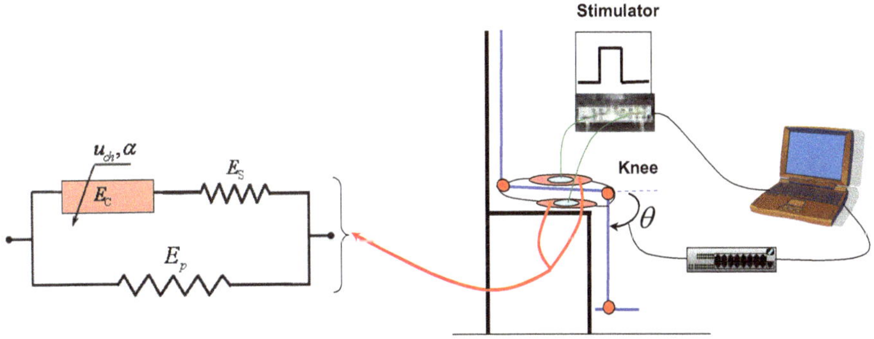

Fig. 1. Functional Electrical Stimulation applied to skeletal muscles.

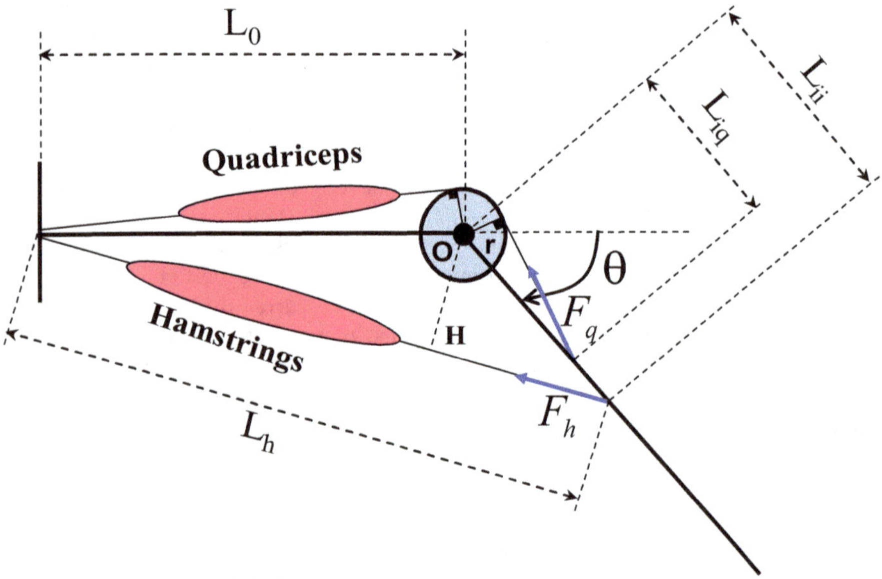

Fig. 2. Biomechanical model of the knee actuated by two groups of antagonistic muscles.

These forces are supposed to be constant along their directions on the whole corresponding muscle (Fig.2), ($\theta = 0$ corresponds to full extension of the knee and $\theta = 90°$ represents the rest position). F_q and F_h are the inputs of the biomechanical model while the angle θ is the corresponding output. The geometric equations allow us to evaluate quadriceps length L_q depending on the knee angle variable theta:

$$L_q(\theta) = \sqrt{L_0^2 - r^2} + r\theta + \sqrt{L_{iq}^2 - r^2} \tag{1}$$

And the hamstrings length $L_h(\theta)$:

$$L_h(\theta) = \sqrt{L_0^2 + L_{ii}^2 + 2L_0 L_{ii}\cos(\theta)} \tag{2}$$

From the above equations, we can deduce the relative elongation of quadriceps and hamstrings.

$$\varepsilon_q(\theta) = \frac{L_q - L_{0q}}{L_{0q}} = \frac{\sqrt{L_0^2 - r^2} + r\theta + \sqrt{L_{iq}^2 - r^2} - L_{0q}}{L_{0q}}$$
$$\varepsilon_h(\theta) = \frac{L_h - L_{0h}}{L_{0h}} = \frac{\sqrt{L_0^2 + L_{ii}^2 + 2L_0 L_{ii}\cos(\theta)} - L_{0h}}{L_{0h}} \tag{3}$$

L_{0q} and L_{0h} correspond respectively to the initial quadriceps and hamstrings lengths. Moment arm of the quadriceps is assumed to be constant and equal to the pulley radius r while the moment arm of the hamstrings depends on theta.

$$OH(\theta) = \frac{L_0 L_{ii} \sin(\theta)}{\sqrt{L_0^2 + L_{ii}^2 + 2L_0 L_{ii} \cos(\theta)}} \tag{4}$$

From the equations (3), (4) and the equation of motion that is a nonlinear second order equation, we obtained the acceleration $\ddot{\theta}$ (Eq. 5) as a function of the inertia about the knee joint I, gravity, joint damping factor F_v and joint elasticity K_e.

$$\ddot{\theta} = \frac{1}{I}\left[rF_q - mg\cos(\theta)\beta L_1 - K_e\theta - F_v\dot{\theta} - \frac{L_0 L_{ii} \sin(\theta)}{\sqrt{L_0^2 + L_{ii}^2 + 2L_0 L_{ii} \cos(\theta)}} F_h \right] \tag{5}$$

Identifications of the above parameters were performed based on experiments and are presented in the next section.

2.1 Muscle model

In previous papers (El-Makssoud et al., 2004-a; b), a physiological skeletal muscle model has been proposed to describe the complex internal physiological mechanism controlled by FES. In order to develop strategies for simulation, motion synthesis and motor control during clinical restoration of movement, we have adopted this model. In (Fig.3) we show the muscle model with the parallel element E_p representing the passive properties of the muscle and two elements in series: the serial element E_s and the contractile element E_c. This model is controlled by two variables: u_{ch}, a chemical control input and α the ratio of recruited fibers. This model has been described by two sets of differential equations (Eq.6) where the outputs are K_c and F_c representing, respectively, the stiffness and force generated by the contractile element. K_0 and F_0 are the maximum values of K_c and F_c. These equations could be expressed as follow:

$$\begin{cases} \dot{K}_c = \left(s_0 \alpha k_0 - s_u K_c + s_v q \dfrac{s_0 \alpha F_0 - s_u F_c}{1 + pK_c - s_v q F_c} K_c \right) u_{ch} - \dfrac{s_v a K_c}{1 + pK_c - s_v q F_c} \dot{\varepsilon} \\ \dot{F}_c = \dfrac{s_0 \alpha F_0 - s_u F_c}{1 + pK_c - s_v q F_c} u_{ch} + \dfrac{bK_c - s_v a F_c}{1 + pK_c - s_v q F_c} \dot{\varepsilon} \end{cases} \tag{6}$$

$$s_u = sign(u_{ch}) = \begin{cases} -1 & if \quad u_{ch} < 0 \\ +1 & if \quad u_{ch} > 0 \end{cases} \qquad s_v = sign(\dot{\varepsilon}_c) = \begin{cases} +1 & if \quad \dot{\varepsilon}_c > 0 \\ -1 & if \quad \dot{\varepsilon}_c < 0 \end{cases} \tag{7}$$

$$s_0 = \frac{1 + s_u}{2} \qquad a = \frac{L_0}{L_{c0}} \qquad b = L_0 \qquad p = \frac{1}{k_s} \qquad q = \frac{1}{L_{c0} k_s}$$
$$\varepsilon_c = \frac{L_c - L_{c0}}{L_{c0}} \qquad \varepsilon_s = \frac{L_s - L_{s0}}{L_{s0}} \qquad \varepsilon = \frac{L - L_0}{L_0} \qquad L = L_c + L_s \tag{8}$$

Where s_u, and s_v are the sign functions related respectively to the control and velocities of the contractile element, L_c and L_s represent respectively the length of the contractile and the elastic elements. The ratio of recruited fibers α is considered as a global scale factor which gives the percentage of the maximal possible force that could be generated by the muscle.

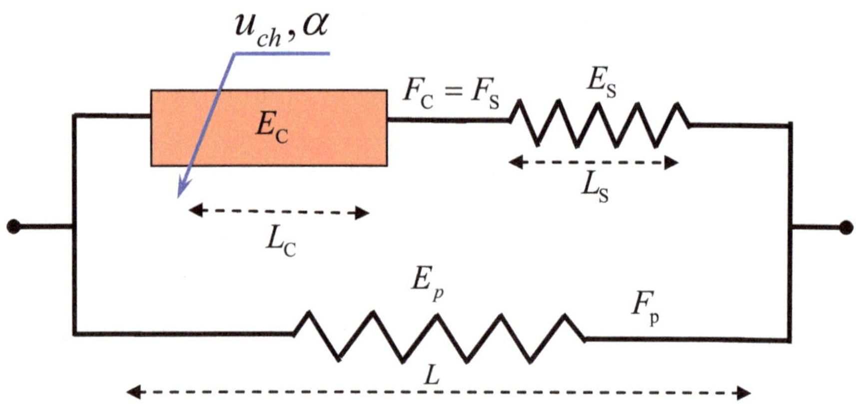

Fig. 3. Muscle model and particularity of E_c (El-Makssoud et al., 2004-a).

2.2 State space model of the muscles-knee

Let us consider the model of the muscles and knee joint as a non-linear state space model:

$$\dot{\mathbf{x}} = f(\mathbf{x}, \mathbf{t}, \mathbf{u}) \tag{9}$$

Where $\mathbf{x} = [x_1 \ldots x_6]^T = [K_{c_1} \quad K_{c_2} \quad F_{c_1} \quad F_{c_2} \quad \theta \quad \dot{\theta}]^T$ is the state vector while the control vector is expressed by $\mathbf{u} = [u_{q_{ch}} \quad \alpha_q \quad u_{h_{ch}} \quad \alpha_h]^T$. The variable θ represents the joint knee angle. The state variables K_{c1}, F_{c1}, u_{qch}, α_q and K_{c2}, F_{c2}, u_{hch}, α_h are respectively the state variables of the quadriceps and hamstrings. Consequently, the state representation of the biomechanical model (knee-muscles) could be expressed as:

$$\dot{x}_1 = \left(s_{0_1}\alpha_1 k_{0_1} - s_{u_1}x_1 + s_{v1}q_1 \frac{s_{0_1}\alpha_1 F_{0_1} - s_{u_1}x_3}{1 + p_1 x_1 - s_{v_1}q_1 x_3} x_1 \right) u_1 - \frac{s_{v_1} a_1 x_1 r x_6}{L_{01}\left(1 + p_1 x_1 - s_{v_1} q_1 x_3\right)}$$

$$\dot{x}_2 = \left(s_{0_2}\alpha_2 k_{0_2} - s_{u_2}x_2 + s_{v_2}q_2 \frac{s_{0_2}\alpha_2 F_{0_2} - s_{u_2}x_4}{1 + p_2 x_2 - s_{v_2}q_2 x_4} x_2 \right) u_2 + \frac{s_{v_2} a_2 x_2 L_0 L_{ii} \sin(x_5)}{L_{02}\sqrt{L_0^2 + L_{ii}^2 + 2L_0 L_{ii}\cos(x_5)}\left(1 + p_2 x_2 - s_{v_2} q_2 x_4\right)}$$

$$\dot{x}_3 = \frac{s_{0_1}\alpha_1 F_{0_1} - s_{u_1}x_3}{1 + p_1 x_1 - s_{v_1}q_1 x_3} u_1 + \frac{\left(b_1 x_1 - s_{v_1} a_1 x_3\right) r x_6}{L_{01}\left(1 + p_1 x_1 - s_{v_1} q_1 x_3\right)}$$

$$\dot{x}_4 = \frac{s_{0_2}\alpha_2 F_{0_2} - s_{u_2}x_4}{1 + p_2 x_2 - s_{v_2}q_2 x_4} u_2 - \frac{\left(b_2 x_2 - s_{v_2} a_2 x_4\right) L_0 L_{ii} \sin(x_5)}{L_{02}\sqrt{L_0^2 + L_{ii}^2 + 2L_0 L_{ii}\cos(x_5)}\left(1 + p_2 x_2 - s_{v_2} q_2 x_4\right)} \tag{10}$$

$$\dot{x}_5 = x_6$$

$$\dot{x}_6 = \frac{1}{I}\left(x_3 r - x_4 \frac{L_0 L_{ii} \sin(x_5)}{\sqrt{L_0^2 + L_{ii}^2 + 2L_0 L_{ii}\cos(x_5)}} - mg\cos(x_5)\beta L_1 - K_e x_5 - F_v x_6 \right)$$

2.3 Model parameters identification

The parameters of the biomechanical system have been identified based on different protocols. The geometric parameters such as the insertion points, the muscle lengths, the moment arms, etc., were identified based on the Hawkins model (Hawkins & Hull, 1990) and using the Levenberg-Marquardt (Levenberg, 1944) algorithm. The knee joint dynamic parameters such as the joint stiffness and viscosity were identified through linear least square algorithm (Gautier & Poignet, 2002). Some muscle parameters such as the maximal muscle force and the force-length relationship were identified using non-linear interpolation. Other muscle parameters not yet identified on humans were taken from literature (El-Makssoud et al., 2004-a), basically the muscle stiffness and the contractile-elastic muscle length distribution.

2.3.1 Knee joint parameters identification

Kinematics data for the knee joint were measured through a motion analysis system and using the passive pendulum test. This test consists in recording the knee joint angle and velocity during a passive movement. The table 1 summarizes the identified knee joint parameters for a given subject. These parameters correspond respectively to the thigh length L_0, the quadriceps moment arm r and the two muscles insertion points L_{iq} and L_{ii} and their standard deviation. The hamstrings moment arm is position dependent (Eq. 4).

Parameter	L_0	r	L_{iq}	L_{ii}
Value (m)	0.3726	0.0397	0.0401	0.0648
Standard deviation (%)	0.335	3.230	3.138	0.441

Table 1. Knee joint parameter identification.

The parameters shown above, have been satisfactory identified and close to those found in literature (Kromer, 1994). The standard deviations were less than 4%. We can notice that the chosen movement trajectories excite sufficiently the unknown parameters. Figure 1 shows the muscle length computed by the Hawkins model and the model described above (Eq. 1, 2).

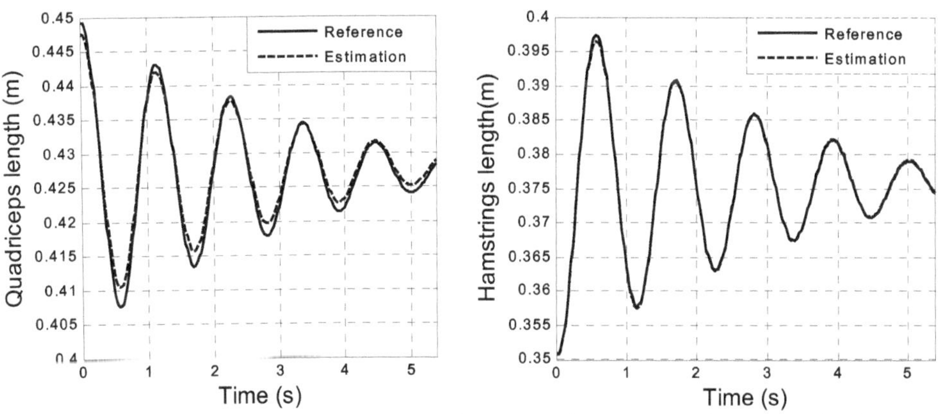

Fig. 4. Cross validation after parameter estimation (data not used during identification processing).

The dynamic parameters of the knee joint such as the knee stiffness and the knee viscosity were identified based on the following equation and using the linear least square method:

$$I\ddot{\theta} = -mgl\cos(\theta) - K_e\theta - F_v\dot{\theta} \tag{11}$$

We should notice that during a passive movement, the active moment produced by the muscles is equal to zero. Different subjects (healthy and paralyzed) have participated in the identification process. This latter was performed with the subject laying semi-supine with the lower legs hanging over the edge of a chair (Fig. 5). The operator raised the shank of the subject to given angle (about 45°) and leave the shank to swing freely until it reached the resting position (90°). The movement was recorded using a video based on motion analysis system (Vicon). Passive markers were fixed on the hip, knee and ankle (Fig. 5-b, 5-c). Kinematic data were acquired at 50 Hz sampling rate. In this application only three markers were sufficient to compute the knee joint angle and velocity. This system has the advantage to not overwhelming the subject by an external sensor that could affect the accuracy of the identification. Several tests were performed for each subject. The EMG signal analysis of the main muscles (quadriceps and hamstrings), serves only to identify any undesired voluntary muscle contractions and then reject the trial.

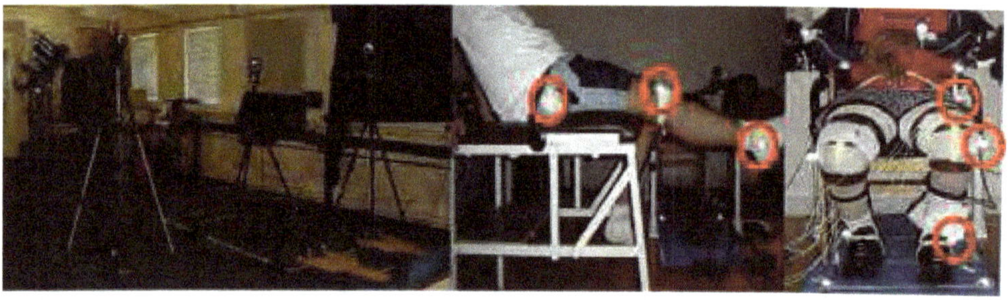

Fig. 5. a) Vicon system – b) Healthy subject - c) Paraplegic patient.

The anthropometric parameters such as the shank mass and inertia were estimated by using the regression equation proposed by DeLeva and Zatsiorsky (DeLeva, 1996), and by measuring the weight and the height of each subject. The anthropometric parameters of the subjects who participated in the identification are shown in table 2.

Subject	I (Kg.m²)	m (Kg)	l (cm)
Healthy	0.1682	4.8852	19.46
Paraplegic 1	0.1536	4.5830	19.2
Paraplegic 2	0.2092	5.6162	20.26

Table 2. Estimation of the anthropometric parameters (Inertial moment, mass and length).

The dynamic parameters of the knee joint such as viscosity and stiffness were identified by means of linear least square methods (Gautier & Poignet, 2002). The knee angle position was extracted from the kinematic data, while velocity and acceleration were computed by numeric derivation using a low-pass filter. The identified parameters as well as their standard deviation (sd) are shown in table 3. These results could be compared to some results in literature (Ferrarin et al., 2001), computed in the same context.

Subject	F_v (N.m.s/rad)	sd (%)	K_e (N.m/rad)	sd (%)
Healthy	0.0838	6.4845	0.17	2.266
Paraplegic 1	0.0659	13.3589	0.1095	6.0050
Paraplegic 2	0.0897	10.6973	0.0529	10.1739

Table 3. Dynamic parameter identification.

2.3.2 Muscle parameters identification

The force-length relation (Riener & Fuhr, 1998) expressed by equation (Eq. 12) as well as the maximal isometric force that could be generated by a muscle were identified using a special experimental platform (Fig. 6)(Mohammed 2006). This latter is equipped by a force sensor, position sensor, a mechanical shank and foot blocking system, allowing force and position measurements during isometric stimulation tests.

$$F(L) = \exp\left[-\left(\frac{\bar{l}-1}{b_l}\right)^2\right] \tag{12}$$

Where $\bar{l} = \frac{L}{L_0}$, L is the muscle length and L_0 the muscle length at the rest position . b_l could be easily identified based on equation (Eq. 12).

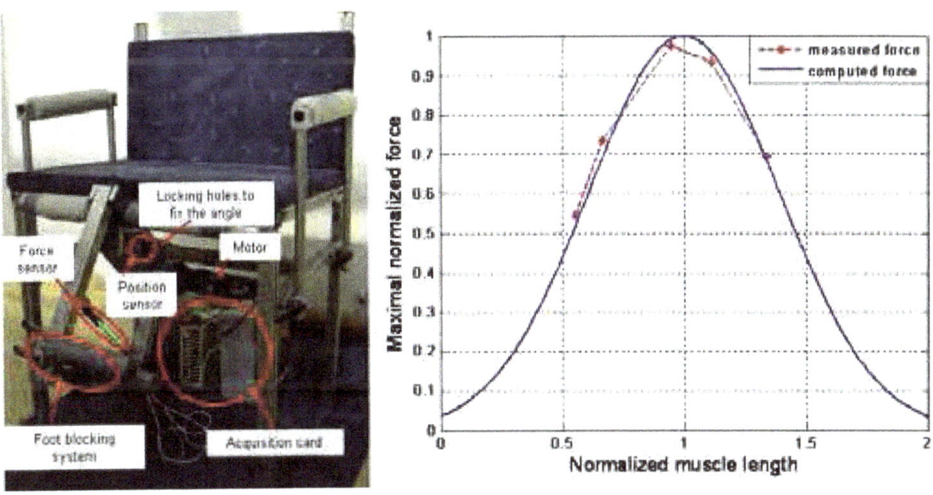

Fig. 6. Experimental platform and muscle parameter identification.

The muscle stiffness and the contractile-elastic muscle length distribution as shown in table (4), were taken from (El-Makssoud et al., 2004-a).

Muscle model parameters	Variable	quadriceps	hamstrings	Unit
Stiffness of the serial element E_s	K_s	1.10^4	1.10^4	N/m
Contractile element length E_c	L_{co}	41.10^{-2}	38.10^{-2}	m
Elastic element length E_s	L_{so}	8.10^{-2}	10.10^{-2}	m

Table 4. Parameters of both muscles: quadriceps and hamstrings

3. Sliding mode control

The nonlinearities of the muscle model and the required robustness regarding parameter variations and external disturbances lead us to adopt a controller relying on the sliding mode theory. This latter became recently widely used due to its high accuracy and robustness with respect to parameters' uncertainty and external disturbances. The control task is to keep a constraint, given by equality of a smooth function called sliding surface, equal to zero. The dynamic smoothness in the vicinity of the sliding surface represents the sliding order of the system. In this study, the goal was to control the muscles-knee biomechanical system under FES by means of high order sliding mode controller (HOSM) (Fridman, & Levant, 2002). The HOSM generalizes the basic sliding mode approach by acting on the higher order time derivatives of the sliding variable instead of influencing the first time derivative as it happens in the standard sliding mode control or first order sliding mode. Consequently, the discontinuity of the control vector does not appear in the first (r-1)th total time derivative (Eq. 13,14). The HOSM has the potential to provide greater accuracy and decrease the chattering phenomenon. A 2-sliding mode control may provide up to second order of sliding precision with respect to measurement interval. In this application, a state model of the knee with two antagonist muscles was derived. Here, the term antagonist will be used for muscles, whose moment in a two-dimensional system about a joint is in the opposite direction as the resulting joint moment. The antagonistic function of a muscle is not necessarily restricted to oppose motion but may give stability and stiffness to a joint. Unknown perturbations were added to the muscle forces generated in order to study the accuracy and robustness of the controller under external disturbances.

$$\frac{\partial s^{(i)}}{\partial \mathbf{u}} = 0, \quad (i = 1, 2, \ldots, r-1), \quad \frac{\partial s^{(r)}}{\partial \mathbf{u}} \neq 0 \tag{13}$$

$$s = \dot{s} = \ddot{s} = \ldots = s^{(r-1)} = 0 \tag{14}$$

Where s, r and **u** represent respectively the sliding surface, the relative degree and the resulting control vector.

3.1 Position control law strategy

The sliding surface used to constraint the dynamic behaviour of the biomechanical model is a first order differential equation chosen as:

$$s = \left(\dot{\theta}_d - \dot{\theta}\right) + \lambda\left(\theta_d - \theta\right) \tag{15}$$

Where $\dot{\theta}_d$ and θ_d are respectively the desired velocity and position, λ is a positive coefficient. Higher values of λ, lead to a faster convergence along the sliding surface to the zero point of the phase-plane. Let us consider the sliding surface (Eq. 15) in order to determine the relative order of the controlled system. We obtain the following result:

$$\frac{\partial \dot{s}}{\partial \mathbf{u}} = 0, \quad \frac{\partial \ddot{s}}{\partial \mathbf{u}} \neq 0 \tag{16}$$

Therefore, the relative degree of the sliding mode control is r = 2. Considering the step response case ($\ddot{\theta}_d$ = $\dot{\theta}_d$ = 0), the second order time derivative of the sliding surface can be written as:

$$\ddot{s} = -\ddot{x}_6 - \lambda \dot{x}_6 \tag{17}$$

The expression of the second order time derivative of the state variable x_6 is given by:

$$\ddot{x}_6 = \frac{1}{J}\left(\begin{array}{l} \frac{rS_{0_1}\alpha_1 F_{01}}{1+p_1x_1-s_{v_1}q_1x_3}u_1 - \frac{rs_{u_1}x_3}{1+p_1x_1-s_{v_1}q_1x_3}u_1 + r\frac{\left(b_1x_1-s_{v_1}a_1x_3\right)rx_6}{L_{01}\left(1+p_1x_1-s_{v_1}q_1x_3\right)} \\ -\frac{s_{0_2}\alpha_2 F_{02}L_0L_{ii}\sin(x_5)}{\left(1+p_2x_2-s_{v_2}q_2x_4\right)\sqrt{L_0^2+L_{ii}^2+2L_0L_{ii}\cos(x_5)}}u_2 + \frac{s_{u_2}x_4L_0L_{ii}\sin(x_5)}{\left(1+p_2x_2-s_{v_2}q_2x_4\right)\sqrt{L_0^2+L_{ii}^2+2L_0L_{ii}\cos(x_5)}}u_2 \\ -\frac{\left(b_1x_1-s_{v_1}a_1x_3\right)rX_6L_0L_{ii}\sin(x_5)}{L_{01}\left(1+p_1x_1-S_{v_1}q_1x_3\right)\sqrt{L_0^2+L_{ii}^2+2L_0L_{ii}\cos(x_5)}} - x_4\frac{L_0L_{ii}x_6\cos(x_5)\sqrt{L_0^2+L_{ii}^2+2L_0L_{ii}\cos(x_5)}}{L_0^2+L_{ii}^2+2L_0L_{ii}\cos(x_5)} \\ -X_4\frac{L_0^2L_{ii}^2\sin^2(x_5)}{\left(L_0^2+L_{ii}^2+2L_0L_{ii}\cos(x_5)\right)\sqrt{L_0^2+L_{ii}^2+2L_0L_{ii}\cos(x_5)}} + mg\beta L_1x_6\sin(x_5) - K_ex_5 - F_vx_6 \end{array}\right) \tag{18}$$

Inserting the expressions of $\dot{x}_6$ and $\ddot{x}_6$ within equation (Eq. 17) allows writing the second order time derivative of the sliding surface as:

$$\ddot{s} = \varphi(\mathbf{x},\mathbf{t}) + \gamma(\mathbf{x},\mathbf{t})\mathbf{u} \tag{19}$$

It is assumed that $|\varphi| \leq \Phi$, $0 < \Gamma_m \leq \gamma \leq \Gamma_M$ (Levant, 1993), where Γ_m, Γ_M and Φ are positive constants. We express the equation (Eq. 19) as:

$$\begin{cases} \dot{y}_1 = y_2 \\ \dot{y}_2 = \varphi(\mathbf{x},\mathbf{t}) + \gamma(\mathbf{x},\mathbf{t})\mathbf{u} \end{cases} \tag{20}$$

Where $y_1 = s$. In that case, the problem is equivalent to the finite time stabilization problem for a second order system.

3.2 Statement of the control algorithm

(Levant, 1993) presented a range of 2-sliding algorithms to stabilise second order uncertain nonlinear systems. In the current study we implemented the algorithm with prescribed law of variation of the sliding surface. This choice has been made based on criteria of relative robustness and finite time convergence (Fridman, & Levant, 2002). The general formulation of such a class of a sliding mode control algorithm is:

$$\dot{u} = \begin{cases} -u & if\ |u| > 1 \\ -V_M\, sign(y_2 - g_c(y_1)) & if\ |u| \leq 1 \end{cases} \tag{21}$$

Where V_M is a positive constant and g_c a continuous function (Fig. 7) as given by Eq. 22. Moreover, this function must verify some specific conditions (Fridman, & Levant, 2002).

$$g_c(y_1) = -\lambda_1 |y_1|^{\rho} sign(y_1), \quad \lambda_1 > 0, \quad 0.5 < \rho \leq 1 \tag{22}$$

The sufficient condition for the finite time convergence to the sliding manifold is defined by the following inequality:

$$V_m > \frac{\Phi + \sup\left[\dot{g}_c(y_1)g_c(y_1)\right]}{\Gamma_m} \tag{23}$$

Larger values of λ_1 accelerate the convergence to reach the sliding surface and provide better robustness and stability. A substitution of y_2 by Δy_1 is theoretically possible if y_2 is not available.

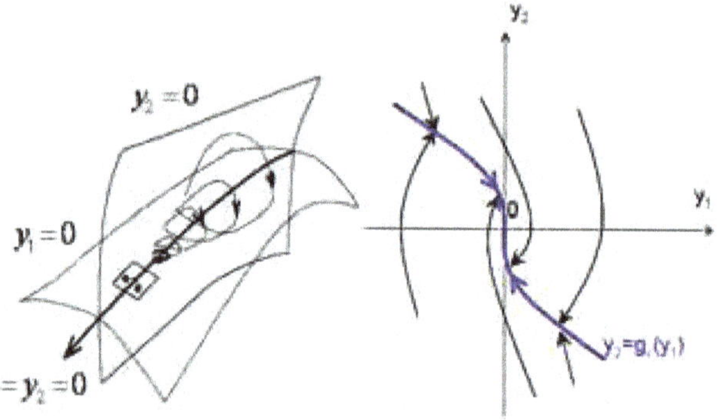

Fig. 7. Phase plot of the prescribed convergence law algorithm (Levant, 1993).

3.3 Simulation results

We have implemented the control algorithm defined by equation (Eq. 21) on the simulator of the knee-muscle biomechanical model (cf. Eq. 10). The components of the control vector **u** are the chemical inputs (u_q, u_h) and the ratio of the recruited fibers (α_q, α_h). These coefficients depend on sliding mode controller output. In our case, the knee joint is controlled by two muscle's groups: quadriceps and hamstrings. Consequently, there are two electrical currents, I_q and I_h as well as two Pulse Width Modulation values, PW_q and PW_h which have to be deduced from the sliding mode control variable u (Mohammed, et al. 2005). According to the sign of the resulting control variable at the output of the HOSM controller, we have chosen to stimulate either the quadriceps or the hamstrings (Eq. 25).

$$u = -\int V_M sign(y_2 - g_c(y_1))\,dt \qquad (\text{if } |u| \le 1) \tag{24}$$

$$\text{If } (u > 0) \Rightarrow \begin{cases} I_q = \dfrac{u}{u_{nom}} I_{\max} \\ I_h = 0 \end{cases} \qquad \text{If } (u < 0) \Rightarrow \begin{cases} I_q = 0 \\ I_h = \dfrac{u}{u_{nom}} I_{\max} \end{cases} \tag{25}$$

Where, u_{nom} and I_{max} represent respectively the nominal value of the sliding control variable u and the maximal value authorized to stimulate a muscle (around 200 mA). The current values for quadriceps I_q and hamstrings I_h and/or the Pulse Width, respectively PW_q and PW_h enable us to evaluate the required ratios of fibers to be recruited (α_q, α_h). The chemical inputs u_q and u_h are automatically activated when the electrical currents are respectively superior to zero. We have implemented this algorithm on a simulator built with the Matlab-Simulink environment. In the following simulations, we have applied two different knee desired positions, starting from the rest position, $\theta_d = 90°$ as:

$$\begin{cases} 1) \quad 1s < t < 4s : \theta_d = 130^\circ \\ 2) \quad 6s < t < 9s : \theta_d = 50^\circ \\ 3) \quad \text{Otherwise} : \theta_d = 90^\circ \end{cases} \tag{26}$$

The coefficients of the 2-sliding controller were chosen to verify the condition equations (Eq. 23). The following values have been used: $\lambda = 10$, $\lambda_1 = 20$, $\rho = 0.7$, $V_M = 1$. Figure 8-a shows the step response for different desired values. Desired and current angle curves match when sliding surface reaches zero. As we can notice, the dynamic of the system is constrained to the dynamic of the sliding surface. The finite time convergence of the sliding surface is about 1sec in knee flexion and extension (Fig.8-b). In Fig.9-a, we present the resulting stimulation currents for both quadriceps and hamstrings I_q and I_h. The control vector **u** computed by the equation (Eq. 24) is shown in Fig.9-b.

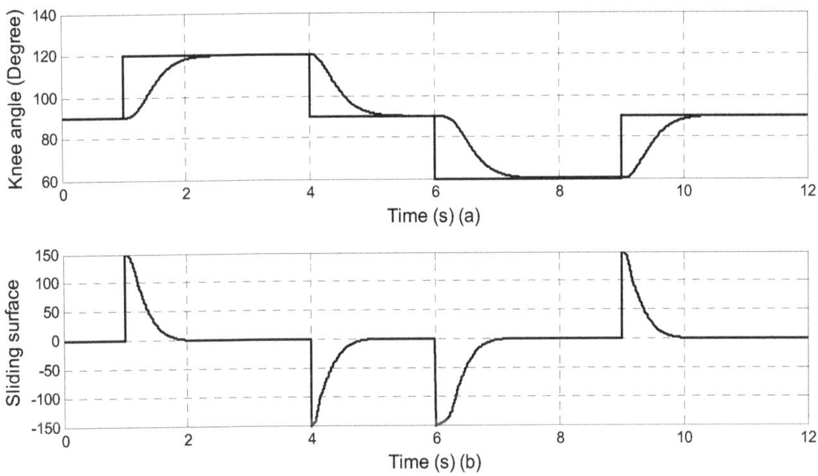

Fig. 8. a) Desired step and actual knee angle variation, b) Stabilization of the sliding surface.

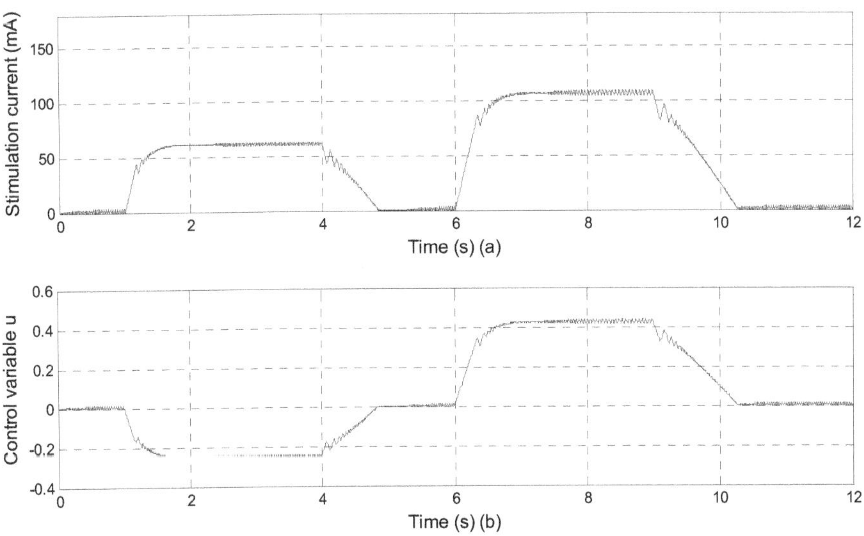

Fig. 9. a) Stimulation currents of both muscles, b) The control vector u.

4. Model predictive control MPC

The ability to handle nonlinear multi-variable systems that are constrained in states and/or control variables motivates the use of Model Predictive Control (MPC), (Allgöwer et al., 1999). This approach proved its efficiency in a large variety of industrial processes, especially in chemical processes. The MPC problem is usually stated as an optimization one subject to physical coherent constraints, and is solved with classical optimization algorithms. The MPC has been widely used in different applications due to their interesting properties (Camacho & Bordons, 1995). In our particular case, the nonlinearities of the muscle model, the constraints on the input stimulation current and on the output knee joint position lead us to adopt a controller relying on MPC. Few studies applied this technique to a musculoskeletal system. Some authors have used MPC with black-box models instead of continuous time physiological models (Schauer & Hunt, 2000).

4.1 Problem formulation

The MPC problem is usually formulated as a constrained optimization problem, (Allgöwer et al., 1999):

$$\min_{u_k^{H_p}} J(x_k, u_k^{H_p})$$

subject to:

$$\begin{aligned} u_{i|k} &\in U, \quad i \in [0, H_u] \\ x_{i|k} &\in X, \quad i \in [0, H_p] \end{aligned} \tag{27}$$

where

$$U := u_k \in \mathrm{R}^m \mid u_{\min} \le u_k \le u_{\max}$$

$$X := x_k \in \mathrm{R}^m \mid x_{\min} \le x_k \le x_{\max}$$

Internal controller variables predicted from time instance k are denoted by a double index separated by a vertical line where the second argument denotes the time instance from which the prediction is computed. $x_k = x_{0|k}$ is the initial state of the system to be controlled at time instance k and: $\hat{u}_k = \left[u_{0|k}, u_{1|k}, \ldots u_{H_u-1}, u_{H_u-1}, \ldots u_{H_u-1}\right]$ an input vector of dimension H_p (prediction horizon). At each sample, a finite optimal control problem is solved over the prediction horizon. We assume that we would like the controlled variables, y_k (Fig.10), to follow some reference trajectory r. Predictive control consists in computing the vector $\hat{u}_k$ of consecutive inputs $u_{i|k}$ over the control horizon H_u by optimizing the objective function J under given constraints (Eq. 27). The control signal is assumed to be constant after H_u samples over a horizon of $(H_p - H_u)$ dimension. When the solution of the optimal control problem has been obtained, the value of the first control variable in the optimal trajectory, $u_{k|k}$, is applied to the process. The rest of the predicted control variable trajectory is discarded, and at the next sampling interval the entire procedure is repeated (Kesson, 2003). These computations are updated at each sampling time.

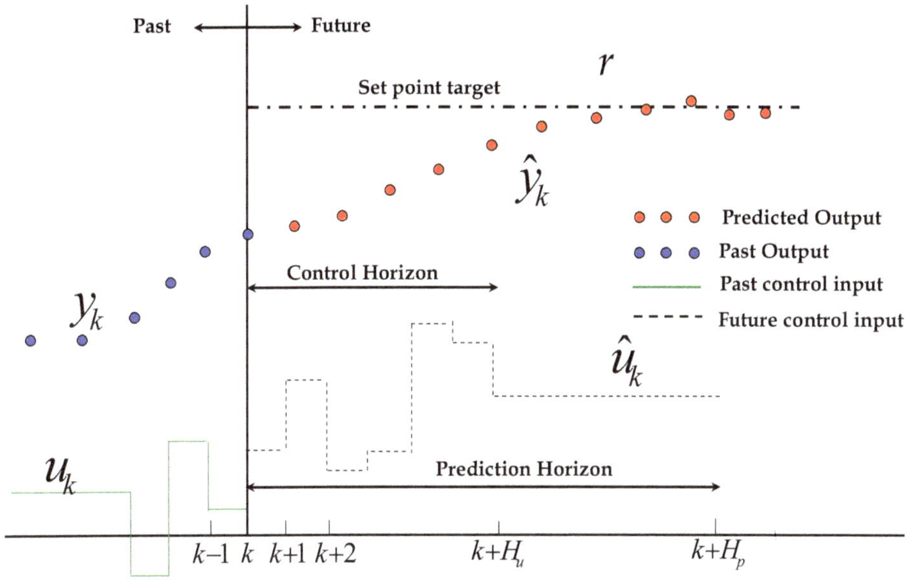

Fig. 10. Principles of the predictive control strategy design (Seborg et al., 2004).

The nonlinear equality constraint on the state represents the dynamic model of the system. Bounding constraints over the inputs $u_{i|k}$ and the state variables $x_{i|k}$ over the prediction horizon H_p are defined through the sets U and X (Eq. 27). The objective function J is usually defined as:

$$J(x_k, u_k^{H_p}) = \phi(x_{H_p|k}) + \sum_{i-0}^{H_u} L(x_{i|k}, u_{i|k}) \tag{28}$$

where Φ is a constraint on the state at the end of the prediction horizon, called state terminal constraint, and L a quadratic function of the state and inputs. The computation of the solution $u_k^{H_p}$ can be divided in two steps: firstly, computation of a solution satisfying the constraints (including the state terminal constraint), and secondly optimization. The first step involves bounding constraints (Eq. 27), and nonlinear constraints expressing the dynamic model of the system (Eq. 9). Simulations were performed in Matlab-Simulink environment using the "ode45" integration algorithm with variable step size. The simulation codes were adapted from MPCtools, (Kesson, 2003).

4.2 Model Linearization

The system (Eq. 9) is a nonlinear multivariable system. In a first step and in order to apply a linear predictive controller, we made some assumptions to the nonlinear system. The goal was to get a feasible solution before applying the controller to the non linear plant. Some hypotheses make this nonlinear system easier:

- We consider that the chemical control u_{ch} is a positive constant indicating a muscular fiber fusion. This hypothesis could be justified in our case by the fact that the stimulation frequency is much greater then the muscular fiber fusion.

Consequently, during stimulation, we have only contractions and no relaxations: $s_u = 1, \quad s_v = -1, \quad |u| = u, \quad |\dot{\varepsilon}_c| = -\dot{\varepsilon}_c$

- Only one muscle, the quadriceps has been taken into account in the following causing knee extension. When no extension, the gravity induces knee flexion to the rest position.
- We suppose that the stiffness of the serial element which represents the tendon is much greater than the stiffness of the contractile element. This hypothesis is true since we are performing only dynamic movements and no isometric stimulations were considered.

$$\dot{\varepsilon}_c = \frac{L_0}{L_{c0}}\dot{\varepsilon} - \frac{1}{L_{c0}K_s}\dot{F}_c$$

In the above conditions, the term $\frac{1}{L_{c0}K_s}\dot{F}$ is less than $10^{-3}\frac{L_0}{L_{c0}}\dot{\varepsilon}$

By taking into account the above assumptions, the plant model will have a reduced nonlinear form where $\mathbf{x} = [x_1\ x_2\ x_3\ x_4]^T = \left[K\ F\ \theta\ \dot{\theta}\right]^T$ is the state vector and $\mathbf{u} = \alpha$ is the control input. The plant model could thus be expressed by the following set of differential equations:

$$\begin{aligned}
\dot{x}_1 &= ax_1 + bx_1x_4 + cf_l(x_3)u \\
\dot{x}_2 &= dx_1x_4 + ax_2 + bx_2x_4 + ef_l(x_3)u \\
\dot{x}_3 &= x_4 \\
\dot{x}_4 &= fx_2 + h\cos(x_3) + lx_4
\end{aligned} \tag{29}$$

Where:

$$a = -u_{ch}, b = \frac{r}{L_{c0}}, c = u_{ch}K_0, d = -r, e = u_{ch}F_0$$

$$f = \frac{r}{I}, h = \frac{-mg\beta L_1}{I}, l = \frac{-F_v}{I}, f_l = \exp\left[-\left(\frac{\overline{l}-1}{b_l}\right)^2\right]$$

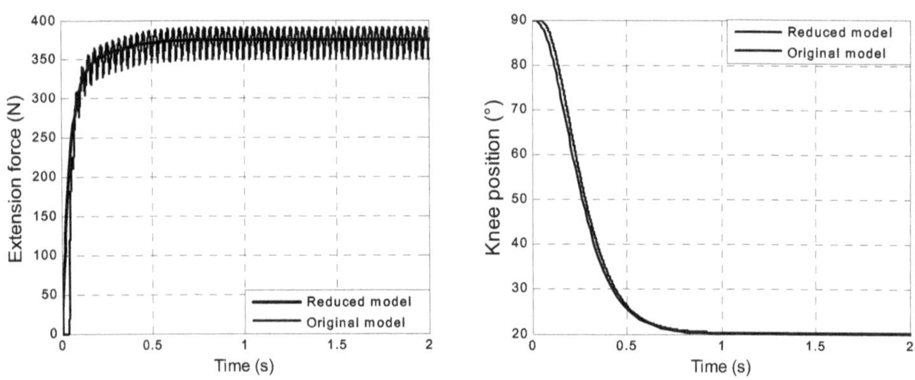

Fig. 11. Non linear models: original and reduced.

The above hypotheses were validated through simulations as shown in figure (11). This latter presents the responses of both, the original non linear model (Eq. 9) and the reduced non linear model (Eq. 29). On the left side, we show the force generated by both models. The original non linear model presents some oscillations reflecting the contraction-relaxation cycle. These oscillations results from the stimulation frequency. On the right side of figure (11), we present the knee position output of both models. We can notice that the linearized model fits well with the original one in terms of force generation as well as knee angular position. A linearization of this system around an arbitrary operating point $(\overline{\mathbf{x}},\overline{\mathbf{u}})$ has been computed using its Jacobian. The linear model could be formulated as follows:

$$\begin{cases} \dot{\mathbf{x}} = \mathrm{A}\,\mathbf{x} + \mathrm{B}\,\mathbf{u} \\ \mathbf{y} = \mathrm{C}\,\mathbf{x} + \mathrm{D}\,\mathbf{u} \end{cases} \tag{30}$$

Where:

$$\mathrm{A}=\begin{bmatrix} a+b\overline{x}_4 & 0 & c\overline{u}\dot{f}_l(\overline{x}_3) & b\overline{x}_1 \\ d\overline{x}_4 & a+b\overline{x}_4 & e\overline{u}\dot{f}_l(\overline{x}_3) & d\overline{x}_1+b\overline{x}_2 \\ 0 & 0 & 0 & 1 \\ 0 & f & -h\sin(\overline{x}_3) & l \end{bmatrix} \quad \mathrm{B}=\begin{bmatrix} c\overline{u}f_l(\overline{x}_3) \\ e\overline{u}f_l(\overline{x}_3) \\ 0 \\ 0 \end{bmatrix} \quad \mathrm{C}=\begin{bmatrix}0 & 0 & 1 & 0\end{bmatrix} \quad \mathrm{D}=0$$

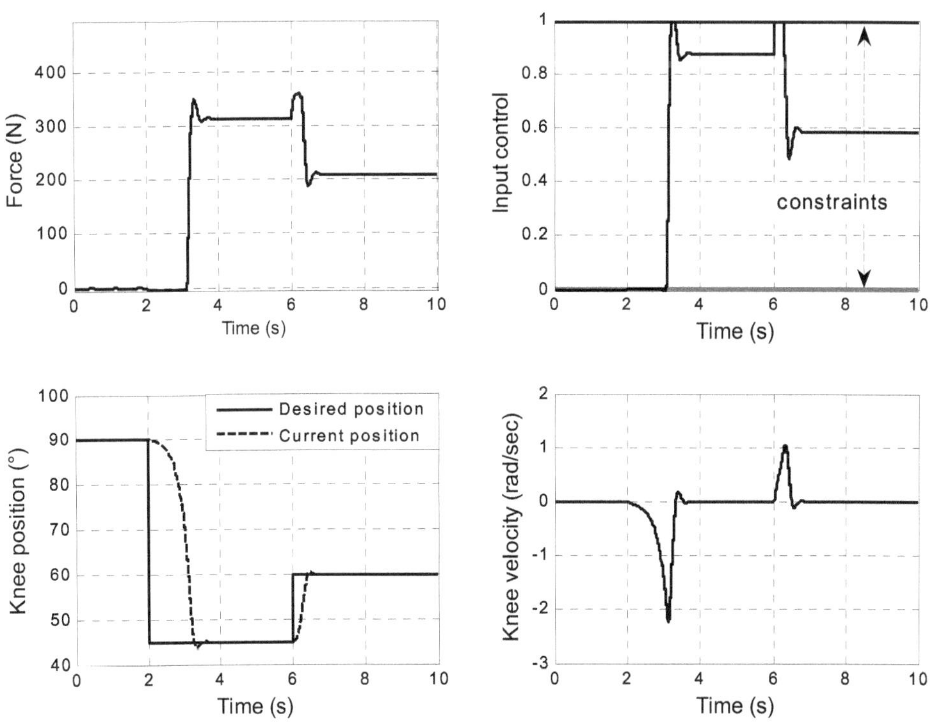

Fig. 12. Tracking knee joint trajectory and controller performance.

4.3 Simulation results (MPC)

Different simulation tests have been carried out. The sample period was set to 0.01 sec, the prediction and control horizon H_p and H_u were computed as a function of the system time constant: H_p =30 and H_u =10. The constrained input u = α was the recruitment variable. Since the recruitment function is static, the optimal pulse width or stimulation amplitude could be easily computed. The recruitment variable has been constrained to be between 0 and 1 representing respectively no fiber recruited and full recruitment. The controlled variable, which is the system output, was constrained to stay between θ = 0° (hyperextension) and θ = 90° (resting position). Only the knee angle was used as feedback to update the control input. Controller parameters were calculated offline. Simulation results are shown in figures 12, 13 and 14.

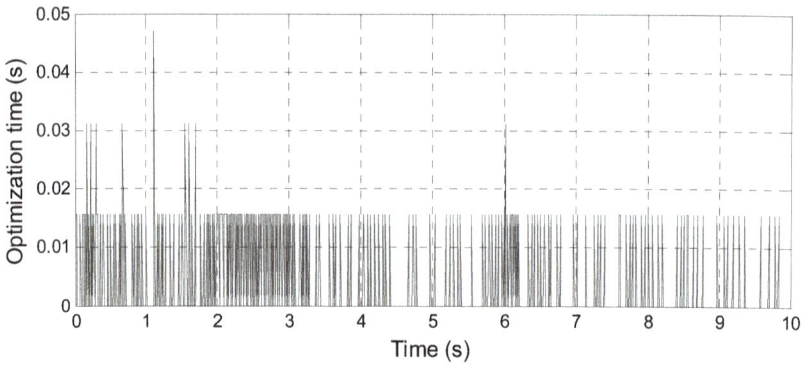

Fig. 13. Predictive control optimization time.

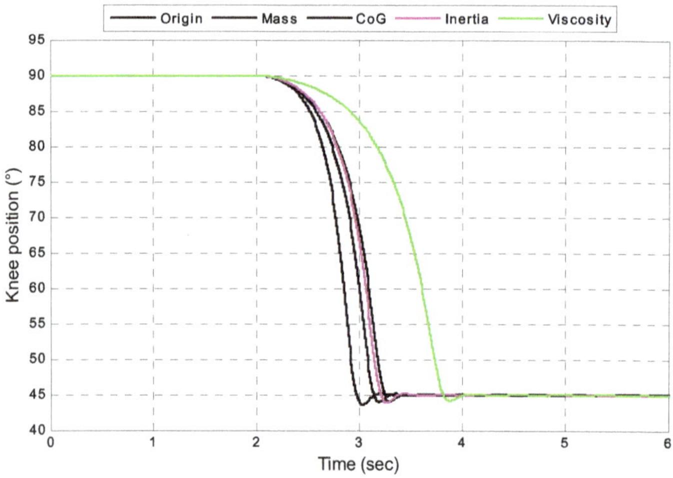

Fig. 14. MPC robustness: uncertainty on mass, position of the centre of gravity, inertia and viscosity.

In figure (12), initial conditions correspond to θ =90°, which means the knee joint is in the rest position. After 2 seconds, the desired trajectory was stepped to θ = 45° which corresponds to medial knee extension. The controller converges to the desired position in a finite time while maintaining the control input between its limits. At time = 6 s, we perform a 15° knee flexion inducing a muscle force and stiffness decrease. The controller managed to converge to the desired position and to fully compensate the position change without need for any feedback observer and respecting at the same time the constraints on input and output. Figure (13) shows the optimization time needed to perform the above simulation. It should be noticed that the muscle parameters used in these simulation relate to a healthy subject (Tables 2 and 3). The inaccuracy that may occur on these parameters when dealing with paraplegic patients could be compensated by the robustness of the (MPC) controller. In figure (14), we studied the controller robustness against parameter variations. In fact, the uncertainty could affect mainly the inertial parameters which have been estimated, based on statistical abacuses and regression equations (De Leva, 1996). Although the parameters uncertainties imposed were relatively important (20% - 25%) from the initial value, the MPC controller showed a satisfactory robustness regardless these uncertainties.

5. Controllers performance – comparative study

In this section, we have drawn a comparison between the controllers' performance (HOSM and MPC) in terms of input control and state regulation. These controllers were simulated under the same conditions. A classical linear controller based on poles placement (PP) serves as a reference controller.

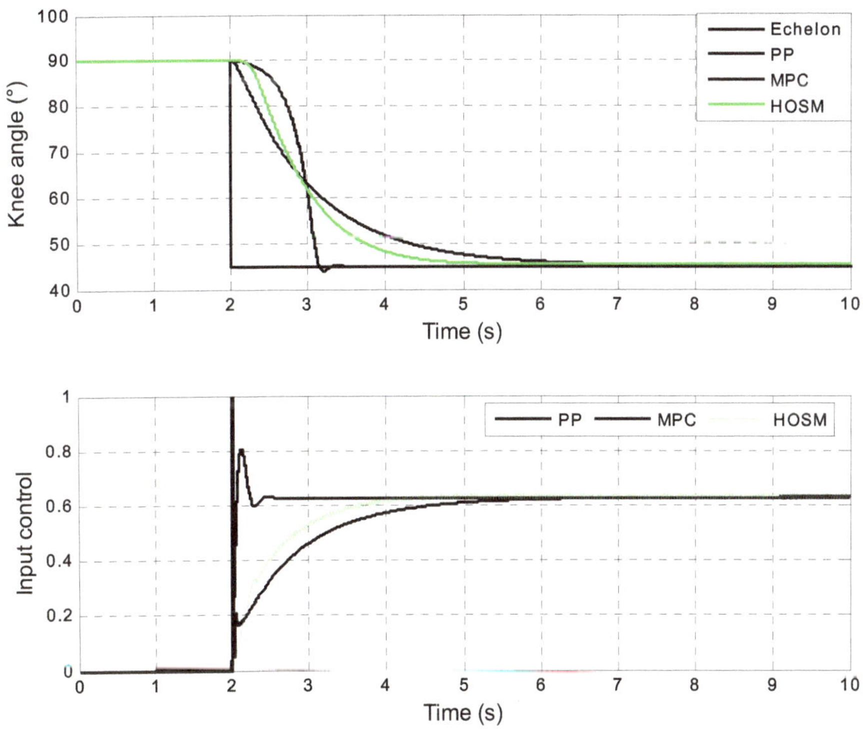

Fig. 15. Comparison of control strategies: desired position corresponds to 45° knee extension. PP for poles placement, MPC for predictive control and HOSM for high order sliding mode.

In figure (15), we have simulated a 45° knee extension by activating the quadriceps muscle. Unlike the PP controller which takes the longest time to converge to the desired position and presents at the same time an input saturation during the transient period, the MPC controller converged to the desired position in a relatively limited time. Saturation of the input control means an important rate of stimulation firing during the transient period. The HOSM controller shows a satisfactory performance in terms of time convergence and position regulation. We can notice that the system dynamics evolution is constrained to the sliding surface dynamic (Eq. 15). Input control does not show also any overshoot, and the chattering effect has been considerably reduced. In order to study the robustness of these controllers, we have induced a position perturbation that corresponds to a quick and limited knee flexion. In terms of position regulation figure (16) shows that the different controllers succeed to converge to the desired position. In terms of input control, the PP controller is very sensitive to this perturbation; the MPC controller is much less sensitive and finally the HOSM controller that showed the best performance against external perturbation.

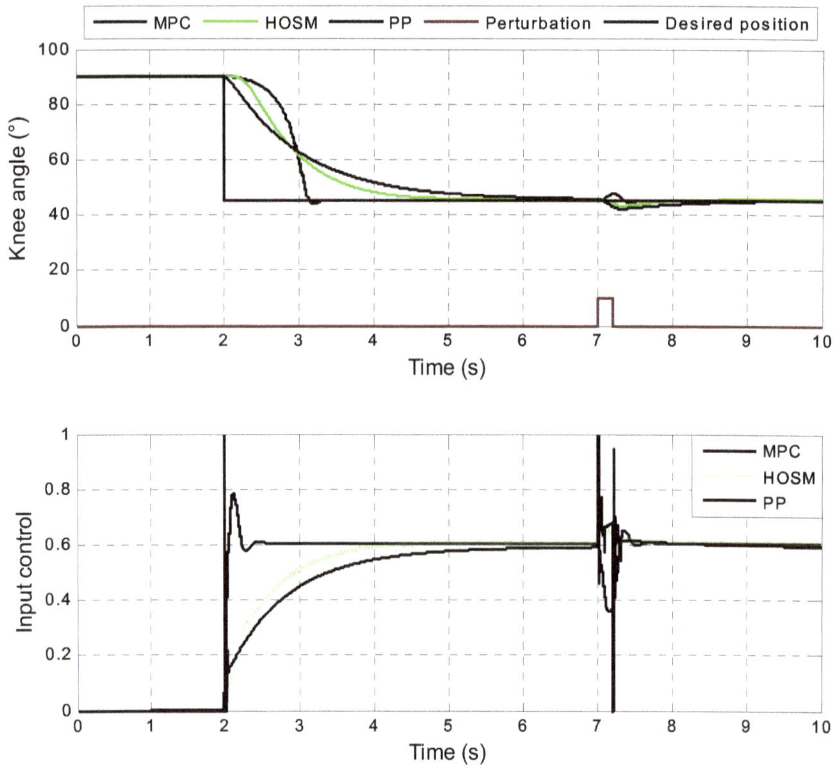

Fig. 16. Controllers behaviors against an external perturbation.

6. Conclusion

The main challenge that we face when applying FES to the paralyzed lower limbs is to avoid hyperstimulation and to defer the muscular fatigue as much as possible. Few studies have treated the human muscle as an entire physiological element in a closed loop system. Known by their robustness against unknown perturbation and their accuracy against model mismatch, we have used robust control techniques such as the High Order Sliding mode (HOSM) and the Model Predictive Control (MPC) in a closed loop control scheme. The MPC offers the possibility to integrate constraints on input, output and measured states explicitly in its formulation. These strategies have ensured, by simulations, a robust control and a safer movement of the paralysed lower extremities. The controllers were applied to a multi-scale muscle model developed within the *DEMAR* project and recently published (El-Makssoud et al., 2004 -a). It is based on internal physiological characteristics assembling two levels: the microscopic one, involving the sliding actin-myosin filaments and the macroscopic part represented by a contractile element and an elastic element. This highly non linear model has been described by a set of differential equations. We have made some realistic assumptions to the biomechanical model of the knee joint actuated by two groups of antagonistic muscles (quadriceps and hamstrings). As a result we obtained a simplified nonlinear version of the knee-muscle formulation. Dynamic and geometric parameters were identified based on experimental kinematics data recorded using a video based motion analysis. Different identification techniques were applied such as the least square, non-linear interpolation, regression equations, etc. We were able to control the quadriceps-hamstrings muscles for the knee flexion-extension in order to track a predefined position trajectory within a large range of movement. Satisfactory stability and tracking error were achieved after a finite time delay. The performance of the closed loop system has been assessed in the presence of external force perturbations. Controller responses to these perturbations vary from the most sensitive (PP) to the MPC controller and finally the HOSM controller which seemed to be the most robust against external perturbations. We should notice that the system dynamic was constrained to follow the sliding surface dynamics. The MPC had shown a better performance in terms of time response than the HOSM. The results show that we respect the constraints on input and output. We are trying to limit the computational effort which is a common deficit of the MPC design. Actually, the optimisation time obtained (Fig.13) is around 20 ms in Matlab environment which is quite encouraging for a real time implementation. Experiments are ongoing to validate the control scheme on paraplegic patients by using the multi-moment platform used during the identification protocol (Fig. 6).

7. References

Allgöwer, F.; Badgwell, T.A.; Qin, S.J.; Rawlings, J.B. & Wright, S.J. (1999). Nonlinear predictive control and moving horizon estimation - an introductory overview, *In: Frank, P.M (edt.), Advances in control: highlights of ECC'99*, Springer, (1999), p. 391-449.

Bajd, T.; Kralj, A.; Sega J.; Turk R.; Benko H. & Strojnik, P. (1981). Use of a two- channel functional electrical stimulator to stand paraplegics, In: *Physical therapy*, 61(4), p.526-7.

Camacho, E. & Bordons, C. (1995). Model Predictive Control in the Process Industry *Springer-Verlag New York, Inc.*

DeLeva, P., (1996) Adjustments to zatsiorsky-seluyanov's segment inertia parameters. *Journal of Biomechanics*, Vol.29, p.1223-1230.

Donaldson, N. & Yu, C. (1996). FES standing control by handle reactions of leg muscle stimulation (CHRELMS), *IEEE Transactions on rehabilitation engineering*, 4(4) p.280-284.

El-Makssoud, H.; Guiraud, D. & Poignet, P. (2004-a). Mathematical muscle model for Electrical Stimulation control strategies, *IEEE International Conference on Robotics and Automation*, p. 1282-1287.

El-Makssoud, H.; Guiraud, D. & Poignet, P. (2004-b). Enhancement of physiological and mechanical modelling of the skeletal muscle controlled by Functional Electrical Stimulation. *International Functional Electrical Stimulation Society (IFESS)*, Bournemouth, UK 6-9 September 2004.

Ferrarin, M.; Palazzo. F & Riener R. (2001). Model-Based Control of FES Induced Single Joint Movements, *IEEE Transactions on Neural systems and rehabilitation engineering*, 9(3), p.245-257.

Fridman, L. & Levant, A. (2002). High-Order Sliding Modes, *in: Sliding Modes Control in Engineering*, Ed. W. Perruquetti, J.P. Barbot, Marcel Dekker, Inc. New-York, p. 53-101.

Gautier, M. & Poignet P., (2002). Closed loop identification by inverse model of physical parameters of mechatronic systems. *Journal européen des systèmes automatisés*, Vol.36, No.3, p.465-480.

Hawkins, D. & Hull, M. (1990). A method for determining lower extremity muscle- tendon lengths during flexion/extension movements. *Journal of Biomechanics*, Vol. 23, p.487-494.

Kesson, J. (2003), Operator Interaction and Optimization in Control Systems, *P.hd thesis*, Department of Automatic Control Lund Institute of Technology.

Kromer, V. (1994). Analyse des forces musculaires au cours de la marche - Approche en corps rigide et simulation en mécanismes plans flexibles par éléments finis, *P.h.d. Thesis*, Institut national polytechnique de Lorraine (INPL).

Levant, A. (1993). Sliding order and sliding accuracy in sliding model control, *International Journal of Control*, Vol.58 No.6, p.1247-1263.

Levenberg, K. (1944). A method for the solution of certain problems in least square. *Quarterly applied Mathematics*, Vol. 2, p.164-168.

Mohammed, S.; Fraisse, P.; Guiraud, D.; Poignet, P. & H. El Makssoud, (2005-a). Robust Control Law Strategy Based on High Order Sliding Mode : Towards a Muscle Control, in: *IROS'05: International Conference on Intelligent Robots & Systems*, p. 2882-2887.

Mohammed, S. (2006), Contribution à la synthèse de movement et à la commande des muscles squelettiques sous Stimulation Electrique Fonctionnelle, *P.h.d. Thesis*, LIRMM-Université de Montpellier II.

Mulder, AJ.; Veltink, PH. & Boom, HB. (1992). On/off control in FES-induced standing up: a model study and experiments. *Medical and Biological Engineering and Computing*, 30(2), p. 205-212.

Poboroniuc, M.; Wood, D.; Donaldson, N.; Fuhr, T. & Riener R. (2003). Closed-loop control for FES-based restoration of standing in paraplegia, *2nd World Congress of the International Society of Physical and Rehabilitation Medicine-ISPRM*, Prague, Czech Republic, May 18-22, p.201-204.

Poboroniuc, M.; Fuhr, T.; Wood, D.; Riener, R. & Donaldson, N. (2002). FES-Induced Standing-Up and sitting down control strategies in Paraplegia", *FESnet Conference*. September 2nd-3rd, Glasgow, UK, p.1-3.

Riener, R. & Fuhr, T. (1998). Patient-Driven Control of FES-Supported standing Up: A simulation study, *IEEE Transactions on rehabilitation engineering*, 6(2), p.113-123.

Schauer, T. & Hunt, K.J., (2000). Nonlinear predictive control of knee-joint angle using FES, *International Functional Electrical Stimulation Society (IFESS)*, Aalborg, Denmark, p. 425-428.

Seborg, D.E.; Edgar, T. F. & Mellichamp, D. A., (2004) Process Dynamics and Control, 2nd edition, John Wiley and Sons, New York.

Veltink, P.H.; Chizeck, H.J.; Crago, P.E. & El-Bialy, A. (1992). Nonlinear joint angle control for artificially stimulated muscle. *IEEE Transactions on biomedical engineering*, Vol. 39 N.4, p. 368-380.

Wood, DE.; Harper, VJ.; Barr, FMD.; Taylor, PN., Phillips, GF. & Ewins, DJ. (1998). Experience in Using Knee angles as part of a closed-Loop Algorithm to control FES-Assisted Paraplegic Standing, *6th Vienna International Workshop on Functional Electrostimulation*, (Vienna, Austria), p.137-140.

11

Robotics and Virtual Reality Applications in Mobility Rehabilitation

Rares F. Boian[1], Grigore C. Burdea[2] & Judith E. Deutsch[3]
[1] *Department of Mathematics and Computer Science, Babeş-Bolyai University, Romania*
[2] *CAIP Center, Rutgers University, New Jersey, USA*
[3] *Rivers Lab SHRP, University of Medicine and Dentistry, New Jersey, USA*

1. Introduction

Gait training is a method to reduce mobility dysfunction. Diverse patient populations exhibit mobility impairments that can be ameliorated with gait training. Two such populations are people post-stroke and post-spinal cord injury.

The ability to walk is one of several functions affected by stroke. Immediately after the stroke only 37% of the survivors are able to walk (Jorgensen et al., 1995). Of the patients with initial paralysis only 21% regain walking function (Wandel et al., 2000).

Another patient population that can benefit from gait training (Dietz et al., 1998; Nicol et al., 1995) is the spinal cord injury victims. According to the Travis Roy Foundation there are currently between 250,000 and 400,000 Americans living with spinal cord injury.

Gait training or locomotion therapy uses several devices to assist the patient move and maintain balance. Canes, crutches, walkers, and platforms are simple ambulatory assistive devices that modify a patient's independence and functional mobility. Treadmills often equipped with un-weighing devices are used for training walking at various speeds on a straight flat surface or small incline. These features, along with treadmills' simple design and affordable costs are sufficient reasons for their popularity. Treadmills, however, cannot render more complex walking surfaces which patients encounter daily, such as: stairs, curves, uneven surfaces (e.g. cobblestone paths), or surfaces with various stiffness or friction coefficients.

Training patients to negotiate complex walking surfaces can be done either through in-vivo training assisted by a physical therapist, or through using devices able to simulate such surfaces. The former approach often takes the patient out of the controlled clinic environment, which is not always feasible and may raise safety concerns. The latter approach may offer an alternative to real environment training. It would allow patients to exercise in controlled and safe conditions in the clinic, which could potentially be more time and personnel efficient than real environment training, In this context, numerous research projects have approached gait simulators trying to create robotic devices that could render complex walking surfaces.

The integration of such robotic systems with virtual environments may, in theory, expand the range of applications to entertainment and real-life task training of patients with walking dysfunction. The appealing reasons for using such systems are the flexibility and transparent data collection offered by virtual environments over real environments (Iwata, 1999; Sveistrup, 2004). In addition, the ability to train for a task in a controlled environment, away from the potential hazards of a real environment makes such simulators viable choices in medical or military applications.

2. Locomotion Simulators

Locomotion simulators, which attempt to simulate the sensations of walking, have been the focus of many researchers due to their applicability in simulating real-life tasks. Beside the medical reasons presented above, gait simulators are an attractive subject due to their applicability for military training or gaming. However, the design of a locomotion simulator for therapeutic purposes must consider and possibly solve several aspects raised by the people using it and by the environment where it will be used.

- *Safety* - The first and most important aspect is safety. Gait simulators are usually complex robotic devices on which the patient stands and moves. To avoid accidents, the simulator must be constrained to move only within the physiological limits of the human body. It also must provide the patient with means to quickly reach safety should anything wrong happen with the simulator.
- *Environment* - A gait simulator must also be suitable for usage in a clinic or home environment. Given the size, these devices are most often used in clinics, but there are research projects (the simulator presented in the last part of this chapter included) that aim to reduce the simulator's size. The environment also imposes restrictions on the actuators. Hydraulic actuators are appropriate for balancing the weight of a person, but they are unsuitable for medical usage, because they are impossible to keep clean, and also pose the risk of dangerous leakages.
- *Interference with patient* - Although not always possible, a simulator should allow the patient to move freely, without constraining him or her. This implies supporting normal step lengths, various locomotion speeds, and changes of direction. Solutions for this requirement usually impose compromises on the size of the simulator.
- *Mechanical bandwidth* - The human haptic sensory capabilities require a force display to rendering bandwidth of about 1 KHz (Burdea, 1996), while the human motor actions require around 10 Hz bandwidth. Thus, a walking simulator needs to render forces at 10 Hz to be able to follow the patient's motion. In order to simulate more complex walking surfaces, forces should ideally be applied at 1 KHz bandwidth. However, these forces are usually felt through shoes, so there is no need of such high fidelity.
- *Surface simulation* - The interaction between a gait simulator and the patient is defined by the surface to be rendered. In order to render complex surfaces realistically, the contact between the simulator and the patient's foot should include multiple active points that define the shape of the surface. Ideally, the simulator should also support changes of walking direction and surface inclination. The solutions to all these issues depend primarily on the design and mechanical limits of the simulator.

- *Assistive mode* - The design of walking simulators for physical therapy also needs to consider assistive mode functioning. As the patients are likely to have difficulty walking, it can be useful to actively guide their feet while walking.
- *Data collection* - One benefit of involving robotics in the rehabilitation procedures is the possibility of collecting data about the patient actions and motions. Data measured during exercises can then be processed and serve as objective base for progress evaluation.

The design of a gait simulator poses numerous issues to be solved, besides those listed above. However, all designs must address one essential requirement: to create the sensation of walking on an infinite surface. The treadmill design solves this problem with a straight forward approach, but is limited to simulating an infinite straight smooth path. To rendered surfaces richer in features, researchers devised several designs, which Hollerbach (Hollerbach, 1999) classifies into three categories: walk-in-place devices, treadmills, and foot platforms.

2.1 Walk-in-Place Devices

These devices require the user to walk in place without advancing while his or her motions are tracked by sensors. The recorded data are then interpreted by a driving workstation that computes the direction and speed of the virtual avatar and changes the view in the virtual environment. These systems do not output any haptic feedback to the user. The only forces the user feels is the contact with the floor.

Templeman et al (Templeman et al, 1999) and Parsons et al. (Parsons et al., 1998) developed such systems using magnetic trackers to measure the user's motion and infer the direction and speed of walking.

Iwata tried the same approach using slippery shoes and asked the user to walk normally (Iwata & Yoshida, 1999). An improved walk-in–place device is presented in Bouguilla et al. (Bouguilla & Sato, 2002). The user walked on a turntable that counteracted the user's change of direction by rotating in the opposed direction.

Compared to a regular treadmill, the walk-in-place systems bring the possibility of changing the walking direction but do not allow the patients to actually walk with normal gait. Iwata's approach with slippery shoes may be risky when dealing with people with disabilities.

2.2 Treadmills

The treadmill category includes devices that allow the user to walk normally on top of a mobile surface that slides in the direction opposed to that of walking.

Such a treadmill is the Sarcos Treadport (Christensen et al., 2000) which can simulate steep up-hill walking and inertial forces.

The Torus treadmill (Iwata, 1999) allowed the user to walk in any direction at a maximum speed of 0.5m/sec.

Another omni-directional treadmill is presented in (Wang et al., 2003). The device developed by Wang et al. used a low friction cloth on top of a rigid board. The cloth was moved in the direction opposite to that of walking by high-friction casters pressed against the board.

The ATR-GSS device presented in (Miyasato, 2000) is a regular treadmill instrumented with mobile plates under the belt. Various walking surface shapes can be simulated by moving the plates up and down.

The advantages brought by these systems when compared with regular treadmills are readily apparent. The change in direction and up-hill walking are frequent daily life scenarios, for which the patients could be trained for. The disadvantage of these devices is that they were not designed for physical rehabilitation, thus their deployment in a clinic is problematic due to size and actuator choices.
The Lokomat System and the Robomedica BWS System are walking simulators developed specifically for clinical usage. Both of them rely on a regular treadmill and provide an actuated systems for dynamically supporting the patient's weight. The Lokomat system, designed for paraplegic rehabilitation, also features an exoskeleton that can guide the patient's legs through the normal gait cycle.

2.3 Foot Platforms

This category includes devices that use one actuated platform for each foot. Depending on the degrees of freedom of the platforms, these systems may be able to simulate complex surfaces, by controlling the position and orientation of the surface at each foot.
Examples of foot platforms are the Sarcos Biport (Hollerbach, 1999) that uses 2DOF platforms and the GaitMaster (Iwata et al., 2001) that uses 3DOF platforms. Just like the treadmills above, the foot platform system presented in this section feature flexibility for rendering more complex surfaces, but their design was not meant for clinical usage.

2.4 Other Walking Simulators

A very realistic simulation of uneven terrain is the Terrain Surface Simulator ALF presented in (Noma et al. 2000). The simulator is a rectangular surface made of small tilt-able plates that can be controlled in real-time. By changing the orientation of the plates, the walking surface can be set in a large variety of shapes. This device is not a treadmill so the user can only walk in any direction within the actuated area.
E-motek Inc. (Amsterdam, Netherlands) has developed the CAREN system, a hydraulically actuated Stewart platform robot supporting a 2-meter diameter board for simulating surfaces with any tilt angle.
VirtuSphere Inc. (Redmond, WA) develops a virtual sphere large enough for a person to fit in. The sphere is made of low-friction material and is supported by a system of casters that allow it to rotate as the user walks.

3. Virtual Environments

The integration of gait simulators with virtual environments makes possible task specific training in the clinic. A patient immersed in a virtual world while exercising may find the therapy less tedious and may also be more motivated (Riva, 2000).
A gait simulator integrated with a VR simulation has to accomplish two main tasks:
map the user's motion into virtual environment navigation and calculate the haptic feedback to be applied to the user's feet or legs as a result of the interactions in the virtual world. The extent to which these tasks are implemented depends mainly on the limitations imposed by the simulator system.
In most situations, the applicability and success of a virtual reality simulation is conditioned by the degree of video and audio feedback. For physical-based simulations, the realism is

also defined by how close the haptic feedback feels compared to the real life experience. In the case of gait simulators, the haptic feedback is calculated from the interaction between a virtual avatar and a virtual surface and applied primarily to the feet.

4. Dual Stewart Platform Mobility Simulator

The main hardware components of the Mobility Simulator are two 6DOF prototype Rutgers Mega-Ankle (RMA) pneumatic robots (see Figure 1). Each robot has a Stewart platform configuration with six dual-acting pneumatic pistons. Each piston is mounted in parallel with a linear potentiometer, which provides information of the smaller mobile platform position vs. the larger fixed one. The mobile platform has a foot attachment plate and a 6DOF force sensor. Force data are used when the Rutgers Mega-Ankle robot is in force control mode. The Mobility Simulator also incorporates an electro-pneumatic control interface, an un-weighting frame (Biodex Co.), a graphical workstation and a large screen custom display. The design of the simulator fits in the "foot platforms" category defined by Hollerbach (Hollerbach, 1999). The user stands with each foot secured with straps to the top of a platform, while the VR simulation (Boian et al., 2004b) is displayed on the large screen facing the user. To improve performance and safety, the user's body is strapped in the un-weighting frame placed above the two platforms. For lightweight users unloading is not necessary, safety being provided by the handlebars mounted on the frame's posts. In this setup, the user can walk on top of the RMA platforms with small steps limited by the platform's workspace (Boian et al., 2003).

During walking, each foot either supports the weight of the body or swings freely while taking a new step. Accordingly, each RMA platform can function in load compensation mode or in free motion mode. In free motion mode the RMA platform follows the swinging foot and compensates for its own mobile platform weight. During this mode, the platform applies very low to zero forces to the foot. In load compensation mode, the platform holds the supporting foot weight and slides backward simulating the behavior of a treadmill. In both modes, the robots can apply additional 6DOF forces or vibrations to the user's foot as commanded by the simulation running on the workstation. The two functioning modes mentioned above are a subset of the actual implementation, sufficient for the purpose of this paper. A more detailed description of the RMA platform's functioning modes can be found in (Boian, 2005).

The simulator software is distributed on two computers: the graphics workstation and the electro-pneumatic control interface (an embedded PC) as illustrated in Figure 2. The graphics workstation handles the graphic and haptic rendering. Based on the information received from the control interface, it calculates the interaction between the virtual feet and the virtual environment and sends back to the control interface commands regarding the forces to be applied or the functioning mode to be used.

The control interface handles the low-level servo control of the two robots, and provides the simulator with the position of each foot calculated through forward kinematics. For performance purposes, the control interface also takes care of switching between certain functioning modes based on the forces applied by the foot as measured by the Rutgers Mega-Ankle 6DOF force sensor. The current functioning mode of each RMA platform is also sent to the graphics workstation. A more detailed presentation of the tasks executed by the control interface can be found in (Boian et al. 2003).

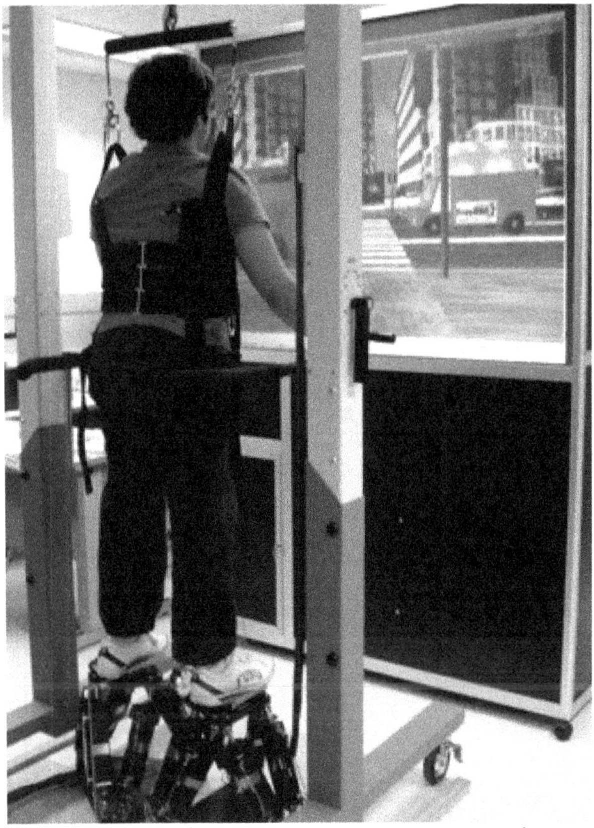

Fig. 1. The Rutgers Mobility Simulator. © Rutgers University and UMDNJ. Reprinted by permission.

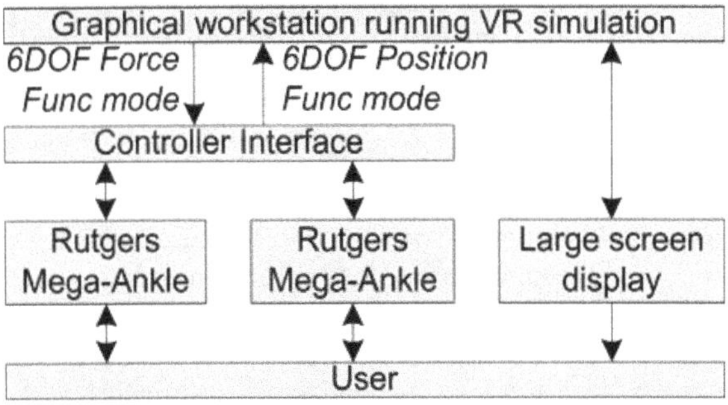

Fig. 2. The Mobility Simulator connection diagram.

4.1 The Rutgers Mega-Ankle servo control

The servo controller design is split over three loops represented as shaded areas in Figure 3. From top to bottom, the loops are: task control loop, dynamics loop, and pressure loop.

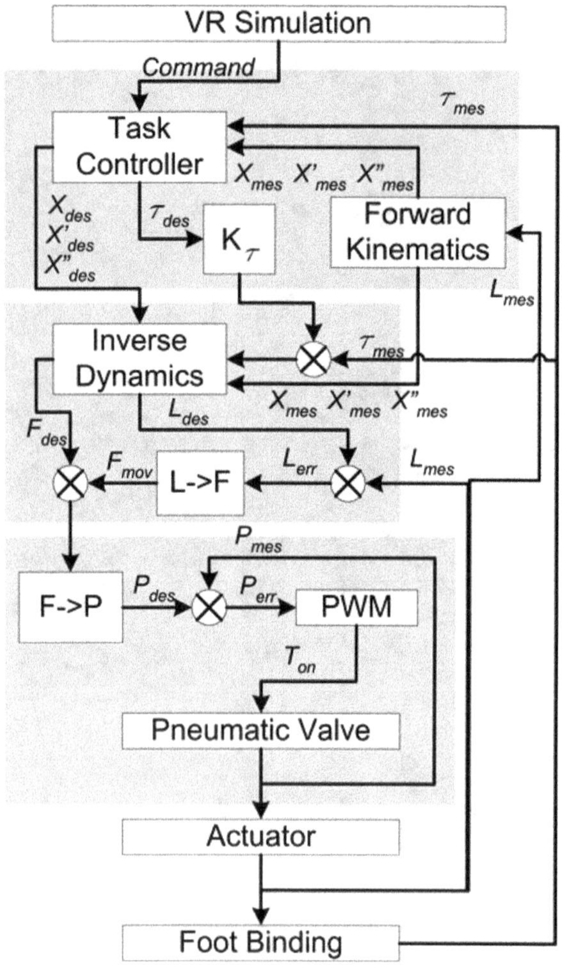

Fig. 3. Controller architecture. © Rutgers University and UMDNJ. Reprinted by permission.

The task control loop is responsible for processing the commands coming from the VR simulation and converting them into Stewart platform desired position, velocity, acceleration and forces. The commands coming from the simulation specify the functioning mode to be used (i.e. weight support mode or free motion mode), and haptic effects and forces to be applied to the users feet. This loop is executed alternatively for each platform. The task controller converts the simulation command using as additional input the measured positions and forces, read by the linear potentiometers and the force sensor of each robot. The dynamics loop transforms the desired Cartesian positions and forces into actuator level forces. The inverse dynamics implementation takes into account the current state of the robot, including position, velocity, acceleration and external forces. The measure external forces T_{mes} are added with the desired forces T_{des} calculated by the task control loop, hence the final force being applied will be the force necessary to counteract the user's action added with the desired force to be applied to the user's foot.

The actuators used by the RMA robots are dual-acting pneumatic pistons, hence the force applied by the cylinder can by controlled by adjusting the air pressure in the upper and lower chambers. The actuator position control transforms the desired change in position into a desired force. The calculated cylinder lengths L_{des} are added with the measured length L_{mes}, and the resulting length difference L_{err} is transformed into a force through the L→F control block. This control uses a proportional derivative (PD) strategy.
Finally, the pressure loop takes the desired actuator force, transforms it into upper and lower chamber pressures. The desired pressures are controlled in Pulse Width Modulation (PWM). The PWM strategy transforms the desired change in pressure P_{err} into the time interval T_{on} during which the valve should be kept open.
F→P is a direct transformation of actuator force into upper and lower pressures designed to minimize the change in pressures in both chambers, hence achieving a better response time. In cases when the desired force cannot be achieved through minimization, the pressures are determined so that they are balanced around the middle of the controllable pressure range. The PWM is implemented using an adaptive strategy. The change in pressure in a cylinder chamber is not linear in time, and the shape of the curve depends on the volume of the actuated cylinder chamber. Another factor taken into consideration is the intake airflow, which is affected by the number of actuator chambers accepting or exhausting air simultaneously. The PWM duty cycle is calculated taken into consideration all these factors using the equation below.

$$T_{on} = kP_{err}(1 + k_V V_{air})(1 + k_N N_{chamber})(1 + k_F F_{flow})$$

V_{air} is the volume of uncompressed air necessary to achieve the change in pressure. $N_{chamber}$ is the number of chambers accepting or exhausting air simultaneously. F_{flow} is the curve of the airflow over time.

4.1.1 Simulator Mechanical Bandwidth

The mechanical bandwidth of the mobility simulator was measured for translations in the horizontal plane and rotations around the front/back axis. The motions are the most commonly used by our system to render haptic effects as discussed in the last section of the paper. The measurements were done with both RMA robots active simultaneously. While the bandwidth of each individual robot is higher when measured separately, when both robots are active the intake airflow is reduced, thus the bandwidth is lowered. The results are presented in Table 1.

X translation 0.1m amplitude	**Y translation** 0.18m amplitude	**Y rotation** 5 deg amplitude
1.56 Hz	1.79 Hz	1.5 Hz

Table 1. RMA robot mechanical bandwidth.

4.1.2 Robot Stability in Foot Support Mode

One of the first problems encountered during the development of the system was the stability of the RMA platforms under load. The robots were stable when subjected to external forces if there was no load attached to them. However, the working regime for which they were developed, involves resisting forces while supporting the weight of the user. Figure 4 shows the response of the robot to sinusoidal input. Under a 50 lbs load, the motion was distorted and the amplitude of the robot increased slowly eventually becoming unstable.

The cause of this problem was the addition of the desired cylinder force F_{des} with the cylinder motion force F_{mov}. Under load, the resulting forces were too high and caused the robot to become unstable. Increasing the derivative gain slowed down the instability but it didn't solve it. The solution was to reduce the proportional gains by a minimum of 42%. With lower gains, the platform was stable under load, but had very little power to move the user's foot backward during the foot support phase, hence making the system unusable. Also, when the system was unloaded, the steady state error was significantly larger. The use of an integrator term was avoided because the usage of the system caused it to windup consistently.

Two adaptive gains were used to bring the robot to respond properly under load. The gains added a fraction of the measured cylinder load to the proportional and derivative gains respectively. The proportional adaptive component helped increase the moving force of the platform when under load, while the derivative adaptive component was increased to compensate for the high proportional gains and insure the stability of the system.

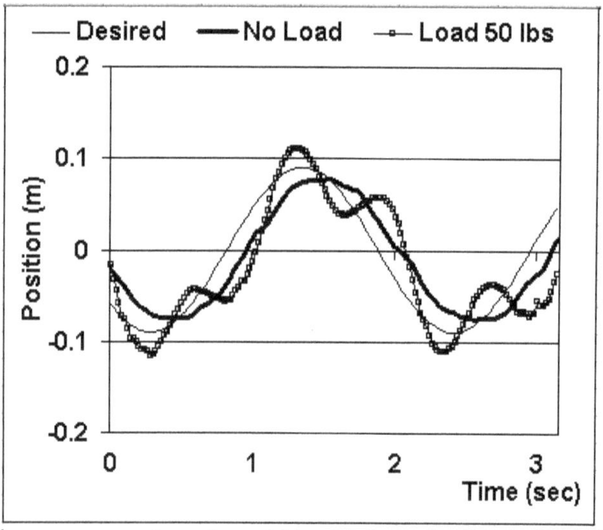

Fig. 4. RMA platform response to a sinusoid input along the Y axis (back-front) with 0.5Hz frequency and 0.18m amplitude. © Rutgers University and UMDNJ. Reprinted by permission.

Figure 5 presents the response of the platform to the same sinusoidal input signal, under a 50 lbs load, with and without the adaptive component added to the lowered proportional and derivative gains. While both the constant and the adaptive response were stable, the adaptive strategy provided the necessary power to move the load closer to the desired position, and reducing the error by approximately half. The adaptive gains did bring a side effect slightly visible in Figure 5; at higher velocity, the adaptive derivative gains increases the damping of the system slowing it down and the releasing it as the load n the robot shifts and the force is reduced. This can be seen as a change in the slope of the adaptive curve in Figure 5.

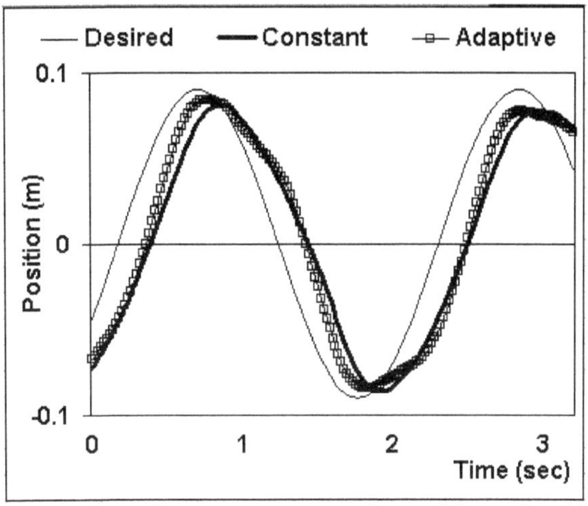

Fig. 5. Response comparison lower constant gains with and without the adaptive component. © Rutgers University and UMDNJ. Reprinted by permission.

4.1.3 Force Minimization in Free Motion Mode.

The second major functioning mode of the RMA robot is following the foot during the swing phase of the gait. In this mode, the platform has to compensate for its own weight and for the forces applied by the user to the end-effector, hence not making itself felt to the foot. To achieve this, the servo controller disables the cylinder position control by canceling out the moving force F_{mov}, and by switching the measured forces signs by changing the value of K_t from 1 to -1. While these changes cause the RMA robot to follow the user's foot, the motion is very slow and large forces are felt at the foot. Figure 6 shows the forces measured at the foot during one swing phase.

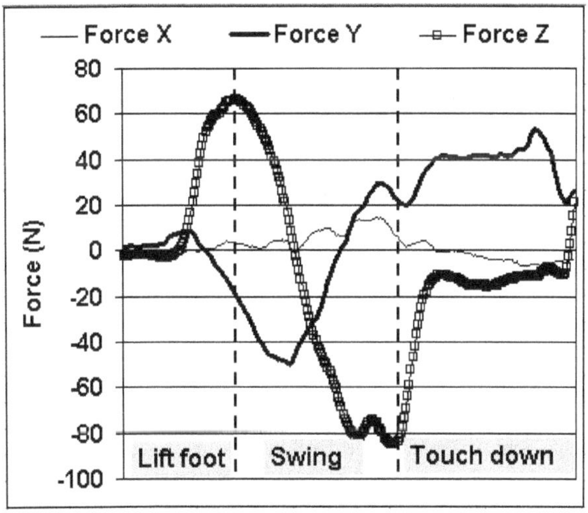

Fig. 6. Free mode forces during swing for K_t = -1.

The source of these large forces has been determined to be the damping created by the pneumatic actuators. While a K_t of 1 is sufficient to resist forces in foot support mode, in free mode, besides responding with a force to the user's force, the robot also has to move, which involves a much large air intake/exhaust activity. The damping is mostly coming from the airflow limitations imposed by the small intake and exhaust sections of the cylinder chambers. To overcome this problem, K_t was increased in absolute value. The increase was done for each of the robot's 6 DOF. The Z-axis (up-down) translation gain was approximately four times larger than the rest of the gains, because the motion on that direction required all the cylinders to either intake or exhaust, hence putting more airflow in a single direction. The measured forces for the increased K_t gains are shown in Figure 7. The forces are now reduced approximately 8 times to a maximum of 11N, which is comparable to the weight of a snow boot.

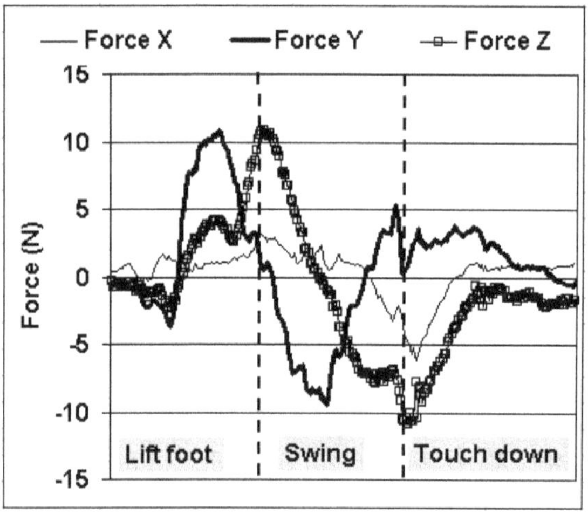

Fig. 7. Free mode forces during swing for larger K_t. © Rutgers University and UMDNJ. Reprinted by permission.

4.2 Haptic rendering for walking over virtual terrain

The Mobility Simulator transforms the input position, force and functioning mode of each RMA platform into haptic feedback to the feet and visual update of the virtual scene using the virtual surface specifications. The virtual ground model is stored on the graphics workstation, as a polygonal mesh with areas characterized by a haptic material. The haptic output data consists of two sets of values specifying the functioning mode to be used by each platform, the 6DOF forces and the vibrations to be applied to the user's foot.

4.2.1 Haptic Material

The ground surface is specified as a polygonal mesh that matches the shape of the visual 3D geometries in the virtual environment. The physical properties of the surface are specified using haptic materials, which are applied in layers that can be either distinct or mixed. The polygonal surface is unbreakable and the haptic materials can be placed on top of it in layers. This approach insures that the foot stepping down will always be supported if it penetrates through all the materials stacked on the surface.

A haptic material is defined as a collection of numerical parameters describing the physical properties of the surface. Given the requirements of an interactive virtual reality simulation, the haptic modeling computations need to be efficient. Thus, the model is not intended to be physically accurate but rather a good approximation of reality. Hence, the set of variables used is limited to stiffness, damping, friction, haptic texture, and breaking coefficient.

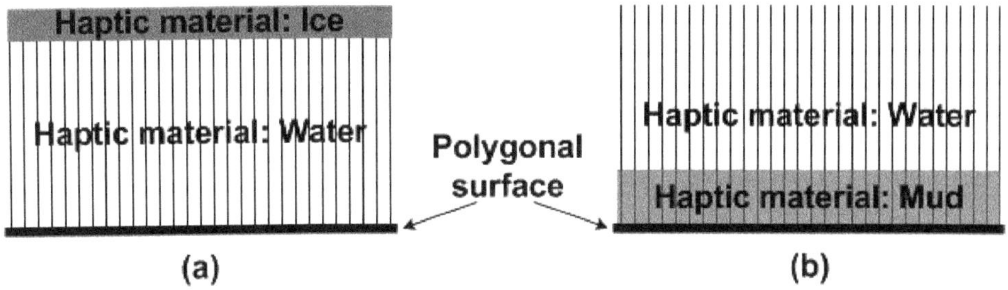

Fig. 8. Layered haptic materials: (a) distinct layers; (b) mixed layers.

The stiffness and damping coefficients are used for defining the material based on Hooke's law. Stepping on elastic materials is very common in every day life, however, the stiffness coefficient can be used to simulate Archimedes's law if considering the foot section constant when stepping into a liquid. The damping coefficient can be used to simulate the slow sinking sensation of walking on a thick carpet. A low friction coefficient can be used for simulating ice. If the foot applies horizontal forces to the material larger than the friction coefficient, the contact will break.

The haptic texture is defined as a vibration with a given amplitude and frequency. The breaking coefficient multiplied with the thickness of the material specifies the maximum force that the material can support. A haptic material is not rendered if the applied force is larger than its breaking force. The breaking coefficient makes it easy to simulate stepping on a thin layer of ice on top of a puddle of water.

4.2.2 Motion Rendering Stages

The processing necessary to calculate the graphics and haptic feedback can be divided into several stages that are executed at every simulation cycle (Figure 9). Only the swinging foot (free motion) is considered for the entire rendering process. The fixed foot (load compensation mode) is addressed only in the last stage of the process.

The process starts by reading the feet positions and functioning modes from the control interface. The functioning mode value is used to decide whether a foot should be moved or not. A foot in load compensation mode is kept fixed although the platform slides it backward.

The next stage requires the calculation of the change in real foot position to be added to the virtual feet. Because the simulator's workspace cannot cover the entire range of motion of the legs, it was necessary to scale the change in each foot's position to increase the virtual walking velocity so that the simulation felt real. The scale is also applied to the vertical displacement making it possible to negotiate realistic virtual obstacles that are visually larger than the platform work envelope.

The next phase updates the positions of the virtual feet with the calculated change. The changes are applied in a frame of reference aligned with the virtual avatar's walking direction calculated in the previous cycle.

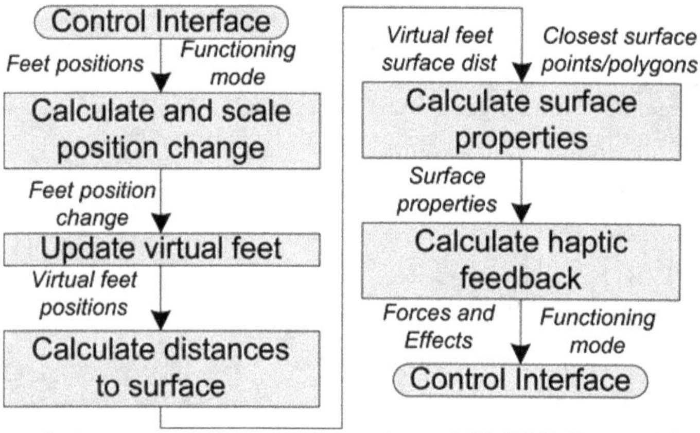

Fig. 8. Haptic rendering stages © Rutgers University and UMDNJ. Reprinted by permission.

After the feet have been mapped into the virtual world, the viewpoint has to be moved accordingly. Positioning the virtual camera above the center of the segment defined by the two feet yields good results although it is not what really happens with the center of gravity of a walking person.

The next stage is calculating the distance between the foot and the surface. This stage will also find the closest surface points to the foot and their corresponding polygons. Similar to the real case, certain surface properties are manifested above the surface (e.g. mud or snow) hence the distance to the surface is relevant to the haptic feedback even if there is no collision with the underlying ground. Based on the results of the previous stage the simulator can find the surface properties around the closest points on the surface.

The last stage of the process is the calculation of forces and haptic effects to be applied to the user's foot, based on the surface properties and the depth of the collision.

4.2.3 Virtual Foot Modeling

The interaction between the virtual foot and the virtual ground surface is based on the haptic mesh concept developed by Popescu (Popescu et al., 1999) as an extension to Ho's simpler haptic point concept (Ho et al., 1997). The virtual foot implemented for the Mobility Simulator is modeled as a mesh of points positioned on the shoe sole. From a haptic point of view, the RMA platforms can only render forces in one point. The use of a mesh of points to calculate the interaction of the foot with the surface is necessary for realistic surface contact calculation.

The number of points in the mesh should be minimized because it is directly proportional to the amount of collision detection calculations, and it increases factorially the number of contact stability calculations. The minimum number of mesh points has been determined to be five. One point is positioned in the center of the mesh, while the rest are positioned on a rectangle around it. The dimensions of the rectangle match the shape of the end-effector foot attachment plate to which the user's foot is secured.

4.2.4 Ground Contact Evaluation

When a foot touches the haptic surface the swinging phase of the foot is over and the support phase is about to begin. The switch between these two phases is tightly connected to the functioning of the servo-controller, which has to be notified to start sliding the support foot backward.

The foot/surface interaction is evaluated by calculating the forces applied by the surface (through the layers of haptic materials) to each of the points in the virtual foot mesh. The vertical components of these forces are then compared with the vertical components of the forces applied by the user's foot to the simulator. The latter forces are calculated by transforming the output of the force sensor mounted on top of the RMA platforms to each point in the mesh. A point of the foot haptic mesh is "supported" if the resultant of these vertical components is pointing upward.

The three contact possibilities that can be differentiated based on the "supported" status of the haptic mesh points are presented in Table 2 and Figure 10.

Contact Status	Description
No contact	None of the mesh points are supported
Stable	Minimum three non-collinear points are supported
Unstable	Remaining cases

Table 2. Contact status based on the haptic mesh point support.

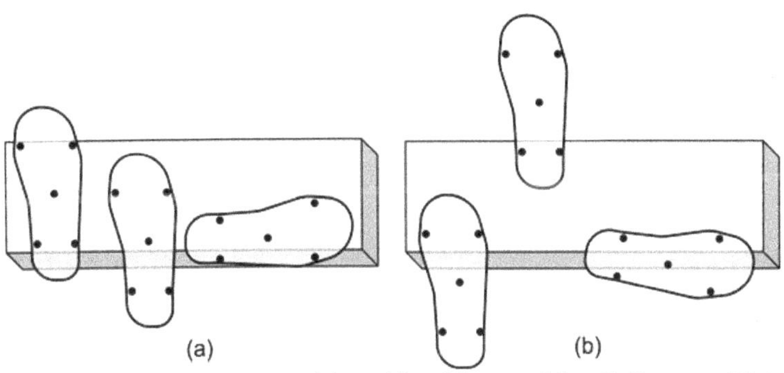

Fig. 10. Foot/surface contact types: (a) stable, (b) unstable. © Rutgers University and UMDNJ. Reprinted by permission.

The resultant of the haptic point forces is transmitted to the control interface to be applied to the swinging foot. If the swinging foot made a stable contact with the surface, the controller is notified to switch the functioning mode. The friction and surface textures are sent to the controller for both feet, regardless of their state.

4.2.5 Low-level Haptic Effects

The mobility simulator system is designed to execute most of the haptic calculations on the workstation, and render the results on the Stewart platforms using a reduced set of basic level effects:

- Apply a 6DOF force
- Change in position (positional jolt)
- Vibrations

These low level haptic effects are extensions of the haptic effects developed for a similar system using smaller Stewart platform robots, and designed for stroke rehabilitation in sitting (Boian et al., 2004a).

The simulation can request the controller to apply a certain force during both free or foot support functioning modes. If the request is made while in free motion mode, the given forces are scaled using positive values of the free mode gains and then applied. The scaling is necessary to counteract the same damping behavior mentioned above. If a force request is made during the foot support mode, the given forces become essentially τ_{des} in Figure 3.
The changes in position are used as an alternative force requests during foot support mode. For instance, to simulate slipping on the ice, a lateral displacement is used instead of applying a lateral force. This is preferred because a known displacement is more controllable and can be adjusted to a comfortable level easier than applying a force which will have a different effect from a user to another, mainly due to differences in weight.
The vibrations are used to simulate surface textures. The frequency and amplitude of the vibrations are calculated on the graphical workstation and sent to the controller. The vibrations are rendered only as changes in orientation around the Y-axis (back-front direction) because it interferes the least with the rest of the foot measurements necessary to calculate the direction of motion, or intersection with the virtual surface.

5. Acknowledgment

The research reported here was supported by grants from the National Science Foundation (BES 0201687 and BES 9708020) and from the New Jersey Commission for Science and Technology.

6. References

Boian, R.F.; Deutsch, J.E.; Lee, C.S.; G.C., Burdea & Lewis J.A. (2003). Haptic Effects for Virtual Reality-based Post-Stroke Rehabilitation. *Proceedings of the Eleventh Symposium on Haptic Interfaces For Virtual Environment And Teleoperator Systems*, pp. 247-253, Los Angeles, CA, March 2003.

Boian, R.F.; Bouzit, M.; Burdea, G.C. & Deutsch, J.E. (2004a). Dual Stewart Platform Mobility Simulator. *Proceedings of IEEE EMBS 2004*, September 2004.

Boian, R.F.; Burdea, G.C.; Deutsch, J.E. & Winter, S. H. (2004b). Street Crossing Using a Virtual Environment Mobility Simulator. *Proceedings of IWVR 2004*, pp. 27-33, Lausanne, Switzerland, 2004.

Boian, R.F. (2005). *Robotic Mobility Rehabilitation System Using Virtual Reality*. Electrical and Computer Engineering, Rutgers University, January 2005.

Bouguilla, L. & Sato, M. (2002). Virtual locomotion system for large-scale virtual environment. *Proceedings of the IEEE Virtual Reality Conference*, pp. 291–292, March 2002.

Burdea, G. (1996). Force and Touch Feedback for Virtual Reality. John Wiley & Sons, New York, NY, USA, 1996.

Christensen, R.R. ; Hollerbach, J.M.; Xu, Y. & Meek, S.G. (2000). Inertial-force feedback for the treadport locomotion interface. *Presence*, vol. 9, no. 1, pp.1–14, February 2000.

Dietz, V.; Wirz, M.; Curt, A. & Colombo, G. (1998). Locomotor pattern in paraplegic patients: training effects and recovery of spinal cord function. *Spinal Cord* 1998; 36: pp. 380-390.

Ho, C.; Basdogan, C. & Srinivasan, M. (1997). Haptic Rendering: Point- and Ray-Based Interactions. *Proceedings of the Second PHANToM Users Group Workshop*, October 2007, Dedham, MA.

Hollerbach, J.M. (1999). Locomotion interfaces. In: *Handbook of Virtual Environments Technology*, Stanney, K.M., (Ed.), pp. 239-254, Lawrence Erlbaum Associates, Inc., 2002.

Iwata, H. (1999). Walking about virtual environments on infinite floor. *Proceedings of IEEE Virtual Reality'99*, pp. 286-293, 1999, Houston, TX.

Iwata, H. & Yoshida, Y. (1999). Path reproduction tests using a torus treadmill. *Presence: Teleoperators and Virtual Environments*, vol. 8, pp. 587–597, 1999.

Iwata, H.; Yano, H. & Nakaizumi F. (2001). Gaitmaster: A versatile locomotion interface for uneven virtual terrain. *Proceedings of the IEEE VR2001 Conference*, pp. 131-137, 2001.

Jorgensen, H.S. ; Nakayama, H.; Raaschou, & Olsen, T.S. (1995). Recovery in walkingcfunction in stroke patients: The copenhagen stroke study. *Archives of Physical Medicine and rehabilitation*, vol. 76, no. 1, pp. 27–32, 1995.

Miyasato T. (2000). Tele-nursing system with realistic sensations using virtual locomotion interface. *Proceedings of the 6th ERCIM Workshop User Interfaces for All*, October 2000, Florence, Italy.

Nicol, D.J.; Granat, M.H.; Baxendale, R.H. & Tuson, S.J. (1995). Evidence for a human spinal stepping generator. *Brain Res* 1995; 684: pp. 230-232.

Noma, H.; Sugihara, T. & Miyasato T. (2000). Development of Ground Surface Simulator for Trl-E-Merge System. Proceedings of IEEE Virtual Reality 2000, pp. 217-224, March 2000.

Parsons, J.; Lampton, D.R.; Parsons, K.A.; Knerr, B.W.; Russell, D.; Martin, G.; Daly, J.; Kline, B. & Weaver. M. (1998) Fully immersive team training: A networked testbed for ground based training missions. *Proceedings of Interservice/Industry Training, Simulation and Education Conference*, Orlando, FL, 1998.

Popescu, V.; Burdea, G. & Bouzit, M. (1999). Virtual Reality Simulation Modeling for a Haptic Glove. *Computer Animation'99*, pp. 195-200, May 1999, Geneva, Switzerland.

Riva, G. (2000). Virtual Reality In Rehabilitation Of Spinal Cord Injuries: A Case Report. *Rehabilitation Psychology*, 45 (1), pp. 1-8, 2000

Sveistrup, H. (2004). Motor rehabilitation using virtual reality, *Journal of NeuroEngineering and Rehabilitation 2004.*

Templeman, J.N.; Denbrook, P.S. & Sibert. L.E. (1999). Maintaining spatial orientation during travel in an immersive virtual environment. *Presence: Teleoperators and Virtual Environments*, Vol 8, pp. 598–617, 1999.

Wandel, A.; Jorgensen, H.S.; Nakayama, H.; Raaschou, H.o. & Olsen, T.S. (2000). Prediction of walking function in stroke patients with initial lower extremity paralysis: the copenhagen stroke. Archives of Physical Medicine and rehabilitation, Vol. 81, No. 6, pp. 736–738, 2000.

Wang, Z.; Bauernfeind, K. & Sugar. T. (2003). Omni-direactional treadmill system. *Proceedings of the Symposium on Haptic Interfaces for Virtual Environment and Teleoperator Systems*, pp. 367–373, Los Angeles, CA, March 2003.

12

Robotic Exoskeletons for Upper Extremity Rehabilitation

Abhishek Gupta and Marcia K. O'Malley
Rice UniversityDepartment of Mechanical Engineering and Materials Science
Houston, Texas 77005 USA

1. Introduction

In 2003, 700,000 persons in the United States suffered a cerebral vascular accident (CVA), or stroke, with the total number of survivors estimated at 5.5 million. The total cost for rehabilitation and lost revenue in 2006 was 57.9 billion (Thom, Haase et al. 2006). Stroke commonly causes significant residual physical, cognitive, and psychological impairment (Gresham 1990). As the geriatric population increases and more effective therapies for acute stroke management emerge, there will be more survivors living with disabilities. In addition to greater numbers of survivors, there has been an increase in the number of more moderately affected survivors (Wolf, D'Agostino et al. 1992), which has increased the demand for stroke rehabilitation in an era of health care cost containment. Efforts to prevent stroke must, therefore, be balanced with pragmatic efforts to prevent disability and maximize quality of life for stroke survivors. Persons with hemiparesis following stroke constitute the largest group of patients receiving rehabilitation services in this country. The current consensus regarding rehabilitation of patients with some voluntary control over movements of the paretic limb is that they be encouraged to use the limb in functional tasks and receive training directed toward improving strength and motor control, relearning sensorimotor relationships, and improving functional performance (Gresham, Alexander et al. 1997). Given such recommendations, the research community has responded with efforts to improve the effectiveness of rehabilitative treatment of motor disability resulting from stroke.

1.1 Robotic devices for rehabilitation

A significant area of focus has been on the use of robotic devices for delivery of consistent and repeatable movement therapy. Indeed, the interest in rehabilitation applications for robotic devices, especially simple one- and two- DOF devices that focus on upper-extremity rehabilitation, has been increasing since the late 1980s and early 1990s (Erlandson 1992;

Reinkensmeyer, Dewald et al. 1996; Reinkensmeyer, Takahashi et al. 2000). For example, Khalili and Zomlefer suggested that a two joint robot system could be used for continuous passive motion and could be programmed to the particular needs of the patient (Khalili and Zomlefer 1988). Goodall et al. used two single degree-of-freedom (DOF) arms to stabilize sway in hemiparetic patients, and suggested the level of assistance could be withdrawn to encourage patients to relearn to balance on their own (Goodall, Pratt et al. 1987). White et al. built a single DOF pneumatically powered orthotic device for elbow flexion that could be used for continuous passive motion, to measure patient strength, and to assist elbow flexion (White, Scneider et al. 1993). Dirette et al. showed that a continuous passive motion (CPM) machine, when used regularly, can effectively reduce edema in the hands of flaccid hemiparetic patients (Dirette and Hinojosa 1994).

A more recent thrust of robotic assisted rehabilitation research has been to focus on the ability of the devices to assist limb movements and facilitate recovery of motor function in subjects with chronic hemiparesis due to stroke, such as with the Mirror-Image Motion Enabler - MIME (Burgar, Lum et al. 2000). In an initial study with MIME including twenty-eight subjects (two groups of 14), all had improved motor function as a result of therapy (Burgar, Lum et al. 2000). Preliminary data from these ongoing clinical efficacy trials suggest that robot-aided therapy has therapeutic benefits. Improvements have been demonstrated in strength and in the Fugl-Meyer (FM) assessment of motor function. Trends in the data suggest that the underlying mechanisms for these results may be increased strength, as well as more appropriate activation and inhibition of muscle groups.

The reader is referred to extensive reviews of robotic therapy for upper and lower extremity for a more complete discussion of the state of the field and results of ongoing clinical trials (Fasoli, Krebs et al. 2004; Hogan and Krebs 2004; Reinkensmeyer, Emken et al. 2004; Stein 2004; Riener, Nef et al. 2005; O'Malley, Ro et al. 2006). The MIME studies together with the cited related work support the conclusions that robotic manipulation of an impaired limb may favorably affect recovery following a stroke. An important additional finding is that improvements in motor control are possible beyond six months following a stroke.

Such findings with shoulder and elbow rehabilitation motivate the extension of robotic-assisted rehabilitation distally for the upper extremity, so that forearm pronation-supination, wrist flexion-extension, radial-ulnar deviation, and ultimately digital manipulation are enabled. Several devices have been presented in the literature to achieve at least a subset of these movements. For example, Charles et al. (Charles 2005) have developed an extension of the MIT-MANUS system to provide three rotational degrees-of-freedom for wrist rehabilitation. Hesse et al. (Hesse, Schulte-Tigges et al. 2003) have also extended the utility of their arm trainer to include wrist motion. In order to improve the applicability of the MIME system for full arm rehabilitation post stroke, the authors have developed a wrist rehabilitation robot, the *RiceWrist*, which interfaces with MIME and provides a variety of interaction modes for the therapist to select for the patient.

1.2 Haptic interfaces

Haptic or force-reflecting interfaces are a specific type of robotic device used to display touch or force-related sensory information from a virtual or remote environment to the user (see, for example, surveys (Boman 1995; Burdea 1996; Lay and Day 2003). The ability to interact mechanically with virtual objects through incorporation of haptic feedback allows users to manipulate objects in the simulated or remote environment with ease when compared to a purely visual display. Added advantages of haptic simulators include increased repeatability, scalability, safety, and control over environmental conditions. It is also possible to simulate additional physical forces and fields, which may or may not be part of a natural environment, to convey information to the user. This makes a haptic display suitable for a variety of applications like remote operation in hazardous environments, simulators for surgical training (Basdogan, Ho et al. 2001; Feygin, Keehner et al. 2002; Carignan and Akin 2003), and rehabilitation research (Todorov, Shadmehr et al. 1997; Prisco, Avizzano et al. 1998; Jack, Boian et al. 2001; Sveistrup 2004). Physical therapy utilizing the resistance offered to a user's motion during haptic interaction can be used for rehabilitation of impaired arm movements in patients. Furthermore, research has shown that augmented feedback presented in virtual environments accelerates the learning of motor tasks (Todorov, Shadmehr et al. 1997). For these reasons, the authors have developed an arm exoskeleton that can be utilized for such training and rehabilitation applications.

1.3 Force feedback exoskeletons

In order to effectively interface with the distal joints of the upper extremity, many groups are turning towards exoskeleton-type robotic devices. Such ungrounded or wearable interfaces permit greater human movement during haptic interactions. However, the increased workspace for an ungrounded (Tsagarakis, Caldwell et al. 1999) device is achieved at the expense of design simplicity when compared to grounded (Bergamasco, Allotta et al. 1994) devices.

A force-feedback exoskeleton is a haptic device worn by the user. Arm exoskeletons can simulate large forces at the hand or arm, like the weight of an object that is held. This is achieved by providing feedback to the various joints of the arm—the shoulder, elbow, and wrist. Although worn by the user, the device itself may be grounded, in which case it restricts user mobility. In the mid 1960s and early 1970s, a group of researchers at Cornell University and later at General Electric developed some of the earliest master-slave teleoperation systems, the Handyman and Hardiman (Mosher 1967). The Hardiman was an anthropomorphic exoskeleton placed inside a larger slave robot, and was used to amplify human power output. Input commands from the user were obtained from both the arms and legs. These early exoskeleton haptic devices were hampered by limitations in actuation, computation, and control systems technology. The reader is encouraged to review (Burdea 1996) for an exhaustive discussion of the early stages of exoskeleton and haptic interface development. In recent years, improvements in sensing and actuation technologies, control systems, and computing resources have led to the development of many successful haptic interfaces.

Although there have been a large number of high-performance hand controllers, research in design of exoskeletons for other parts of the body is still in an early phase. The first modern exoskeleton arm/glove was designed and developed at ARTS laboratory for the replication of sensations of contacts and collisions (Bergamasco, Allotta et al. 1994). The ARTS arm, also known as the PERCRO exoskeleton, is a 7-DOF ungrounded device, attached to the operator's shoulder and torso. The operator holds onto the device with his/her palm. Hence, the device can only exert forces at the palm of the user. It uses DC motors with a cable transmission system for actuation. A 9-DOF under-actuated exoskeleton arm developed at the Korea Institute of Science and Technology (KIST) by Lee et al. addressed the workspace issues associated with the PERCRO exoskeleton. Their device allows for full reproduction of the human arm's workspace when operating the exoskeleton (Lee, Park et al. 1998). A revised exoskeleton device from the same group employs electrical brakes in place of pneumatic actuators for improved bandwidth (Kim, Lee et al. 2005). An alternate arm exoskeleton developed at KIST addresses the limited wearability issues of previous designs by using parallel mechanisms and pneumatic actuators (Jeong, Lee et

al. 2001). The wearable Salford arm addresses some of the issues and limitations of earlier designs (Tsagarakis, Caldwell et al. 1999). For example, nearly 90% of the human arm's workspace can be replicated with their device. Pneumatic muscle actuators (pMAs) were selected to power the robot due to their high power-to-weight ratio. A drawback of this choice is the highly nonlinear behavior and slow response of the pMAs, presenting additional control challenges.
In recent years, robotic exoskeletons are being developed specifically for rehabilitation applications, such as the ARMin system. This six-DOF device was designed to enable training for specific activities of daily living (Nef, Mihelj et al. 2006). Kousidou et al. have incorporated the Salford arm into the Rehab Lab system for virtual rehabilitation of complex three-dimensional trajectories in the workspace (Kousidou, Tsagarakis et al. 2006). Carignan et al. (Carignan and Liszka 2005) present a prototype five-DOF exoskeleton system currently under development that focuses on shoulder rehabilitation. Finally, Gupta et al. have incorporated their lower-arm exoskeleton device (Gupta and O'Malley 2006) into the MIME system, creating a full upper-extremity robotic rehabilitation system (Gupta, Patoglu et al. 2007). A review of exoskeleton devices for rehabilitation applications was compiled by Ruiz et al., and contains images of many of these devices (Ruiz, Forner-Cordero et al. 2006).

1.4 Exoskeleton control

Force control of arm exoskeletons is traditionally implemented under the assumption of pseudostatic operation (see, for example, (Bergamasco, Allotta et al. 1994)). In this approach, the robot Jacobian can be used to compute required actuator torques for some desired force at the end-effector. Recently, Rosen et al. presented some interesting results with the use of myosignals, command signals sent to the human muscles by the brain, in predicting human arm motion during operation of a single-DOF arm exoskeleton (Rosen, Brand et al. 2001). They demonstrated that the prediction of operator motion can be used to improve upon the force control and overall quality of the haptic device. The group has since expanded their design to include the full seven-DOF of the arm (Perry and Rosen 2006).

1.5 Exoskeleton design

Many exoskeleton interfaces attempt to optimize one or more of the following characteristics of the haptic system, namely power-to-weight ratio (Lee, Park et al. 1998; Tsagarakis, Caldwell et al. 1999; Jeong, Lee et al. 2001), workspace (Lee, Park et al. 1998), wearability (Jeong, Lee et al. 2001) or stability, and control bandwidth (Bergamasco, Allotta et al. 1994; Nakai, Oshashi et al. 1998; Williams II 1998). Individual designs, however, achieve these optimizations at the expense of other useful features, usually workspace (Bergamasco, Allotta et al. 1994; Nakai, Oshashi et al. 1998; Jeong, Lee et al. 2001) or control bandwidth (Lee, Park et al. 1998; Tsagarakis, Caldwell et al. 1999; Jeong, Lee et al. 2001). In this chapter, the authors present work towards the design of a high-quality haptic interface with a workspace comparable to that of human arm workspace. This is achieved at the expense of added weight and decreased mobility due to device grounding.

2. Design Challenges

Haptic feedback aids an operator to reliably complete a remote or virtual task. Primary requirements for such a system are the ability to convey commands to the remote or virtual plant and to reflect relevant sensory information, specifically forces in the remote or virtual environment, back to the operator. In essence, the dynamics of the device must not interfere with the interaction between the operator and environment. An ideal haptic interface behaves as a rigid body, through which the user interacts with the environment, over the complete range of frequencies of forces in the virtual environment.

In practice, however, performance is limited by physical factors, such as actuator and sensor quality, device stiffness, friction, device workspace, force isotropy across the workspace, backlash, and computational speed. Force isotropy, which refers to the equality of force exertion capability of the device in all directions, is important to ensure consistent device performance across the workspace. The desired size and shape of the workspace itself is typically dependent on the target application, and serves as an important factor in determining the overall device size and mechanism. Increased workspace is only achieved at the expense of a larger and heavier device, since the force output requirements scale with the workspace size. Also of consideration in the design of haptic arm exoskeletons is the biomechanics of the human arm. The arm imposes a force/position constraint on the device, thus affecting the system behavior and performance. These design factors are discussed in detail in the following sections.

2.1 Biomechanics of Human Arm

A haptic arm exoskeleton places kinematic constraints on the human arm. The human arm has seven DOF: abduction/adduction and flexion/extension of the shoulder; rotation of the upper arm; flexion/extension of the elbow; rotation of the forearm; and radial/ulnar deviation and flexion/extension of the wrist. It is desirable that the haptic exoskeleton does not compromise the natural arm motion and workspace of the operator. The device should also have torque capabilities to match and enhance human abilities. Table I shows the workspace and torque capabilities of the human arm for reference.

2.2 Performance-Related Design Parameters

A high-quality haptic interface is characterized by stability robustness and transparency. The stability bandwidth refers to the range of frequencies of forces that can be reflected to the operator with the device, while ensuring stable system behavior. Research has shown that stability of a haptic simulation is related to the simulation rate, virtual wall stiffness, and device viscosity (Elllis, Ismaeil et al. 1996). Transparency is a measure of the degree of distortion between the force at the human-robot interface and the desired contact force as commanded through the virtual environment. Transparency can be degraded by such things as backlash, inertia, or friction in the haptic device, sensor resolution, and computational delay (Colgate and Brown 1994). Often with haptic interfaces, the quality of the device is characterized by the maximum virtual wall stiffness that can be stably displayed.

Joint	Human Isometric Strength (Nm)	Human Joint Workspace Limits (degrees)
Elbow Flexion/Extension	72.5	Flexion: 146 Extension: 0
Forearm Supination/Pronation	9.1	Supination: 86 Pronation: 71
Wrist Palmer/Dorsal Flexion	19.8	Palmer Flexion: 73 Dorsiflexion: 71
Wrist Abduction/Adduction	20.8	Adduction: 33 Abduction: 19

Table 1. Workspace and torque limits of human arm.

Research has shown that fairly low stiffness and force values are sufficient for object detection (O'Malley and Goldfarb 2002; O'Malley and Goldfarb 2004). Therefore, if a haptic exoskeleton is designed for teaching arm movements using virtual force fields, a low force output interface would suffice. In this case, as the authors intend for the device to be used as a general purpose training tool for arm movements, it is required that the device be able to simulate high-quality virtual surfaces. As a result, emphasis is placed on the design of a high-performance interface, which encompasses the human arm workspace. In addition, for rehabilitation applications, the ability to control feedback to individual human arm joints is desirable and has been addressed through this design.

2.3. Control-Related Design Parameters

As mentioned earlier, a haptic system applies trajectory-dependent forces to the operator's body. This is typically implemented in one of two modes—the impedance control mode or the admittance control mode. Impedance control techniques measure position at the human-machine interface and in turn adjust the commanded force at the human-machine interface depending on the virtual environment model to be displayed. It is desirable that an impedance-controlled haptic device allows free movement in response to the operator's motion commands, so that when the human is moving in free space (not in contact with any virtual objects), there is no resistance to motion. This requirement translates to a need for backdrivability in impendence-controlled haptic devices. In this control mode, it is also desirable for the device to have minimal inertia to facilitate maneuvering. Furthermore, low inertia and friction improve interface performance by reducing the forces required to compensate for device dynamics. Alternatively, admittance control methods rely on measurement of forces at the human-machine interface and controlled robot motion based on the virtual environment model. An admittance controlled haptic device should prevent movement of the robot in response to operator-generated forces to allow for consistent force measurement and motion control.

It is apparent that haptic exoskeleton design involves various tradeoffs, which limit the achievable performance of the device since, in all instances, stability must be maintained. To summarize these tradeoffs, mechanism design choices may limit or affect human motion abilities; sensor and actuator selection is directly related to device weight, force output range, system stability, and cost; and actuator placement and inclusion of transmissions affects the apparent inertia of the device. All of these design decisions are greatly influenced by the intended application for the device.

The MAHI exoskeleton, named for the Mechatronics and Haptic Interfaces Lab at Rice University, has been designed primarily for training and rehabilitation in virtual environments. These applications typically require the use of virtual force fields for guidance (Rosenberg 1993) or active assistance (Gillespie, O'Modhrain et al. 1998; O'Malley and Gupta 2003). The exoskeleton device must therefore allow natural human arm movements, with minimal reduction in workspace of the human arm. Because the device is to be worn, special care must be taken to ensure safety of the wearer. Furthermore, mobility of the interface is not normally a requirement for such a system. Hence, the device can be grounded to support excessive weight, and gravity compensation can be implemented through the controller. Additionally, the low accelerations and velocities associated with human movements ensure that the inertia of the device plays a small role in its operation (Shimoga 1992; Bergamasco, Allotta et al. 1994). Therefore, when designing the MAHI exoskeleton, the kinematic design of the robot was given prime consideration.

3. MAHI arm exoskeleton

3.1 Basic Mechanism Design

The basic kinematic structure of the 5-DOF MAHI exoskeleton is depicted in Fig. 1. The exoskeleton is comprised of a revolute joint at the elbow, a revolute joint for forearm rotation, and a 3-revolute-prismatic-spherical (RPS) serial-in-parallel wrist.

The 3-RPS platform, mentioned by Lee and Shah (Lee and Shah 1988), consists of a base plate, three extensible links l_1, l_2, and l_3, and a moving platform, as shown in Fig. 2. The moving platform houses the end-effector that is affixed to the operator during operation. The moving platform is connected to the three extensible links by means of spherical joints spaced at 120° along the circumference of a circle of radius r. The other end of the links connects to the base platform via revolute (pin) joints, which are also spaced 120° along a circle of radius R. The axes of rotation of the revolute joints are oriented along the tangents to the circle of radius R. Linear actuators placed along the link are used to change the link length, thereby moving the top platform. It should be noted that the platform has limited movement transverse to the vertical axis through the base and no singularities for $\theta_i \in (0, \pi)$ (Lee and Shah 1988).

The choice of a parallel mechanism for the design of the exoskeleton wrist over a serial mechanism was motivated primarily by the compactness of the parallel mechanism. Furthermore, use of a parallel mechanism allows for higher torque output, stiffness, and decreased inertia compared to a similar serial mechanism. During operation, the robot is worn so that the axis elbow joint of the robot aligns with the operator's elbow joint, and the top plate of the wrist of the robot aligns with the wrist joint of the operator. This configuration aids in preserving natural arm movements by aligning the robot's kinematic structure with that of the human arm. Velcro strapping and an ergonomic palm splint are used to maintain this alignment. The mapping between the robot configuration and arm position is further simplified by the use of the 3-RPS kinematic structure for the robot. The equivalence between the human wrist joint angles and the xyz Euler angle representation for the orientation of the platform is shown in Section 3.4.

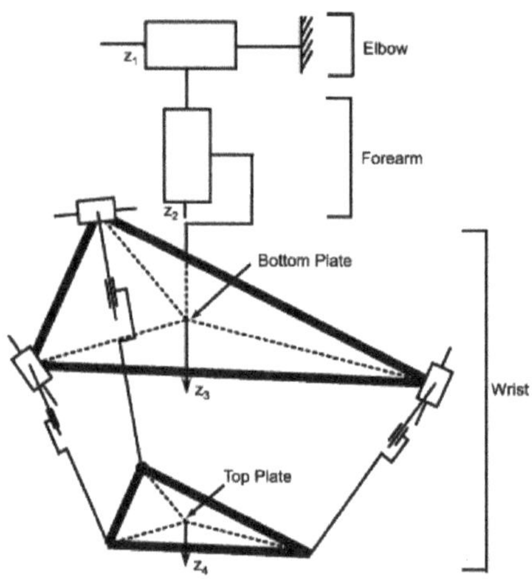

Fig. 1. Exoskeleton mechanism: A 3-RPS platform is used as the wrist of the robot. Joints R1, R2, and R3 and B1, B2, and B3 are located at vertices of equilateral triangles.

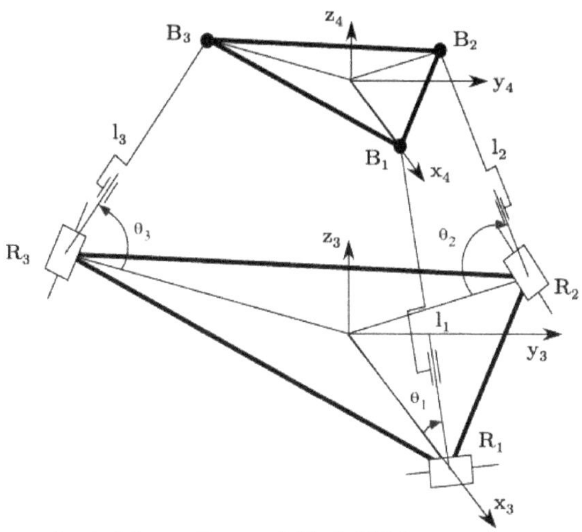

Fig. 2. 3-RPS platform, adapted from (Lee and Shah 1988).

3.2 Sensing and Actuation

Sensor Selection Sensor resolution affects the range of frequencies of forces that can be displayed by the haptic interface (Colgate and Brown 1994). Consider, for example, the simulation of a thin virtual wall. If the sensor resolution or the computational speed is not high enough, then there exists a possibility that the human can pass his/her arm through the wall without feeling the force. Furthermore, during simulation of stiff virtual surfaces, reduction in sensor resolution increases the delay in sensing the human's actions in the virtual environment, and this delay can decrease system stability. With these considerations, high resolution optical encoders were selected for the device.

Actuator Selection The actuators for a haptic device determine the range of magnitude and frequencies of forces that can be displayed with the interface. To reproduce real-life environments, it is desirable that the device be able to display forces in a large range of magnitudes as well as frequencies. In general, the use of high-power actuators is accompanied with an increase in weight, thereby increasing the inertia of the device. Thus, high power-to-weight ratio and high bandwidth are desirable qualities for actuators used in a haptic interface. The bandwidth refers to the dynamic response of the actuator; a low-bandwidth actuator fails to display high-frequency forces to the operator, reducing system transparency in such situations. This gains importance in that human kinesthetic/proprioceptic sensing bandwidth is 20-30 Hz and tactile sensing bandwidth is 0-400 Hz (Shimoga 1992).

No single actuator technology provides the benefit of both high power-to-weight ratio and high bandwidth. Pneumatic actuators are inexpensive and provide the benefit of high power-to-weight ratio. However, pneumatic actuators have a low bandwidth, which limits their utility as actuators for haptic interfaces. Tsagarakis et al. used pMAs for their exoskeleton (Tsagarakis, Caldwell et al. 1999). However, these actuators have highly nonlinear dynamics in addition to low bandwidth, making them unsuitable for application in haptic devices. Hence, electrical actuation was chosen for the MAHI exoskeleton. Electrical actuators have a lower power-to-weight ratio than pneumatic actuators but have very high bandwidth. This increases the weight of the device but allows for better force reflection through the interface.

Transmission and Actuator Placement A transmission can be used to increase the torques or forces delivered by the device, but at the expense of speed of operation. The bandwidth of human motor output, which represents the ability of the hand and fingers to exert forces, is 10-15 Hz (Shimoga 1992), thus making the use of a transmission in haptic interfaces advantageous. Furthermore, use of a transmission allows the actuators themselves to be placed closer to the base of the robot, reducing rotational inertia. Use of transmissions, however, is associated with tradeoffs like backlash, nonlinear dynamics, and complex cable routing. For example, gears introduce backlash into the system, whereas belt drives introduce nonlinearities. Friction, backlash, backdrivability, and size were key considerations in designing the transmission. A cable drive, which, by design is backdriveable and free of backlash, is used as the transmission for elbow and wrist. In contrast, the forearm joint is direct drive actuated. For the elbow joint, a large cable drive with an approximate 10:1 transmission ratio was used, allowing backlash-free motion that is fully backdriveable (See Fig.3). High torque rotary electric motors with a cable-driven mechanism are employed for the robot wrist (Fig. 4), whereas the forearm joint is directly driven using a frameless electrical motor.

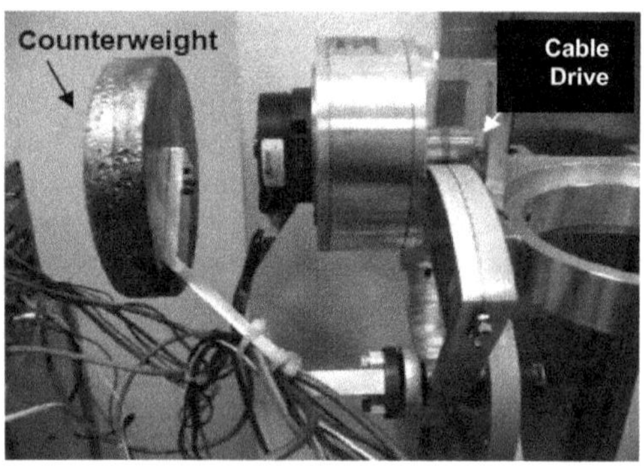

Fig. 3. Elbow joint with a cable drive and counterweight for gravity compensation.

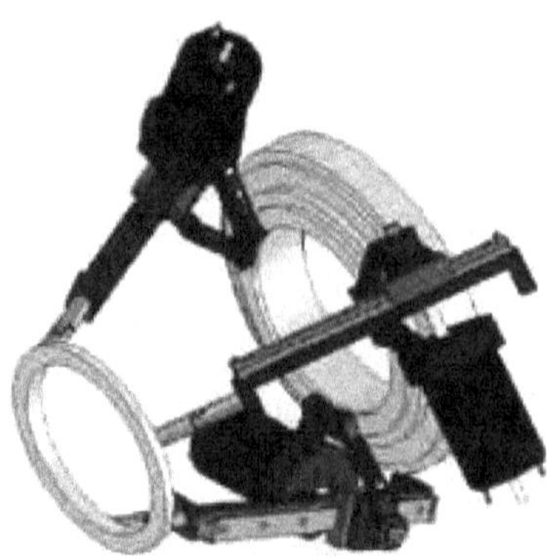

Fig 4. Wrist component of the MAHI arm exoskeleton employing electrical motors with a cable drive.

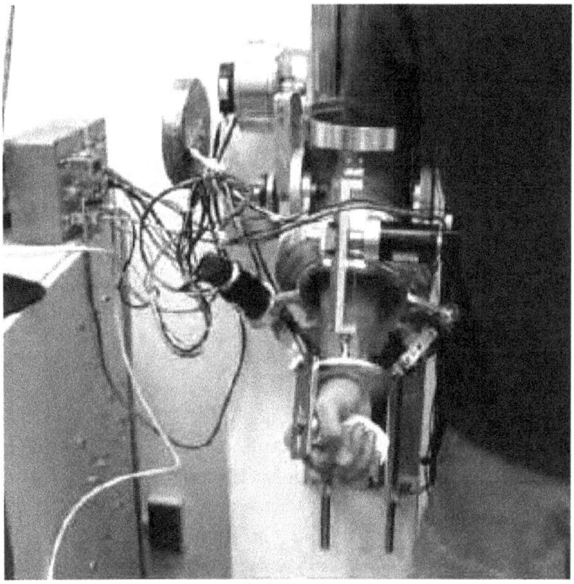

Fig. 5. User operating the MAHI arm exoskeleton.

3.3 Mechanical Design of MAHI Exoskeleton

Fig. 5 depicts a user operating the MAHI arm exoskeleton. The forearm joint employs a frameless brushless DC motor with direct actuation. Due to the use of frameless actuators, the amount of material required for construction was minimized thus reducing the weight of the device. The wrist platform is actuated through high torque rotary electric motors and a cable drive transmission. The range of motion of the spherical joint at the movable plate of the platform limits the workspace of platform. Equations developed by Lee and Shah were used to compute the range of rotations required from the spherical joint in order to meet our workspace criteria (Lee and Shah 1988). It was found that commercially available spherical joints do not suffice to meet the workspace requirements. Hence, the spherical joint was replaced by a 4 DOF spherical joint between the top plate of the platform and the corresponding linear joint links. This joint consisted of a universal-joint attached at either end to the link and the moving platform via rotary joints. This adds redundancy to the system and permits larger rotations. For the purpose of kinematic analysis, the redundancy does not affect any of the geometric relations or equations. Mechanical stops at workspace limits, soft software stops and an emergency stop switch are employed to ensure operator safety. For a detailed discussion of the design of the exoskeleton, the reader is referred to (Gupta and O'Malley 2006; Sledd and O'Malley 2006).

3.4 Kinematic Properties of MAHI Arm Exoskeleton

Table 2 shows the workspace for the MAHI arm exoskeleton in terms of the range of motion about each of the three primary degrees of freedom and corresponding human joint workspace limits. The device is singularity-free and the forward and kinematics of the device have a unique solution within the workspace. For a detailed discussion of the kinematics of the robot refer to (Gupta and O'Malley 2006).

Joint	Peak Torque Output Limits (Nm)	Joint Workspace Limits (degrees)
Elbow Flexion/Extension	55	Flexion: 90 Extension: 0
Forearm Supination/Pronation	5.08	Supination: 90 Pronation: 90
Wrist Palmer/Dorsal Flexion	5.26	Palmer Flexion: 45 Dorsiflexion: 45
Wrist Abduction/Adduction	5.26	Adduction: 45 Abduction: 45

Table 2. Workspace and torque output limits of MAHI arm exoskeleton.

The workspace of the MAHI arm exoskeleton is 100% of the average human joint range of motion except for palmar flexion and dorsiflexion where it is 60%. As shown in Fig. 6, compound movements of the wrist remain singularity-free, albeit with some reduction in the range of motion similar to the case of a human wrist. Thus the MAHI arm exoskeleton provides adequate range of motion for a human operator. It should also be noted that the device is backlash- free due to the use of direct-drive and cable-driven actuation and is highly backdriveable. Furthermore, the 3-RPS platform allows for compact design, centered on the human arm, which increases wearability and maximizes the achievable workspace of the exoskeleton.

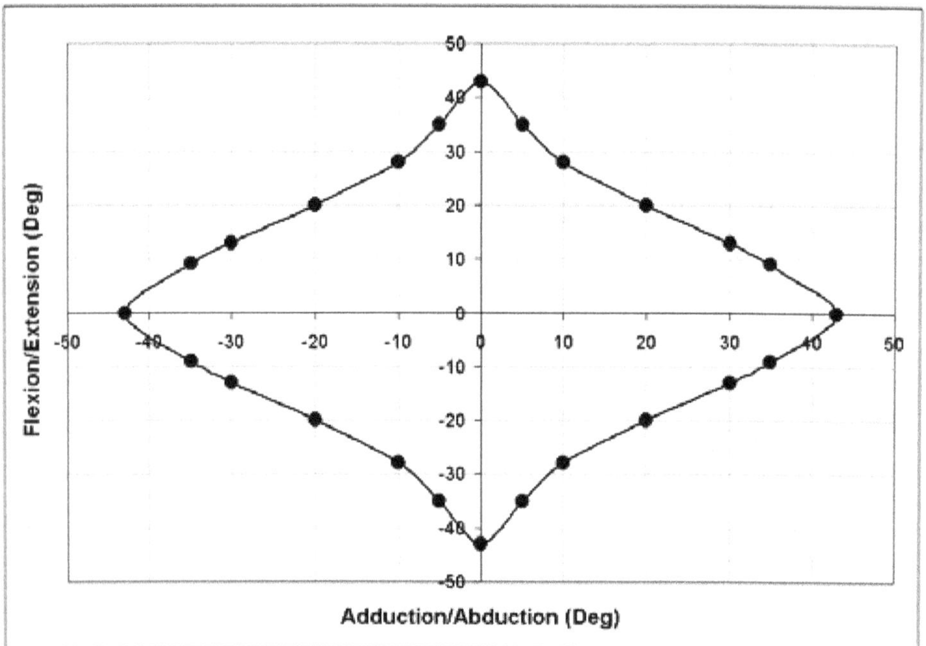

Fig. 6. Range of motion of MAHI arm exoskeleton wrist.

Fig. 7 shows the manipulability of the MAHI arm exoskeleton measured as the absolute determinant of the inverse Jacobian (Yoshikawa 1985). Manipulability of a robot is a quantitative measure that captures the ease with which the device can arbitrarily change position and orientation from a given posture. For the MAHI arm exoskeleton, the manipulability measure is greatest in the center of the workspace, with the wrist at 0° of abduction/adduction, (a) and flexion/extension, (b). Manipulability, as expected, is low at the extents of each joint range of motion, although more so during flexion/extension. For the tasks of rehabilitation and training, it is expected that most useful interactions via the haptic device will take place away from the joint limits, and so manipulability should not limit device performance.

Measurement of Human Motion A simplified kinematic model of the human lower arm and the wrist is shown in Fig. 8. Notice that axes x_4 of the platform (see Fig. 2) and z_2 of the human wrist joint coincide when the exoskeleton is worn by an operator. Similarly, axes y_4 of the platform and z_3 of the arm coincide for any rotation, α, of the top plate of the platform about x_4, or of the human wrist about z_2 (Fig. 8). Furthermore, {3} of the platform has a fixed orientation with respect to {1} of the human arm.

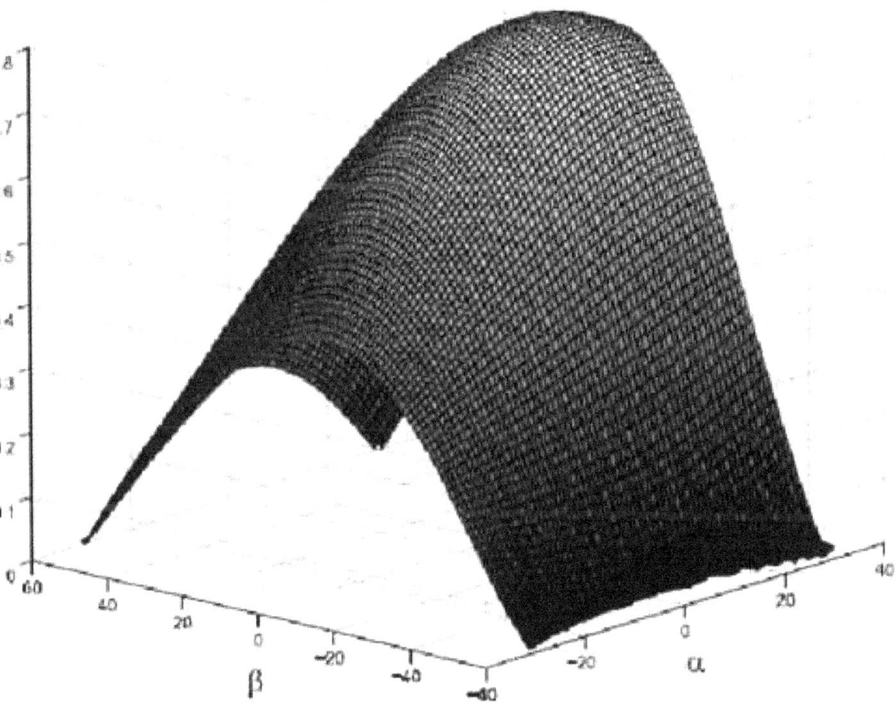

Fig. 7. Manipulability of the wrist mechanism.

Hence, a rotation of the top plate of the platform about axis x_4 (Fig. 2) followed by another rotation about axis y_4 (Fig. 2), is equivalent to a transformation from {3} to {1} of the arm. This implies that with the top plate of the platform centered at the operator's wrist joint, the measurement of the orientation of the top plate with respect to the base of the platform in terms of xyz-Euler angles corresponds to measurement of the flexion/extension and abduction/adduction of the human wrist joint. Thus, the Euler angle of rotation α about axis x_4 corresponds to abduction/adduction of the wrist while the rotation angle β about y_4 corresponds to flexion/extension. With the forearm joints of the robot and human being coincident, the measurement of position of operator's elbow and forearm from robot coordinates and vice versa is trivial.

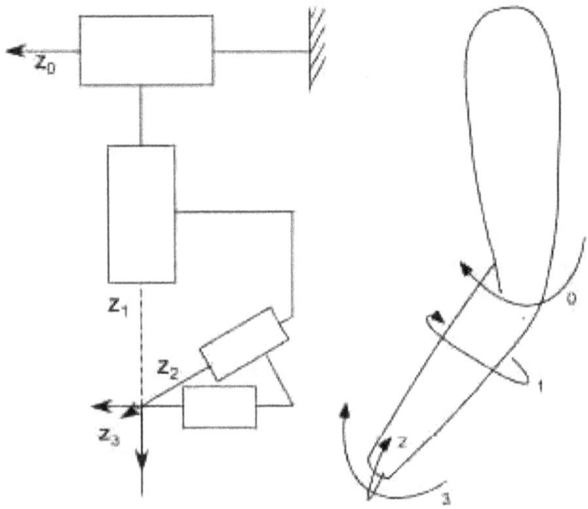

Fig. 8. Simplified kinematic model of the human arm: Other axes have not been shown for clarity. Axes 0 through 3 represent elbow rotation, forearm rotation, wrist adduction/abduction and wrist flexion/extension respectively.

4. Control and Dynamic Performance

The MAHI arm exoskeleton is controlled via a 3.2 GHz Pentium 4 PC with 2GB of RAM. The hardware is controlled through the MATLAB Real Time Workshop Toolbox from Mathworks, and WinCon from Quanser Consulting. All data I/O is handled by the Q8 board from Quanser. Position and force controllers were designed for the elbow, forearm and the wrist platform. Separate joint-space and task-space controllers were designed and tested for the wrist platform. Note that the task-space of the wrist platform refers to the three degrees of freedom corresponding to flexion/extension and abduction/adduction of the wrist, and the height of the platform. The following sections describe controller design in detail.

4.1 Controller Implementations

Joint level control for the MAHI exoskeleton is implemented via a joint-space proportional derivative (PD) trajectory controller. In addition, an inverse kinematics based task-space position controller was designed for the wrist, as shown in Figure 9. The commanded task-space positions and velocities were used to generate reference commands for the aforementioned joint-space controller. The performance of the device under joint-space position control was verified through step responses, set joint control and trajectory following control.

A task-space PD position controller for the wrist platform was also implemented as shown in Figure 10. As compared to the inverse kinematics based controller described in the previous section, this controller allows for independent control of wrist degrees of freedom, namely abduction/adduction, flexion/extension, and platform height. This is critical as during operation it is desirable to constrain the height of the platform to be a constant dependent upon the length of the subject's forearm. Furthermore, this provides the ability to selectively provide guidance and/or feedback to individual human wrist joints. The performance of the controller is discussed in Section 4.2.

Force control for the exoskeleton is implemented as a task-space impedance force controller, as shown in Fig. 10. It is assumed that the velocities of motion are small enough to ignore the dynamic terms in the equations of motion of the device. It should be noted that in the case of the elbow and forearm, the task-space and the joint-space are the same and hence, the impedance controller is simply a joint-space controller. The results of force control are discussed in Section 4.2 through haptic display of virtual walls.

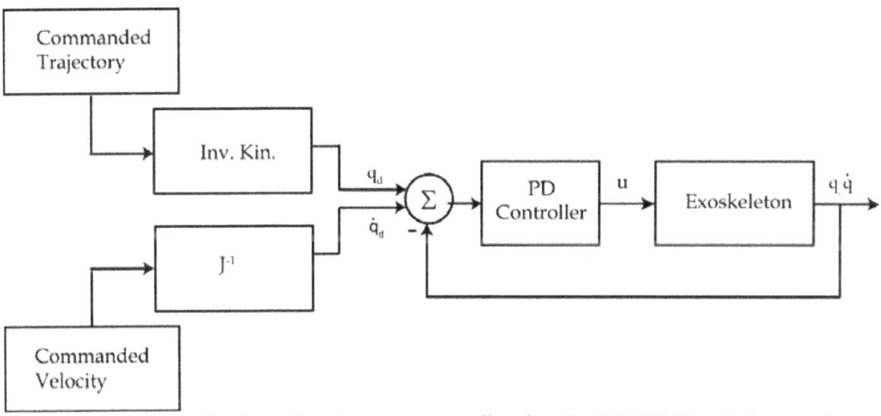

Fig. 9. Inverse kinematics based trajectory controller for the MAHI Exoskeleton where, J is the Jacobian of the device; q_d, $\dot{q}_d$ are the desired joint position and velocities; q, $\dot{q}$ are the current joint position and velocities; and u is the control input.

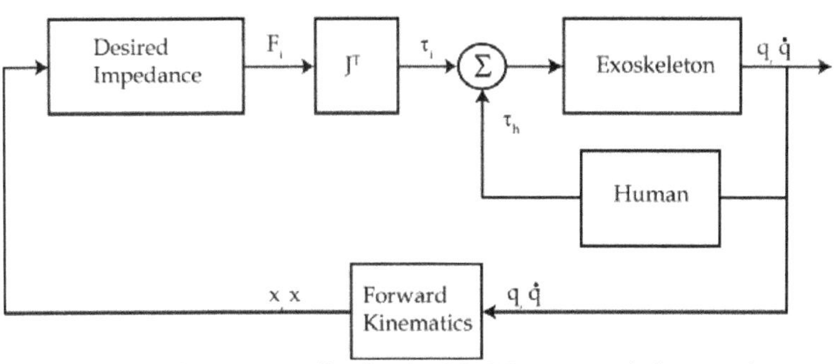

Fig. 10. Task-space impedance controller for the MAHI arm exoskeleton, where, q, $\dot{q}$ are the current joint position and velocities; x, $\dot{x}$ are the current task-space position and velocities; F_i is the desired environment force; J is the Jacobian of the MAHI exoskeleton; τ_i is the desired joint torques; and F_h is the human induced joint torque.

4.2 Dynamic Performance

Tables 1 and 2 list the human isometric strength and the peak torque output capabilities of the MAHI arm exoskeleton for the corresponding joints, respectively. The torque capabilities lag behind human abilities due to practical considerations owing to the power-to-weight characteristics of electrical actuators. Coulomb friction was measured to be 0.041 Nm and 1.134 Nm in the forearm and wrist joints respectively. Viscous friction was found to be negligible.

Position Control As described in Section 4.1, the position control for the wrist and forearm was implemented through a PD controller. Figure 11(a) shows the closed loop step response of the forearm. It can be easily seen that the device reaches steady state position of 1 rad in less than 1 s with no overshoot or oscillations. There is a small steady state error (< 1%) in position due to friction in the bearings, motor cogging and the gravitational torque acting on the joint. The steady state error can be eliminated with the use of a PID controller instead of the PD controller employed. The trajectory following behavior of the forearm tracking a sinusoidal reference signal at a frequency of 4 rad/s is depicted in Figure 11(b). This further verifies that the bandwidth of the controller is over 4 rad/s and matches human actuation bandwidth. Similar results were obtained for the wrist controller.

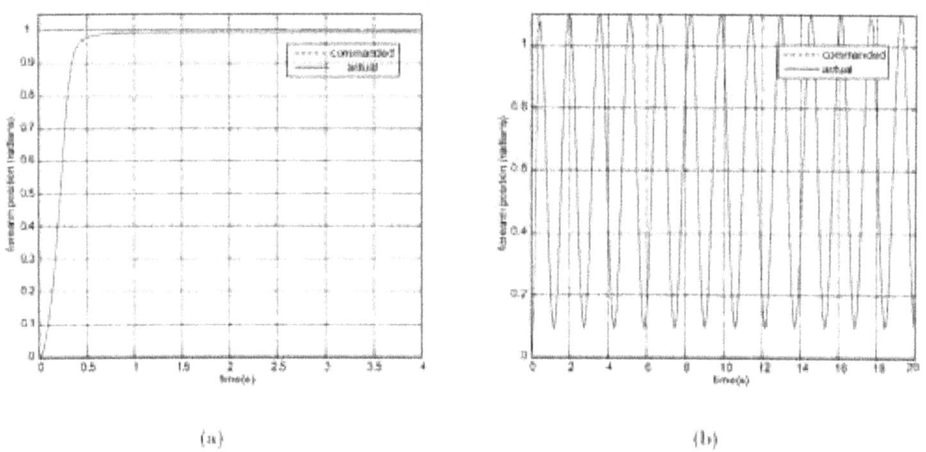

Fig. 11. Position control of the forearm position controller: (a) Step response to a reference signal with a step of 1 rad shows no overshoot and quick, non-oscillatory response. (b) Trajectory following behavior when tracking a 4 rad/s sinusoidal reference signal of amplitude 0.5 rad centered at 0.6 rad demonstrates that the device bandwidth matches human capabilities.

Joint level position control for the wrist was implemented via independent PD controllers acting on each joint, as discussed in Section 4.1. Control results demonstrated that there is negligible structural coupling between the actuated joints. The low structural coupling between the linear joint axes also serves to verify the mechanical design process showing that the axes could be independently controlled as theoretically predicted. A task space PD controller for the wrist platform was also implemented as described in Section 4.1. Trajectory following behavior of the task-space controller tracking sinusoidal trajectories in abduction/adduction and flexion/extension at 4 rad/s is shown in Figure 12. Note the quick system response with little overshoot when tracking sinusoidal trajectories of amplitude 0.15 rad at a frequency of 4 rad/s. Note that the platform height was constrained when testing responses in abduction/adduction and flexion/extension as we start at the boundary of the workspace where it is not possible to change orientation of the top plate of the platform without changing platform height. Trajectory following capability is useful for guidance during training or rehabilitation. These results also serve to verify adequate system performance throughout the workspace of the wrist. For a detailed discussion of the performance of the device under position control please refer to (Gupta, Patoglu et al. 2007).

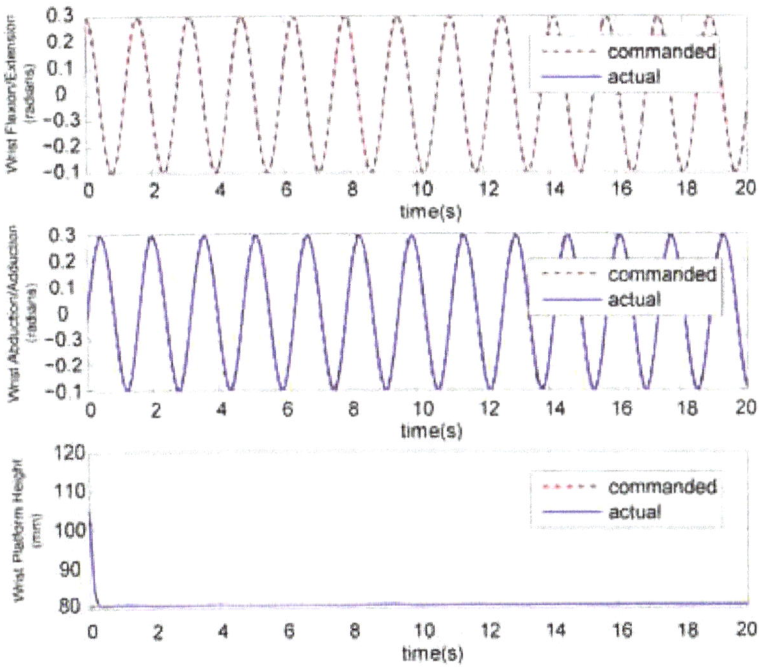

Fig. 12. Task space trajectory tracking control of the wrist platform (reference: height– 80 mm; abduction/adduction and flexion/extension - sinusoids of amplitude 1.5 rad at 4 rad/s).

Force Control As described in Section 4.1 force control for the exoskeleton was implemented through an impedance controller. Figure 13 depicts a subject's interaction with a virtual wall at the forearm joint, implemented as a spring-mass system of stiffness 150 Nm/rad and damping of 10 Nm/rad/s, located at 1 rad. Regions (a), (b) and (c) demonstrate the approach, steady contact and penetration into the wall, respectively. Note that due to torque limitations of the forearm motor, the user can overcome the wall force, thereby saturating the motor. Larger motor output is desired for simulating stronger walls, but device torques that exceed human limits could compromise user safety.

Figure 14 depicts a typical user interaction with two virtual walls located at a rotation of 0.2 rad in flexion/extension and abduction/adduction respectively. The virtual wall was implemented as a spring-damper system. Although slight chattering is noticed upon contact, the device successfully constrains the operator. Upon decreasing the wall gain, it is noted that chatter occurs at larger user penetration depths into the wall. The platform torque output does not match the limits of the human joints and hence, the human operator can saturate the motor output. We believe this actuator saturation along with the low stiffness of the cable drive transmission to be responsible for the chatter.

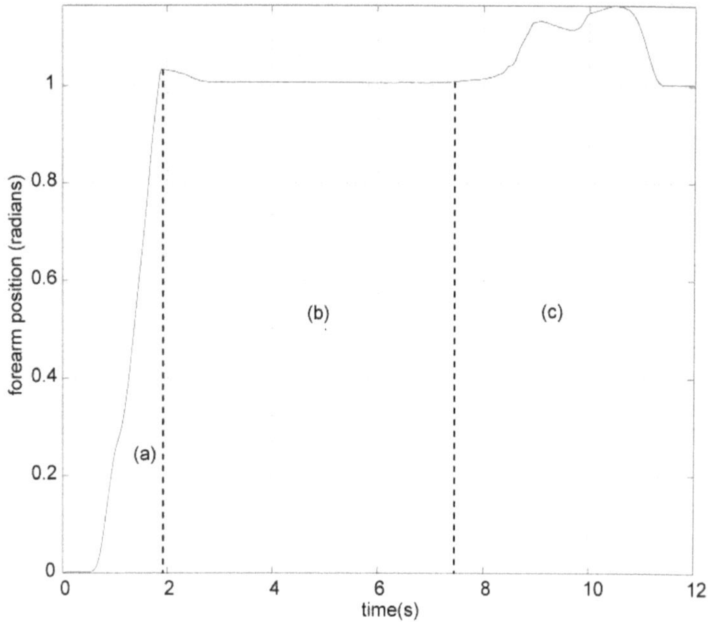

Fig 13. User interaction with virtual wall located at 1 rad for the forearm joint. Regions (a), (b) and (c) demonstrate the approach, steady contact and penetration into the wall. 0.5 mm from their initial position. This demonstrates that there is negligible structural coupling between the actuated joints. The low structural coupling between the linear joint axes also serves to verify the mechanical design process showing that the axes could be independently controlled as theoretically predicted.

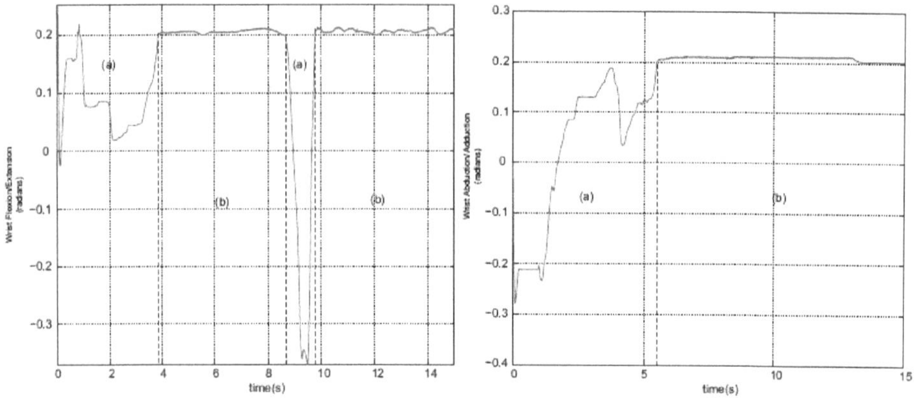

Fig. 14. (a) A virtual wall located at 0.2 rad wrist flexion/extension; (b) A virtual wall located at 0.2 rad wrist abduction/adduction.

5. Integration of MAHI exoskeleton with MIME

Prior work has studied the ability of a device (Mirror-Image Motion Enabler – MIME) (Burgar, Lum et al. 2000) to assist limb movements and facilitate recovery of motor function in subjects with chronic hemiparesis due to stroke. MIME incorporates an industrial robot and operates in three unilateral modes and one bimanual mode. In unilateral operation, passive, active-assisted, and guided movements against a resistance are possible. The bimanual mode enables the subject to practice bilateral, coordinated movements with rate and range under his or her control.

In the current version of MIME, subjects are seated in a wheelchair modified to improve seating support and reduce movements of the upper body. They can sit close to either the front or rear of an adjustable height table. A PUMA-560 robot is mounted beside the table. It is attached to a wrist-forearm orthosis (splint) via a 6-axis force transducer, a pneumatic breakaway overload sensor set to 20 Nm torque, and a quick-release coupling mechanism. The subject's arm is strapped into the splint with the wrist in neutral position. Robot/forearm interaction force and torque measurements from the transducer are recorded and archived by a personal computer. The control program monitors these data and the motion of the robot in order to prevent potentially hazardous situations from occurring. Switches and mechanical stops are strategically placed to permit rapid de-activation of the robot, if necessary.

Preliminary data from clinical efficacy trials using MIME suggest that robot-aided therapy has therapeutic benefits. Improvements have been demonstrated in strength and in the FM assessment of motor function. Trends in the data suggest that the underlying mechanisms for these results may be increased strength, as well as more appropriate activation and inhibition of muscle groups (Burgar, Lum et al. 2000).

Such findings with shoulder and elbow rehabilitation motivate the extension of robotic-assisted rehabilitation distally for the upper extremity, so that forearm pronation-supination, wrist flexion-extension, radial-ulnar deviation, and ultimately digital manipulation are enabled. The MAHI exoskeleton wrist (*RiceWrist*) has been integrated with the Mirror-Image Motion Enabler (MIME) (Burgar, Lum et al. 2000) system (see Figure 15). Velcro strapping and a molded splint are used to attach the subject's arm to the device. MIME and *RiceWrist* communicate through the serial port. Communication is mainly for synchronization of start and end of trials.

5.1 MIME-*RiceWrist* Rehabilitation Setup

Figure 16 shows the overall setup for the MIME-*RiceWrist* rehabilitation system. The therapist maintains high level supervisory control over the therapy session. The therapist can customize the physical therapy sessions according to the needs of individual patients. The *RiceWrist* extends the three unilateral operation modes of MIME to include forearm supination and pronation, wrist flexion and extension, and radial and ulnar deviation.

The three unilateral modes of MIME are:

- Passive mode: the robot guides the user to a predetermined goal position.
- Active-assisted mode: similar to passive mode, but the robotic assistance does not begin until the patient overcomes some preset force threshold.
- Constrained mode: the patient moves his/her arm against a viscous field to a goal position. A moving virtual wall prevents the patients from retracting their arm.

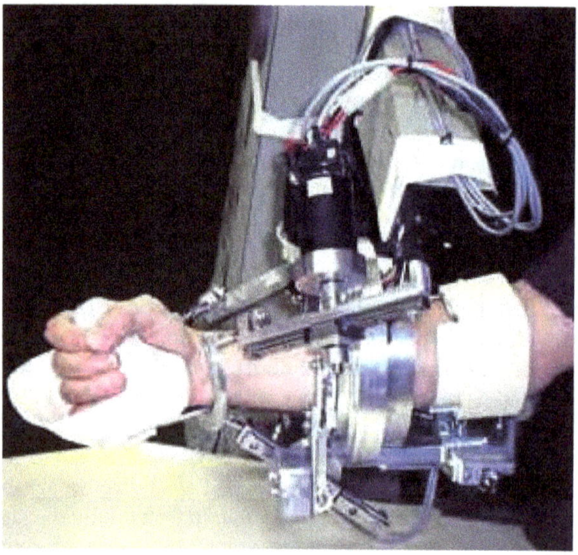

Fig. 15. Subject operating the integrated MIME-*RiceWrist* System.

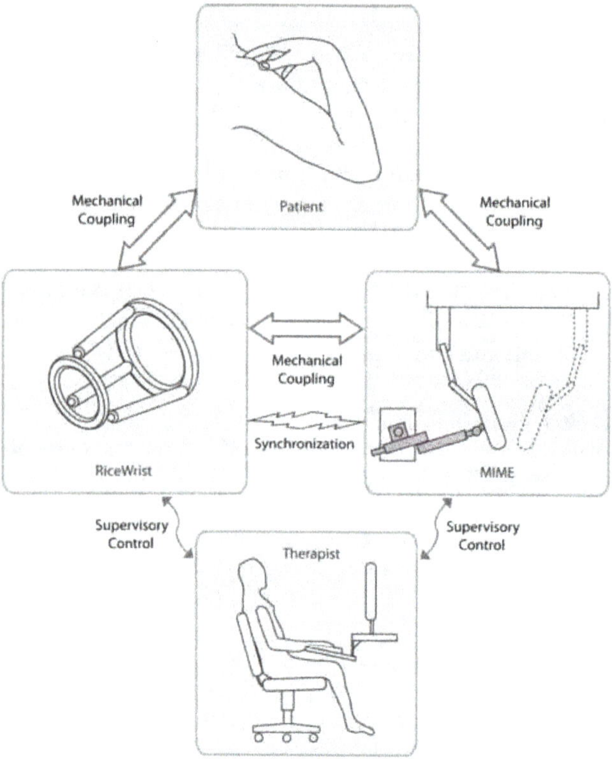

Fig. 16. MIME-*RiceWrist* rehabilitation system setup.

A graphical user interface (GUI), as shown in Fig. 17, is provided to the therapist to facilitate customization of the sessions. The GUI provides an interface to record patient information and individual session details. Prior to a therapy session, the therapist can record the joint limits of the patient to plan the desired start and end positions for reaching movements. This information is also stored on a local file for future reference and updates. For each trial, the therapist can then choose the desired trajectory by selecting start and end positions, number of repetitions and the speed of travel. Three different modes of operation – passive, triggered and constrained – are implemented on the system. Through the GUI, the therapist can also select the mode of operation and associated parameters.

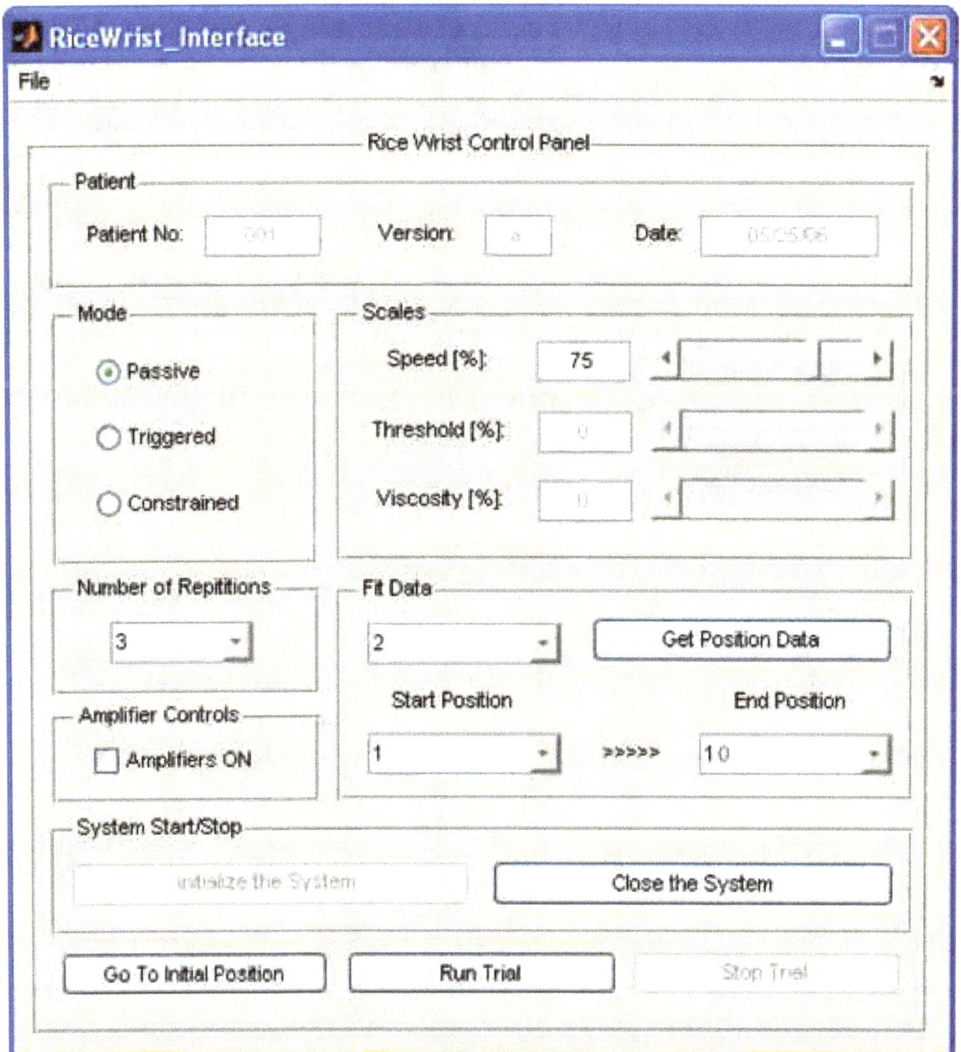

Fig. 17. Graphical user interface for the therapist

5.2 Control Modes

Three control modes that match the control modes of the MIME system – passive, triggered or constrained, have been implemented on the *RiceWrist*. Figure 18 depicts the structure of the controller for the MIME-*RiceWrist* system. The system has five modes of operation, three of which are the aforementioned control modes. The other modes are GoTo and Wait. When operating in the GoTo mode, the system moves to an initial position, which is specified by the therapist. On reaching the desired position, the system switches to the Wait mode, in which a virtual fixture is used to restrict arm movement, until the therapist initiates or resumes the trial. Following the command from the therapist, the system switches to one of the three control modes until the desired end position for the trial is reached. Upon reaching this position, the system switches back to the Wait mode until the therapist commands to initiate the return motion. This process can be repeated for the desired number of repetitions. The **GoTo mode** is implemented as a joint-space trajectory controller, as described in section 4.1. The desired trajectory is computed through linear interpolation using the current and specified initial positions. The **Wait mode** is implemented as a task-space impedance force controller. A high stiffness virtual wall prevents arm motions until a new mode is activated. **Passive** and **Triggered** modes are also implemented through joint-space controllers, whereas the **Constrained mode** is implemented as a task-space impedance force controller as used for the Wait mode. Unlike the Passive and Triggered modes, which are passive, this is an active mode where the patient is required to actively move his arm to the end position. Once movement has been initiated along the trajectory motion reversal is restricted by implementation of a virtual wall in that direction. Resistive impedance can also be displayed to the patient along the trajectory to provide strength training.

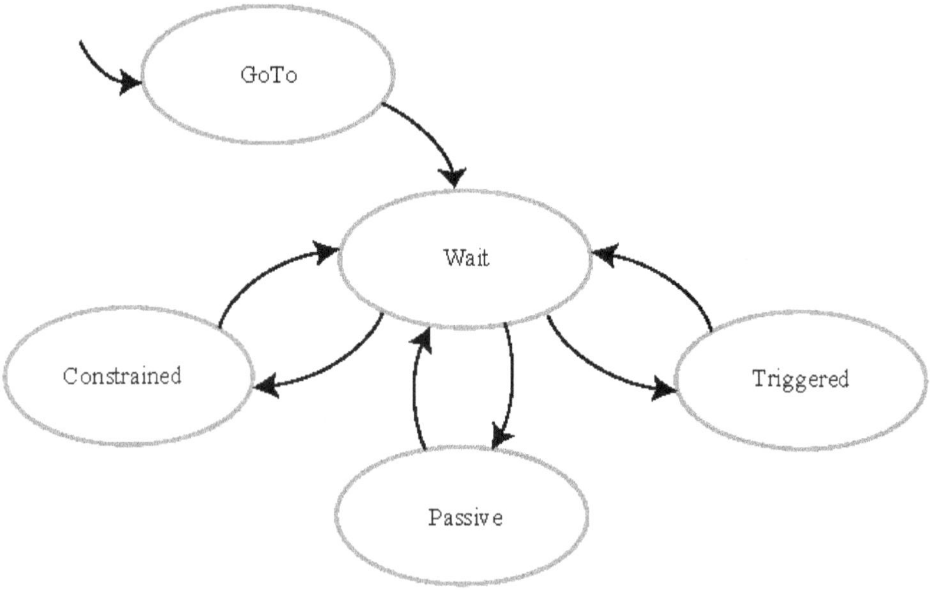

Fig. 18. Structure of the switching controller for the MIME-*RiceWrist* System.

5.3 Controller Performance of the *RiceWrist*

Figure 19 presents the experimental results when the *RiceWrist* is operating in the Passive Mode. Subfigures 19 (a)—(d) depict the trajectories for the four different joints, namely the wrist axes I, II, III, and forearm. Passive mode employs decoupled joint level trajectory controllers for each actuated axis. The solid lines in the figures represent the desired (commanded) trajectories, which are computed through linear interpolation between the specified initial and final joint positions. The dashed lines represent the experimentally recorded trajectories when the *RiceWrist* is operating freely. Finally, the dotted lines represent the experimentally recorded trajectories when the *RiceWrist* is worn by a human subject. The close match among the desired and experimentally observed trajectories imply adequate disturbance rejection characteristics of the implemented controllers.

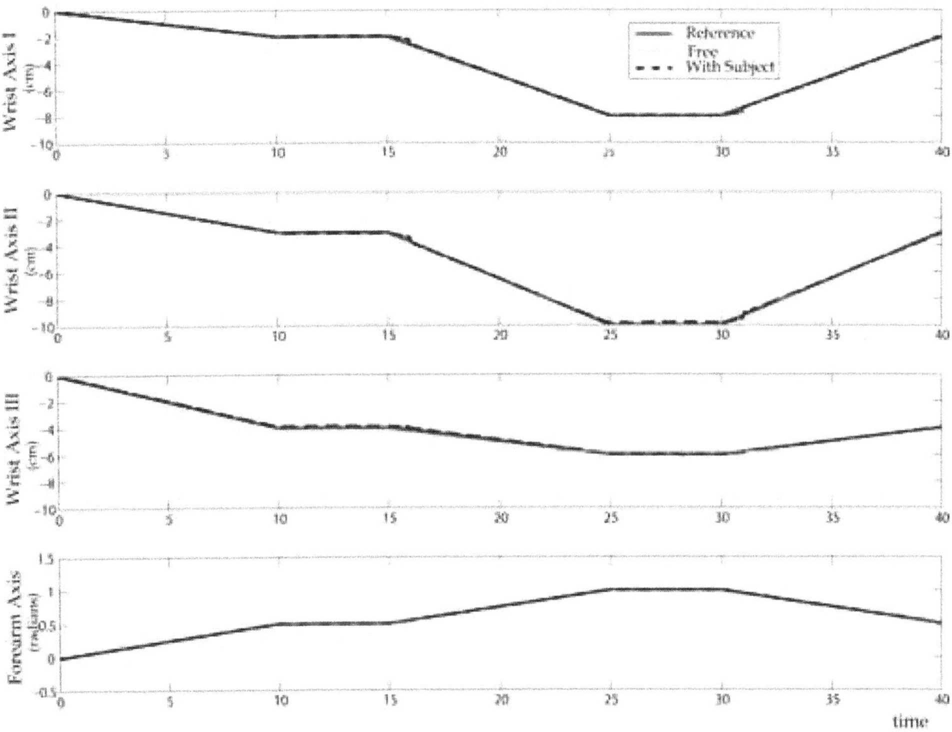

Fig. 19. Experimental results for the *RiceWrist* operating in the Passive mode.

6. Conclusions and Future work

This chapter has presented an overview of existing arm exoskeleton robotic devices, with a focus on those aimed at upper-extremity rehabilitation. The design and control of the MAHI arm exoskeleton was presented as a case study in exoskeleton design for rehabilitation applications. The device is compact, low-friction and backlash-free with high manipulability in the workspace of interest. Additionally, the MAHI exoskeleton allows unconstrained human arm movements over a large workspace and provides for easy measurement of elbow, forearm and wrist joint angles. The device exhibits excellent behavior under position control with a fast response time, very small oscillations, little overshoot and small steady state errors. Furthermore, there is little structural coupling between various controlled degrees-of-freedom of the device (forearm rotation, wrist flexion/extension and wrist abduction/adduction). The ability of the device to independently provide accurate guidance or kinesthetic feedback to individual human joints is critical during motor learning. It is demonstrated that the device is able to simulate sufficiently stiff virtual surfaces although, the quality of the surface is limited by maximum torque output of the robot.

The chapter concludes by presenting the *RiceWrist*, a sub-set of the MAHI exoskeleton identical in design yet lacking the elbow joint, which has been integrated with the Mirror-Image Motion Enabler (MIME). The *RiceWrist* extends the three unilateral operation modes of MIME to include forearm supination and pronation, wrist flexion and extension, and radial and ulnar deviation. Currently, preliminary trials with healthy patients are underway in order to tune the experimental protocols of the MIME- *RiceWrist* system. Future work will focus on clinical trials with hemiparetic stroke patients to study the efficacy of the approach in forearm/wrist rehabilitation. The device will also be used as a test bed for studying mechanisms of human motor learning and development of training methodologies.

7. References

Basdogan, C., C.-H. Ho, et al. (2001). "Virtual Environments for Medical Training: Graphical and Haptic Simulation of Laproscopic Common Bile Duct Exploration." *IEEE/ASME Trans. Mechatron.* **6**(3): 269-285.

Bergamasco, M., B. Allotta, et al. (1994). *An Arm Exoskeleton System for Teleoperation and Virtual Environment Applications.* IEEE Int'l Conf. Robot. Automat.

Boman, D. K. (1995). "International Survey: Virtual-Environment Research." *Computer* **28** (6): 57-65.

Burdea, G. C. (1996). *Force and Touch Feedback for Virtual Reality*, John Wiley Inc.

Burgar, C. G., P. S. Lum, et al. (2000). "Development of Robots for Rehabilitation Therapy: The Palo Alto VA/Stanford Experience." *Journal of Rehabilitation Research and Development* **37**(6): 663-673.

Carignan, C. and M. Liszka (2005). *Design of an arm exoskeleton with scapula motion for shoulder rehabilitation.* IEEE Conference on Advanced Robotics.

Carignan, C. R. and D. L. Akin (2003). Using Robots for Astronaut Training. *IEEE control syst. mag.* **23:** 46-59.

Charles, S. K. K., H. I.; Volpe, B. T.; Lynch, D. & Hogan, N. (2005). *Wrist Rehabilitation Following Stroke: Initial Clinical Results.* International Conference on Rehabilitation Robotics.

Colgate, J. E. and J. M. Brown (1994). *Factors Affecting the Z-Width of a Haptic Display.* IEEE Int'l Conf. Robot. Automat.

Dirette, D. and J. Hinojosa (1994). "Effects of Continuous Passive Motion on the Edematous Hands of Two Persons with Flaccid Hemiplegia." *American Journal of Occupational Therapy* **48**(5): 403-409.

Elllis, R. E., O. M. Ismaeil, et al. (1996). "Design and Evaluation of a High-Performance Haptic Interface." *Robotica* **14**: 321-327.

Erlandson, R. F. (1992). "Applications of Robotic/Mechatronic Systems in Special Education, Rehabilitation Therapy." *IEEE Trans. Rehab. Eng.* **3**(1): 22-34.

Fasoli, S. E., H. I. Krebs, et al. (2004). "Robotic Technology and Stroke Rehabilitation." *Topics in Stroke Rehabilitation* **11**: 11-19.

Feygin, D., M. Keehner, et al. (2002). *Haptic Guidance: Experimental Evaluation of a Haptic Training Method for a Perceptual Motor Skill.* Int'l Sympo. Haptic Interfaces for Virtual Environ. Teleop. Syst.

Gillespie, B., S. O'Modhrain, et al. (1998). *The Virtual Teacher.* ASME Int'l Mech. Eng. Congress Expo.

Goodall, R. M., D. J. Pratt, et al. (1987). "Enhancing Postural Stability in Hemi-Plegics Using Externally Applied Forces." *Intl. J. of Rehab. Research (suppl 5)* **10**(4): 132-140.

Gresham, G. E. (1990). "Past Achievements and New Directions in Stroke Outcome Research." *Stroke* **21 (9 Suppl):II**: 1-2.

Gresham, G. E., D. Alexander, et al. (1997). "Rehabilitation." *Stroke* **28**(7): 1522-1526.

Gupta, A. and M. K. O'Malley (2006). "Design of a Haptic Arm Exoskeleton for Training and Rehabilitation." *IEEE/ASME Trans. Mechatron.* **11**(3).

Gupta, A., V. Patoglu, et al. (2007). "Design, Control and Performance of RiceWrist: A Force Feedback Wrist Exoskeleton for Rehabilitation and Training." *Int'l J. Robot. Research.*

Hesse, S., G. Schulte-Tigges, et al. (2003). "Robot Assisted Arm Trainer for the Passive and Active Practice of Bilateral Forearm and Wrist Movements in Hemiparetic Subjects." *Archives of Physical Medicine and Rehabilitation* **84**(6): 915-920.

Hogan, N. and H. I. Krebs (2004). "Interactive Robots for Neurorehabilitation." *Restorative Neurology and Neuroscience* **22**: 349-358.

Jack, D., R. Boian, et al. (2001). "Virtual Reality Enhanced Stroke Rehabilitation." *IEEE Trans. Neural Syst. Rehab. Eng.* **9**(3): 308-318.

Jeong, Y., Y. Lee, et al. (2001). *A 7 DOF Wearable Robotic Arm using Pneumatic Actuators.* Int'l Symp. Robot.

Khalili, D. and M. Zomlefer (1988). "An Intelligent Robotic System for Rehabilitation of Joints and Estimation of Body Segment Parameters." *IEEE Trans. Biomed. Eng.* **35**(2): 138-146.

Kim, Y. S., J. Lee, et al. (2005). "A force Reflected Exoskeleton-Type Masterarm for Human-Robot Interaction." *IEEE Trans. Syst., Man, Cybern. A* **35**(2): 198-212.

Kousidou, S., N. Tsagarakis, et al. (2006). *Assistive Exoskeleton for Task Based Physiotherapy in 3-Dimensional Space.* IEEE/RAS-EMBS International Conference on Biomedical Robotics and Biomechatronics.

Lay, S. D. and A. M. Day (2003). "Recent Developments and Applications of Haptic Devices." *Comp. Graph. Forum* **22**(2): 117-132.

Lee, K. M. and D. K. Shah (1988). "Kinematic Analysis of a Three Degrees-of-Freedom in-Parallel Actuated Manipulator." *IEEE Trans. Robot. Automat.* **4**(3): 354-360.

Lee, S., S. Park, et al. (1998). *Design of a Force Reflecting Master Arm and Master Hand using Pneumatic Actuators.* IEEE Int'l Conf. Robot. Automat.

Mosher, R. S. (1967). From Handyman to Hardiman, SAE paper no.670088.

Nakai, A., T. Oshashi, et al. (1998). *7DOF Arm Type Haptic Interface for Teleoperation and Virtual Reality Systems.* Int'l Conf. Intell. Robots Syst.

Nef, T., M. Mihelj, et al. (2006). *ARMin – Robot for Rehabilitation of the Upper Extremities.* IEEE International Conference on Robotics and Automation.

O'Malley, M. K. and M. Goldfarb (2002). "The Effect of Force Saturation on the Haptic Perception of Detail." *IEEE/ASME Trans. Mechatron.* **7**(3): 280-288.

O'Malley, M. K. and M. Goldfarb (2004). "The Effect of Virtual Surface Stiffness on the Haptic Perception of Detail." *IEEE/ASME Trans. Mechatron.* **9**(2).

O'Malley, M. K. and A. Gupta (2003). *Passive and Active Assistance for Human Performance of a Simulated Underactuated Dynamic Task.* Int'l Sympo. Haptic Interfaces for Virtual Environ. Teleop. Syst.

O'Malley, M. K., T. Ro, et al. (2006). "Assessing and Inducing Neuroplasticity with TMS and Robotics." *Archives of PMR, Special Issue on Neuroplasticity and Neuroimaging in Acquired Brain Injury: Measurements, Concepts, and Applications.*

Perry, J. C. and J. Rosen (2006). *Design of a 7 Degree-of-Freedom Upper-Limb Powered Exoskeleton.* IEEE Conference on Biomedical Robotics and Biomechatronics.

Prisco, G. M., C. A. Avizzano, et al. (1998). *A Virtual Environment with Haptic Feedback for the Treatment of Motor Dexterity Disabilities.* IEEE Int'l Conf. Robot. Automat.

Reinkensmeyer, D. J., J. P. A. Dewald, et al. (1996). "Robotic Devices for Physical Rehabilitation of Stroke Patients: Fundamental Requirements, Target Therapeutic Techniques, and Preliminary Designs." *Technology and Disability* **5**: 205-215.

Reinkensmeyer, D. J., J. L. Emken, et al. (2004). "Robotics, Motor Learning and Neurologic Recovery." *Annual Reviews in Biomedical Engineering* **6**: 497-525.

Reinkensmeyer, D. J., C. D. Takahashi, et al. (2000). "Design of Robot Assistance for Arm Movement Therapy Following Stroke." *Advanced Robotics* **14**(7): 625-637.

Riener, R., T. Nef, et al. (2005). "Robot-Aided Neurorehabilitation of the Upper Extremeties." *Medical and Biological Engineering and Computing* **43**: 2--10.

Rosen, J., M. Brand, et al. (2001). "A Myosignal-Based Powered Exoskeleton System." *IEEE Trans. Syst., Man, Cybern. A* **31**(3): 210--222.

Rosenberg, L. (1993). *Virtual Fixtures: Perceptual Tools for Telerobotic Manipulation.* IEEE Int'l Symp. Virt. Reality.

Ruiz, A. F., A. Forner-Cordero, et al. (2006). *Exoskeletons for Rehabilitation and Motor Control.* Biomedical Robotics and Biomechatronics, 2006. BioRob 2006. The First IEEE/RAS-EMBS International Conference on.

Shimoga, K. (1992). *Finger Force and Touch Feedback Issues in Dexterous Telemanipulation.* NASA-CIRSSE Int'l Conf. Intel. Robot. Syst. for Space Expl.

Sledd, A. and M. K. O'Malley (2006). *Performance Enhancement of a Haptic Arm Exoskeleton.* Int'l Sympo. Haptic Interfaces for Virtual Environ. Teleop. Syst.

Stein, J. (2004). "Motor Recovery Strategies after Stroke." *Topics in Stroke Rehabiliation* **11**: 12-22.

Sveistrup, H. (2004). "Motor Rehabilitation using Virtual Reality." *J. NeuroEng. and Rehab.* **1**(10).

Thom, T., N. Haase, et al. (2006). "Heart disease and stroke statistics-2006 update: a report from the American Heart Association Statistics Committee and Stroke Statistics Subcommittee." *Circulation* **113**(6): e85-151.

Todorov, E., R. Shadmehr, et al. (1997). "Augmented Feedback Presented in a Virtual Environment Accelerates Learning of a Difficult Motor Task." *J. Motor Behav.* **29**(2): 147-158.

Tsagarakis, N., D. G. Caldwell, et al. (1999). *A 7DOF Pneumatic Muscle Actuator Powered Exoskeleton.* Int'l Workshop Robot and Human Interact. Commun.

White, C. J., A. M. Scneider, et al. (1993). *Robotic Orthosis for Stroke Patient Rehabilitation.* IEEE Intl. Conf. Eng. Med. Biol.

Williams II, Robert L.; Murphy, Mark A.; North, Debra; Berlin, James & Krier, Michael (1998). *Kinesthetic Force/Moment Feedback via Active Exoskeleton.* Image Society Conf.

Wolf, P. A., R. B. D'Agostino, et al. (1992). "Secular Trends in Stroke Incidence and Mortality: The Framingham Study." *Stroke* **23**: 1551--1555.

Yoshikawa, T. (1985). "Manipulability of Robotic Mechanisms." *Int'l J. Robot. Research* **4**(2): 3-9.

Permissions

All chapters in this book were first published in RR, by InTech Open; hereby published with permission under the Creative Commons Attribution License or equivalent. Every chapter published in this book has been scrutinized by our experts. Their significance has been extensively debated. The topics covered herein carry significant findings which will fuel the growth of the discipline. They may even be implemented as practical applications or may be referred to as a beginning point for another development.

The contributors of this book come from diverse backgrounds, making this book a truly international effort. This book will bring forth new frontiers with its revolutionizing research information and detailed analysis of the nascent developments around the world.

We would like to thank all the contributing authors for lending their expertise to make the book truly unique. They have played a crucial role in the development of this book. Without their invaluable contributions this book wouldn't have been possible. They have made vital efforts to compile up to date information on the varied aspects of this subject to make this book a valuable addition to the collection of many professionals and students.

This book was conceptualized with the vision of imparting up-to-date information and advanced data in this field. To ensure the same, a matchless editorial board was set up. Every individual on the board went through rigorous rounds of assessment to prove their worth. After which they invested a large part of their time researching and compiling the most relevant data for our readers.

The editorial board has been involved in producing this book since its inception. They have spent rigorous hours researching and exploring the diverse topics which have resulted in the successful publishing of this book. They have passed on their knowledge of decades through this book. To expedite this challenging task, the publisher supported the team at every step. A small team of assistant editors was also appointed to further simplify the editing procedure and attain best results for the readers.

Apart from the editorial board, the designing team has also invested a significant amount of their time in understanding the subject and creating the most relevant covers. They scrutinized every image to scout for the most suitable representation of the subject and create an appropriate cover for the book.

The publishing team has been an ardent support to the editorial, designing and production team. Their endless efforts to recruit the best for this project, has resulted in the accomplishment of this book. They are a veteran in the field of academics and their pool of knowledge is as vast as their experience in printing. Their expertise and guidance has proved useful at every step. Their uncompromising quality standards have made this book an exceptional effort. Their encouragement from time to time has been an inspiration for everyone.

The publisher and the editorial board hope that this book will prove to be a valuable piece of knowledge for researchers, students, practitioners and scholars across the globe.

List of Contributors

Hyun Seok Hong, Jung Won Kang and Myung Jin Chung
KAIST Republic of Korea

Yasuhisa Hirata, Asami Muraki and Kazuhiro Kosuge
Department of Bioengineering and Robotics, Tohoku University Japan

Peralta H., Monacelli E., Riman C., Baklouti M., Ben Ouezdou F. and Mougharbel I.
LISV, Engineering Systems Laboratory of Versailles, Versailles Saint Quentin en Yvelines University, France

Laffont I. and Bouteille J.
Lebanon University, Lebanon New Technologies Platform, Raymond Poincaré Hospital France

Christian Martens
Rheinmetall Defence Electronics Germany

Oliver Prenzel
University of Bremen, Institute of Automation Germany

Artem Kargov, Stefan Schulz, Christian Pylatiuk and Georg Bretthauer
Institute for Applied Computer Science, Forschungszentrum Karlsruhe, Germany

Oleg Ivlev
Institute of Automation, University of Bremen, Germany

Rüdiger Dillmann and Tamim Asfour
Institute of Computer Science and Engineering, University of Karlsruhe, Germany

Michelle J Johnson
Medical College of Wisconsin, Marquette University Milwaukee
Clement Zablocki VA, Milwaukee, Wisconsin, USA

Dominic Nathan
Marquette University SA Milwaukee, Wisconsin, USA
Clement Zablocki VA, Milwaukee, Wisconsin, USA

Kimberly J Wisneski and Jayne Johnston
Clement Zablocki VA, Milwaukee, Wisconsin, USA

John Anderson and Judith Kosasih
Medical College of Wisconsin Milwaukee, USA
Clement Zablocki VA, Milwaukee, Wisconsin, USA

Elaine Strachota
Concordia University, Milwaukee, Wisconsin, USA

Roger O. Smith
University of Wisconsin, Milwaukee, BWisconsin, USA

Michael Bailey-Van Kuren
Miami University USA

Rares F. Boian
Department of Mathematics and Computer Science, Babes-Bolyai University, Romania

Juan-Manuel Belda-Lois, Álvaro Page, José-María Baydal-Bertomeu, Rakel Poveda and Ricard Barberà
Instituto de Biomecánica de Valencia, Spain

Samer Mohammed, Philippe Poignet, Philippe Fraisse and David Guiraud
LIRMM - CNRS/INRIA - Université de Montpellier II France

Axel Gräser
Institute of Automation, University of Bremen, Germany
University of Bremen, Institute of Automation Germany

Patrick Métrailler, Roland Brodard, Yves Stauffer, Reymond Clavel and Rolf Frischknecht
Fondation Suisse pour les Cyberthèses, Monthey, Switzerland
Laboratoire de Systèmes Robotiques, EPFL, Lausanne, Switzerland
Unité de Neuroréhabilitation, CHUV, Lausanne, Switzerland

Grigore C. Burdea
CAIP Center, Rutgers University, New Jersey, USA

Judith E. Deutsch
Rivers Lab SHRP, University of Medicine and Dentistry, New Jersey, USA

Abhishek Gupta and Marcia K. O'Malley
Rice University Department of Mechanical Engineering and Materials Science Houston, Texas

Index